FUNDAMENTALS OF NURSING

Caring and Clinical Judgment

Mary Ann Hogan, MSN, RN, CS
Clinical Assistant Professor
University of Massachusetts Amherst
Amherst, Massachusetts

Marshelle Thobaben, MS, RN, PHN, APNP, FNP
Professor and Community Health and Psychiatric Nursing Consultant
Department of Nursing
Humboldt State University
Arcata, California

Helen Harkreader, PhD, RN
Professor
Austin Community College
Austin, Texas

W.B. Saunders Company
A Harcourt Health Sciences Company
Philadelphia   London   Toronto   Montreal   Sydney   Tokyo

W.B. SAUNDERS COMPANY
A Harcourt Health Sciences Company
The Curtis Center
Independence Square West
Philadelphia, PA 19106-3399

NOTICE

Nursing is an ever-changing field. Standard safety precautions must be followed, but as new research and clinical experience broaden our knowledge, changes in treatment and drug therapy become necessary or appropriate. Readers are advised to check the product information currently provided by the manufacturer of each drug to be administered to verify the recommended dose, the method and duration of administration, and the contraindications. It is the responsibility of the licensed prescriber, relying on experience and knowledge of the patient, to determine dosages and the best treatment for the patient. Neither the publisher nor the editor assumes any responsibility for any injury and/or damage to persons or property.

The Publisher

Study Guide for

FUNDAMENTALS OF NURSING: CARING AND CLINICAL JUDGMENT   ISBN 0-7216-8749-0

Printed in the United States of America

Last digit is the print number: 9 8 7 6 5 4 3

CONTENTS

PREFACE

The *Study Guide* for Harkreader's *Fundamentals of Nursing: Caring and Clinical Judgment* was developed to assist you, the nursing student, to understand and apply important concepts presented in the textbook. As a beginning nursing student, you will probably be expected to learn a tremendous amount of material in a relatively short time. The *Study Guide* was written to help you make good use of your valuable study time.

Each *Study Guide* chapter follows a specific format:

- **Purpose:** Each chapter begins with a brief purpose statement that summarizes in a few sentences the content of the corresponding textbook chapter.
- **Learning Objectives:** The learning objectives from the textbook are reproduced to help you focus on the critical elements of each chapter as you study.
- **Matching:** Matching exercises allow you to test your recall of basic terminology from each chapter.
- **True or False:** True or false exercises allow you to test your understanding of factual information presented in the text of the chapter. The answer key at the end of the book corrects the false statements.
- **Fill-in-the-Blanks:** Fill-in-the-blanks exercises help you master comprehension of important fundamental concepts and apply them in a specific context.

- **Exercising Your Clinical Judgment:** "Exercising Your Clinical Judgment" sections use a case study (often the familiar one presented in the textbook chapter) and NCLEX-style multiple-choice questions to give you practice in applying clinical reasoning skills.
- **Test Yourself:** The "Test Yourself" sections present a series of freestanding NCLEX-style multiple-choice questions to give you practice in test-taking and help you prepare for exams.

The answers to all of the exercises are provided at the end of the book for immediate feedback on the degree to which you have mastered the chapter contents.

Following the answer section, you'll find **Performance Checklists** that correspond to the Procedures in the textbook. Each one presents the essential elements of the corresponding Procedure. The checklists are designed for use in two ways. First, you may use them for individual review as you practice performing Procedures. Second, an instructor may use them to test your mastery of the Procedures. The format allows the instructor not only to rate your performance, but also to provide specific comments that will enhance your learning and help you to refine your skills.

We hope you find the *Study Guide* to be not only useful but also enjoyable for study. We also wish you success as you begin your career, and we hope that you will quickly discover all the richness, fulfillment, and satisfaction that nursing has to offer!

Mary Ann Hogan, MSN, RN, CS
Marshelle Thobaben, MS, RN, PHN, APNP, FNP
Helen Harkreader, PhD, RN

The Nursing Profession as a Context for Practice

PURPOSE

This chapter provides a broad overview of the nursing profession. It describes significant events in history and how they have affected the evolution of the nursing profession. The chapter also examines the various roles you will have as a nurse, professional nursing practice standards, advanced education options, and current issues of concern to those in the nursing profession.

LEARNING OBJECTIVES

After studying this chapter, you should be able to:

1. describe the evolution of nursing from ancient civilizations to the present, including the influence of religious, scientific, and political developments.
2. compare the different educational programs in nursing.
3. describe at least four specializations in advanced-practice nursing.
4. define and discuss nursing knowledge.
5. identify the effects of professionalism, standards of nursing practice, and Nurse Practice Acts on the profession of nursing.
6. describe the contribution of at least three professional nursing organizations to the advancement of nursing.
7. identify nursing roles, components of the health care system, and health care settings.
8. discuss the social issues affecting nursing's political agenda.
9. list the major predictions for contemporary nursing practice in the 21st century.

MATCHING

1. __C__ professionalism
2. __d__ continuing education
3. __a__ nursing
4. __b__ client advocate

a. an accountable discipline guided by science, theory, a code of ethics, and the art of care and comfort to treat human responses to health and illness

b. the nurse who assists clients in expressing their rights whenever necessary

c. behavior that upholds the status, methods, character, and standards of a given profession

d. informal courses that assist professional nurses in developing and maintaining clinical expertise and knowledge that promotes the quality of nursing care

TRUE OR FALSE

5. ___T___ Nursing has been defined in many different ways, but the care-giving focus has remained humanistic and holistic.

6. ___F___ Nursing as a profession is under the domain of medicine and is regulated by medicine. *governed by law - standards set forth by the profession*

7. ___T___ The American Nurses Association is the representative professional association for nurses in the United States.

8. ___T___ Florence Nightingale is considered by many to be the founder of nursing.

9. ___T___ Isabel Hampton Robb founded the organization that later became the American Nurses Association.

10. ___F___ A doctoral degree program is considered entry level education in nursing. *advanced practice education*

11. ___F___ A nurse who is planning the best method of care delivery for a client is engaged in the nursing role of rehabilitator. *critical thinker*

12. ___T___ Specialty nursing organizations often offer certification for nurses practicing in that specialty.

13. ___F___ The nursing profession has consistently tried to be removed from the political arena.

14. ___T___ By the year 2020, it is estimated that 75% of nurses will be employed in community settings.

FILL-IN-THE-BLANKS

15. During the ___Middle___ ___Ages___, the bubonic plague contributed to the founding of many nursing orders, including the Augustinian sisters.

16. The book *Notes on Nursing: What It Is and What It Is Not* was written by ___Florence Nightengale___.

17. The value of primary prevention became understood in America during the American ___Civil___ War.

18. The first nurse to be appointed a university professorship at Columbia University Teachers College was ___Mary___ ___Adelaide Nutting___.

19. In 1893, Lillian Wald founded ___Public health___ nursing when she opened the Henry Street Settlement Service in New York City.

20. *Nursing's Agenda for Health Care Reform* focuses on ___primary care___, ___prevention___, and ___community outreach___.

21. A nurse practitioner, nurse educator, or nurse administrator often completes a two-year ___masters___ ___degree___ program.

22. Continuing education is mandatory in some states to maintain ___professional licensure___.

23. A Nurse Practice Act defines the scope of nursing practice in a ___state___.

24. In the United States, the ___health care delivery system___ is one of the nation's largest industries.

EXERCISING YOUR CLINICAL JUDGMENT

Kate Lorraine is a 22-year-old nursing graduate. She has just taken her first job in a sub-acute unit of a local rehabilitation nursing center. Kate is highly motivated to grow in her professional practice, and to deliver quality nursing care to her clients.

25. To be aware of her specific legal responsibilities in her daily nursing practice, Kate should become familiar with which of the following?
    a. state Nurse Practice Act
    b. National League for Nursing (NLN) accreditation criteria
    c. Association of Rehabilitation Nurses (ARN) guidelines
    d. American Nurses Association (ANA) standards of nursing practice

26. As Kate is working on the evening shift, she observes one client looking through the bedside table drawer of another client. Kate intervenes, knowing which of the following nursing roles assumes the highest priority at this moment?
    a. caregiver
    b. communicator
    c. client advocate
    d. manager

27. Kate takes a supper break with a nursing colleague. They talk about some of the flyers for continuing education programs that are hanging on the break room bulletin board. Kate begins to think about the importance of beginning to acquire continuing education units (CEUs) to maintain:
    a. opportunities for future pay increases.
    b. professional licensure.
    c. status among her colleagues.
    d. membership in the American Nurses Association (ANA).

28. Kate overhears that another nurse has just received generalist certification from the American Nurses Credentialing Center (ANCC). She is aware that this nurse has which of the following as a minimum educational degree?
    a. associate's degree
    b. bachelor's degree
    c. master's degree
    d. doctorate degree

TEST YOURSELF

29. Nursing can best be defined as a discipline that focuses on:
    a. human responses to health and illness.
    b. a wide variety of disease states.
    c. the interaction between nurses and other disciplines.
    d. the women's movement in the United States.

30. The nurse's role as a case manager, who reviews and coordinates care in various health settings, developed as a result of which of the following recent trends in health care?
    a. increased technology
    b. concern for quality regardless of cost
    c. managed care
    d. computerization

31. The official publication by the American Nurses Association for registered nurses is:
    a. RN.
    b. American Journal of Nursing.
    c. Nursing.
    d. Nursing Research.

32. With the changing health care delivery system, the most common setting for nursing practice is shifting away from:
    a. rehabilitation centers.
    b. home care.
    c. ambulatory care centers.
    d. hospitals.

33. Experts predict that, in the future, which of the following is most likely to take place in the health care arena and affect the practice of nursing?
    a. Nurses will work in 24-hour physician-managed clinics.
    b. Hospital stays will become longer once again.
    c. The focus of nursing will revert back to illness rather than health.
    d. Nurse practitioners will provide services traditionally provided by physicians.

The Legal Context of Practice

PURPOSE

This chapter discusses the legal foundation for your nursing practice. It provides information about the legal and professional regulation of nursing practice, client rights, quality of care improvement initiatives, and methods to safeguard your nursing practice against legal threats.

LEARNING OBJECTIVES

After studying this chapter, you should be able to:

1. discuss various sources and types of law that directly or indirectly affect nursing practice.
2. describe four organizations or mechanisms that influence the professional regulation of nursing practice.
3. discuss a variety of legal regulations that influence nursing practice.
4. discuss client rights and their influence on nursing practice.
5. describe two initiatives to improve the quality of nursing care delivered to clients.
6. summarize actions that can be taken to safeguard one's own nursing practice.

MATCHING

1. __g__ accreditation
2. __l__ advance directive
3. __h__ assault
4. __w__ battery
5. __aa__ certification

a. comprises standards and rules applicable to our interactions with one another, which are recognized, affirmed, and enforced through judicial decisions

6. __ee__ civil law
7. __a__ common law
8. __f__ confidentiality
9. __m__ contract
10. __r__ credentialing
11. __x__ criminal law
12. __bb__ defamation
13. __b__ defendant
14. __u__ false imprisonment
15. __dd__ fraud
16. __c__ informed consent
17. __h__ invasion of privacy
18. __n__ law
19. __z__ liability
20. __cc__ license
21. __d__ malpractice
22. __i__ negligence
23. __o__ plaintiff
24. __s__ private law
25. __y__ procedural law
26. __e__ professional misconduct
27. __j__ public law

b. the individual against whom a lawsuit is filed

c. involves the legal right of a client to receive adequate and accurate information about his or her own medical condition and treatment

d. acts of negligence by a professional person as compared to the actions of another professional person in similar circumstances

e. violations of a Nurse Practice Act that can result in disciplinary action against a nurse

f. the client's right to privacy in the health care delivery system

g. a process that monitors an educational program's ability to meet predetermined standards for student outcomes

(Continued on p. 6)

28. ___P___ registration

29. ___K___ statutory law

30. ___T___ substantive law

31. ___V___ tort

h. can occur when the client's private affairs are unreasonably intruded upon by the nurse

i. occurs when harm or injury is caused by an act of either omission or commission; the nurse is judged against what an ordinary, reasonable layperson would do or not do in similar circumstances.

j. regulates the relationship of individuals to government agencies, and may be administrative, constitutional, or statutory

k. law enacted by the legislative branch of government

l. a written document that provides direction for health care when a person is unable to make his or her own treatment choices

m. an agreement between two or more individuals creating certain rights and obligations in exchange for goods or services

n. a body of rules of action or conduct prescribed by a controlling authority

o. the party bringing a lawsuit

p. a process requiring the applicant to provide specific information to the state agency administering the nursing registration process

q. an attempt or threat to touch another person unjustly

r. the methods by which the nursing profession attempts to ensure and maintain the competency of its practitioners

s. controls the relationships between private individuals and/or private organizations

t. stipulates one's rights and duties

u. involves the restraining, with or without force, of another person against his or her wishes

v. a civil wrong by one person against another person or his or her property

w. the actual willful touching of another person that may or may not cause harm

x. defines specific behaviors determined to be inappropriate in the orderly functioning of society

y. establishes a manner of proceeding to enforce a specific legal right or obtain redress

z. the legal obligation or responsibility to provide care to a client that meets the standards of care

aa. a voluntary process by which a nurse can be granted recognition for meeting certain criteria established by a non-governmental association

bb. either a false communication or a careless disregard for the truth which results in damage to one's reputation; can take two forms—libel and slander

cc. grants the owner formal permission from a constituted authority to practice a particular profession

dd. the false representation of some fact with the intention that it will be acted upon by another person

ee. regulates disputes between individuals and/or individuals and groups

TRUE OR FALSE

32. __T__ A nurse overheard making vicious untrue comments about a coworker could be charged with defamation.

33. __F__ False imprisonment does not include refusing to let clients leave the hospital against their wishes, as long as it is in their best interests to stay.

34. __T__ A person who has been declared incompetent by the court is considered to lack the capacity for entering into a contract.

35. __F__ A nurse who diverts and sells narcotics can be tried in the court system under civil law. *criminal law*

36. __T__ Failing to practice within legal boundaries of nursing practice could result in professional discipline, civil or criminal lawsuits, or employer disciplinary action.

37. __F__ The American Nurses Association is the body that has the power to change a Nurse Practice Act. *Individual State*

38. __T__ A nursing school that is accredited meets predetermined standards for student outcomes.

39. __T__ The process of registration or the renewal of registration helps to ensure that a state has the most current information about a person granted a nursing license.

FILL-IN-THE-BLANKS

40. A nurse who administers an injection to a client despite the client's refusal has committed ___battery___.

41. A nurse who is threatened with loss of license is given the right to a fair hearing under ___procedural___ law.

42. A nurse who sits for an examination administered by a specialty nursing organization is seeking ___certification___.

43. The process whereby a union negotiates with an employer for nurses' salaries is termed ___collective___ ___bargaining___.

44. Before undergoing any invasive procedure, the client must give ___informed___ ___consent___.

45. By avoiding conversations about clients in elevators and hallways, a nurse is protecting the client's right to ___privacy/confidentiality___.

46. A nurse would fill out an ___incident___ ___report___ if a client slipped and fell on a wet floor on the nursing unit.

47. When making an entry in the client's medical record, the first two items to enter are the ___date___ and ___time___.

EXERCISING YOUR CLINICAL JUDGMENT

The registered nurse has arrived on the clinical unit in the hospital to begin the shift. The nurse will be assigned to a group of seven clients, and has been designated as the charge nurse for the day as well.

48. While beginning to listen to inter-shift report at the nurses' station, a nurse notes that a client is within earshot. The client states that he would like a cup of coffee until the meal trays arrive. The most appropriate action by the nurse would be to:
    a. ask the client to wait until after report.
    b. tell the client that coffee is unavailable at this time.
    c. ask a nursing assistant to bring coffee to the desk for the client, and continue with report.
    d. ask someone to bring coffee to the client's room, and continue with report after the client leaves.

49. A nurse receives a telephone call stating that a client will be admitted with suspected tuberculosis in the infectious stage. The nurse would plan care for this client using infection control guidelines from the:
    a. Centers for Disease Control.
    b. Occupational Safety and Health Administration.
    c. state Nurse Practice Act.
    d. American Nurses Association.

50. A nurse is documenting care given to an assigned client. The nurse would do which of the following to make an appropriate legal entry in the client's medical record?
    a. use descriptive words such as "good" or "angry"
    b. record measurable and factual information about the client's condition
    c. use correcting fluid after making a mistake
    d. sign each entry using initials and license number

TEST YOURSELF

51. A nurse is being charged with malpractice. The element of malpractice that is proven by determining that the nurse did not meet the standard of care is:
    a. duty.
    b. breach of duty.
    c. causation.
    d. damages.

52. A nurse has not performed a scheduled nursing procedure in some time. The nurse should look to which of the following most important resources before completing the procedure for the client?
    a. agency policy and procedure book
    b. an old nursing textbook
    c. a nurse floating to the unit for the shift
    d. the risk management department

53. A nurse is admitting a client who wishes to have "do not resuscitate" status. The nurse determines whether the client has a copy of which of the following items to add to the client's record?
    a. letter of intent
    b. physician letter of approval
    c. advance directive
    d. last will and testament

54. A nurse is uncertain whether the client understood information about an upcoming invasive diagnostic procedure as presented by a physician. Which of the following factors may invalidate this client's consent?
    a. emotional status only
    b. intelligence
    c. educational level
    d. emotional or physical barriers

55. A nurse who works with a client population with a high incidence of hypertension (high blood pressure) attends a full-day workshop providing information on nursing management of this disorder. This nurse is striving to maintain which of the following types of competency in nursing practice?
    a. technical
    b. cognitive
    c. interpersonal
    d. global

The Ethical Context of Practice

PURPOSE

This chapter explores the theories and principles of ethics. It provides guidelines for ethical decision making that can be applied systematically to nursing practice.

LEARNING OBJECTIVES

After reading this chapter, you should be able to:

1. compare and contrast the concepts of ethics, morals, and values.
2. compare and contrast three theories of ethics: teleology, deontology, and virtue theory.
3. identify ethical principles.
4. discuss the elements of ethical decision making.
5. discuss the contents of the American Nurses Association Code for Nurses.
6. discuss the concepts of nursing advocacy, accountability, and responsibility.
7. describe some guides to ethical decision-making, including advance directives, informed consent, and ethics committees and forums.

MATCHING

1. __D__ autonomy
2. __l.__ beneficence
3. __f.__ deontology
4. __c__ durable power of attorney for health care
5. __J__ ethics

6. __d__ fidelity
7. __h__ justice
8. __m__ living will
9. __b__ morals
10. __o__ nonmaleficence
11. __i__ teleology
12. __g__ values
13. __p__ values clarification
14. __a__ veracity
15. __k__ virtue
16. __n__ virtue theory

a. adhering to the truth

b. standards of conduct that represent the ideal in human behavior to which society expects its members to adhere

c. a document that designates a person to make decisions about the client's medical treatment in the event that the client becomes unable to do so

d. honoring agreements and keeping promises

e. refers to a person's right to make individual choices; to self-determine

f. a theory that is not concerned with the consequences of an act but rather with the obligation or duty to perform the act

g. ideals, beliefs, and patterns of behavior that are prized and chosen by a person, group, or society

h. moral rightness, fairness, or equity

(Continued on p. 10)

i.   a set of theories that postulate that the outcomes or consequences of an action determine its goodness

j.   the branch of philosophy that attempts to determine what constitutes good, bad, right, and wrong in human behavior

k.   a practice of conforming life and conduct to moral and ethical principles

l.   the promotion of good

m.   a document that provides written instructions about when life-sustaining treatment should be terminated

n.   focuses on characteristics that are intrinsic to the person performing an action

o.   requires the practitioner to do no harm

p.   allows you to identify your personal values and develop self-awareness

TRUE OR FALSE

17. ___F___ Applied ethics is the development of systems, theories, principles, and rules that provide guidance when deciding whether an action is right or wrong. *Normative ethics*

18. ___T___ Values shape decisions in everyday life, from the clothes we wear to movies we prefer.

19. ___T___ Maintaining client confidentiality means not discussing client issues in hallways, elevators, hospital parking lots, or at home with family and friends.

20. ___F___ An example of applying the principle of veracity is not telling a terminally ill client her prognosis. *should be told prognosis*

21. ___F___ When two or more principles are in conflict or when choices are favorable, you have an ethical dilemma. *Unfavorable*

22. ___T___ In the United States, the American Nurses Association Code for Nurses is the document governing ethical nursing practice.

23. ___T___ A common ethical problem you may encounter is unit staffing patterns that negatively influence the provision of safe nursing care.

FILL-IN-THE-BLANKS

24. The study of ___ethics___ entails the examination of human behavior in terms of what ought to be done in the course of human interactions, and it seeks to provide guidelines or principles as a way to direct human interaction.

25. The imprinting of ___moral___ conduct begins early in childhood.

26. Values are learned behaviors that are influenced by ___culture___, ethnicity, education, and ___life___ ___experiences___

27. Confidentiality means maintaining another's ___privacy___ by safeguarding information that is entrusted to you.

28. ___Nonmalificence___ is the complement of beneficence.

29. All codes for professional nursing address respect for human dignity, ___rights___, ___confidentiality___, competence, and responsibilities of the nurse in the delivery of health care.

30. Durable powers of attorney for health care and living wills are both included in the client's ___medical___ record.

EXERCISING YOUR CLINICAL JUDGMENT

31. You and your classmate discuss your clients in the parking lot. You think that others are not listening to your conversation. Which of the following principles did you breach?
    a. autonomy
    b. fidelity
    c. confidentiality
    d. beneficence

32. You tell your client that you will give her pain medication at 10 a.m. You follow through and give the medication when you stated. You are supporting which ethical principle when you follow through on your commitment?
    a. autonomy
    b. beneficence
    c. nonmaleficence
    d. fidelity

33. Your client, who has a terminal illness and is expected to live for six months, is alert, oriented, and competent. She has very definite wishes about when life-sustaining treatment should be terminated. To support the client's self-determination, the best advice to give her is to:
    a. tell her primary care provider about her wishes.
    b. have a living will.
    c. have a durable power of attorney.
    d. talk with the institution's ethics committee.

TEST YOURSELF

34. Three components of a moral conflict include:
    a. personal values, uncertainty, and distress.
    b. choosing, prizing, and acting.
    c. uncertainty, dilemma, and distress.
    d. identifying, examining, and evaluating solutions.

35. What theory focuses on characteristics that are intrinsic to the person performing the action? Theorists ask, "How should I be in order to behave ethically?"
    a. virtue
    b. deontology
    c. teleology
    d. beneficence

36. You answer the client's questions about his diabetes, even though it would have been more comfortable for you to tell the client "not to worry" about the disorder. Which ethical principle applies in this situation?
    a. autonomy
    b. virtue
    c. veracity
    d. beneficence

37. Using the six-step ethical decision-making process, step 2 is gathering pertinent data. Which of the following questions should you ask to attempt to gather data about an ethical dilemma?
    a. Do institutional values and systems support the nursing decisions made?
    b. With whom must the final decision be made, and is that person competent or empowered to make decisions?
    c. Is the situation truly an ethical dilemma?
    d. What is the effect on those involved?

38. The American Hospital Association's Patient's Bill of Rights supports the client's right to refuse a recommended treatment or plan of care to the extent permitted by law and hospital policy. Which ethical principle does the bill of rights support?
    a. nonmaleficence
    b. autonomy
    c. beneficence
    d. veracity

4

The Cultural Context of Practice

PURPOSE

This chapter discusses concepts of culture and ethnicity as they relate to nursing care. It provides an overview of transcultural nursing and gives suggestions for performing a transcultural assessment. It also explores basic aspects of selected cultures and their effect on the successful delivery of nursing care.

LEARNING OBJECTIVES

After studying this chapter, you should be able to:

1. discuss culture and ethnicity as they relate to the delivery of nursing care.
2. define humanistic care.
3. outline the elements and objectives of transcultural nursing.
4. describe the dangers of stereotyping.
5. list and explain the six concepts included in transcultural assessment.
6. understand basic aspects of the Irish-American, African-American, Mexican-American, Chinese-American, and Navajo cultures.
7. anticipate the effects of cultural characteristics on the successful delivery of health care.

MATCHING

1. _e_ cultural competence
2. _i_ culture
3. _j_ diversity
4. _a_ ethnic
5. _f_ ethnicity

6. _h_ ethnocentrism
7. _k_ humanistic care
8. _c_ multicultural society
9. _d_ stereotyping
10. _b_ transcultural nursing
11. _g_ universality

a. groups of people of the same race or national origin within a larger cultural system who are distinctive based on traditions of religion, language, or appearance

b. culturally competent nursing care focused on differences and similarities among cultures, with respect to caring, health, and illness, based on the client's cultural values, beliefs, and practices

c. a society composed of more than one culture or subculture

d. the assumption that an attribute present in some members of a group is present in all members of a group

e. having enough knowledge of cultural groups that are different from your own to be able to interact with a member of a group in a manner that makes the person feel respected and understood

(Continued on p. 14)

13

f. reflects the characteristics a group may share in some combination

g. a common mode or value of caring or a prevailing pattern of care across cultures

h. the belief that one's own ethnic beliefs, customs, and attitudes are the correct and thus superior ones

i. a patterned behavioral response that develops over time as a consequence of imprinting the mind through social and religious structures and intellectual and artistic manifestations

j. the differences in modes or patterns of care among cultures; includes specific patterns of care within cultural groups

k. includes understanding and knowing a client in as natural or human a way as possible while helping or guiding the client to achieve certain goals, make improvements, reduce discomfort, or face disability or death

TRUE OR FALSE

12. __T__ One benefit of providing care within the framework of the client's culture is that it can improve compliance with the health regimen.

13. __F__ The majority of Asian-Americans would prefer acupuncture to Western approaches to analgesia.

14. __T__ The nurse who wishes to provide culturally competent care must have a willingness to compromise with the client about some aspects of care.

15. __T__ The cultural phenomenon of space in the transcultural assessment model refers to personal space.

16. __F__ A person who is future-oriented in terms of time often has difficulty accepting a plan of care that conflicts with traditional treatments. has no trouble if the are clear (past oriented)

17. __T__ When communicating with a client from another culture, it is helpful to use eye contact, touch, and seating arrangements that are comfortable for that client.

18. __T__ The African-American culture as a group values religion and the power of prayer.

19. __F__ Mexican-Americans are more likely to believe in an internal locus of control. external

20. __T__ Husbands and elders have authority over wives and children in the social organization of the Chinese-American culture.

21. __F__ Native Americans subscribe to the germ theory of medicine.

FILL-IN-THE-BLANKS

22. A nurse who helps a client to continue an important cultural practice during illness is engaged in cultural care __preservation__ or __maintenance__.

23. A nurse who changes personal behavior or actions to be more fully understood or accepted by the client is engaged in cultural care __accomodation__ or __negotiation__.

24. __Awareness__ is the attribute of cultural competency in which the health care provider recognizes the values and beliefs of both the client and self.

25. __Environmental control__ is the element of transcultural assessment that indicates clients' beliefs about their ability to control disease.

26. The __Irish__-American cultural group has readily assimilated into the cultural mainstream of U.S. society.

27. Sickle cell disease is a genetic disorder that is prevalent in the __African__-American population.

28. __Hispanic__-Americans are the fastest growing minority group in the United States.

29. The cultural group that adjusts personal diet to meet the *yin-yang* quality of a disease is the __Chinese__-American group.

30. Type II diabetes mellitus has high prevalence and tends to occur in the teens and twenties among the __Navajo Indians__.

31. In the Navajo culture, personal __space__ is very important and has no imaginary boundaries.

EXERCISING YOUR CLINICAL JUDGMENT

Mrs. Haygood is a 50-year-old African-American client who has been hospitalized for cardiovascular surgery. She has three grown children and works part time as a receptionist for a local business. The nurse has been assigned as the primary nurse for this client during her postoperative course of recovery.

32. A certified nursing assistant (CNA) tells the nurse that the client speaks "Black English" when conversing with family and friends, and reverts to standard English when speaking with nursing staff. The nurse helps the CNA to understand this behavior by indicating that it most likely represents:
    a. a rejection of American culture by the client.
    b. a dislike of American school systems and the standard English language.
    c. a means of maintaining cultural identity.
    d. a permanent learning disability due to uncertain socioeconomic background.

33. The nurse goes into the room to assess Mrs. Haygood. The nurse interacts with her keeping in mind that individuals of African-American descent are more likely to require how much personal space?
    a. none at all
    b. a smaller amount
    c. a moderate amount
    d. a large amount

34. Using knowledge of the social organization phenomenon of the African-American culture, the nurse places highest priority on accommodating visits to Mrs. Haygood by which of the following individuals?
    a. religious leader
    b. local politician
    c. a new coworker
    d. a friend of a cousin

35. Using knowledge of biologic variations of African-American clients, the nurse would take which of the following into consideration when assessing the health status of Mrs. Haygood?
    a. inflammation is best detected by observation
    b. jaundice is best seen in the nail beds
    c. the client is at very low risk of developing keloid tissue near the incision line
    d. pallor is best seen in the conjunctiva or oral mucosa

TEST YOURSELF

36. Which of the following is not a characteristic shared by people within an ethnic group?
    a. religious faith or faiths
    b. external perception of distinctiveness
    c. food preferences
    d. loose or distant ties to others in the group

37. A culturally competent practitioner has which of the following attributes?
    a. lack of awareness
    b. sensitivity
    c. lack of respect
    d. ability to hold firm to one's viewpoint

38. A nurse who is speaking with a client from a different culture would find which of the following communication strategies to be least helpful?
    a. asking the client about the meaning of health, illness, and planned care
    b. finding out how the illness is likely to affect life, relationships, and self-concept
    c. trying to anticipate the client's responses
    d. asking the client how he or she prefers to manage the illness

39. A Mexican-American client tells the nurse about seeking the help of a curandero before coming to the health clinic. The nurse understands that, in the Mexican-American culture, this type of folk healer is a:
    a. holistic healer.
    b. healer who uses only herbs.
    c. male witch.
    d. female witch.

40. A hospitalized Chinese-American client states a preference for eating foods that have a *yang* quality. The nurse would offer the client which of the following food items?
    a. cucumbers
    b. oranges
    c. watermelon
    d. chicken

CHAPTER 5

The Health Care Delivery System as Context for Practice

PURPOSE

As you begin your professional career in nursing, you will need to identify the components of the health care delivery system, identify the roles of members of the health care team, and understand the effects of social and political forces that will affect your practice. In this chapter you will be introduced to the providers, services, and financing methods that make up the health care delivery system in the United States. You will also explore some of the issues and opportunities facing health care delivery in the 21st century. You will want to further explore these issues as you learn more about health care delivery.

LEARNING OBJECTIVES

After studying this chapter, you should be able to:

1. compare and contrast the four types of health care services.
2. identify health care personnel and describe their training, roles, and responsibilities.
3. discuss inpatient, outpatient, and community settings for the delivery of health care.
4. compare and contrast the various types of health care financing, including private insurance, managed care organizations, and government insurance plans.
5. discuss the effect of demographic and economic factors on the delivery of effective and affordable health care.
6. identify legal and ethical issues in health care delivery.
7. discuss various opportunities in health care delivery, including health care reform, technological progress, environmental challenges, and quality improvement.

MATCHING

1. _b_ access
2. _a_ ambulatory care center
3. _e_ exclusive provider organization (EPO)
4. _d_ diagnosis-related group (DRG)
5. _f_ health maintenance organization (HMO)
6. _h_ independent practice association (IPA)
7. _i_ managed care
8. _j_ Medicaid
9. _c_ continuous quality improvement
10. _k_ Medicare
11. _m_ prospective payment system

a. provides health services on an outpatient basis to those who visit a hospital or other health care facility and depart after treatment on the same day

b. a complex construct representing the personal use of health care services and the structures or processes that facilitate or impede that use

c. work to improve quality while increasing efficiency and productivity so that less costly ways of providing services are identified and implemented

d. a group of patients classified for measuring a medical facility's delivery of care

(Continued on p. 18)

12. ___ preferred provider organization (PPO)

13. ___ hospice

e. a type of group health care practice in which enrollees are restricted to the list of preferred providers of health care, called "exclusive providers"

f. a type of group health care practice that provides basic and supplemental health maintenance and treatment services to voluntary enrollees who prepay a fixed periodic fee that is set without regard to the amount or kind of services received

g. a cluster of special services that address the special needs of dying people and their families

h. a legal entity that physicians in private practice can join so that the organization can represent them in negotiation of managed care contracts

i. a system that combines the functions of health insurance and the actual delivery of care, in which costs and utilization of services are controlled

j. a welfare program providing partial health care services for indigent people; supported jointly by federal and state governments

k. a federally funded national health insurance program in the United States for people over 65 years of age

l. an organization of physicians, hospitals and pharmacists whose members discount their health care services to subscriber patients; may be organized by a group of physicians, an outside entrepreneur, an insurance company, or a company with a self-insurance plan

m. the predetermination of how much will be paid for a specific service

TRUE OR FALSE

14. ___ Health promotion and illness prevention are mutually exclusive concepts.

15. ___ The majority of health care workers are employed by hospitals.

16. ___ Physician assistants and nurse practitioners are the same.

17. ___ Alternative practitioners are irrelevant to a discussion of health practices in the United States.

18. ___ Because of the strict regulation of hospitals, all Americans have equal access to high-quality hospital services.

19. ___ Because long-term care is primarily financed by the government, nursing homes are not-for-profit agencies.

20. ___ Emergency medical technicians are trained to provide critical early treatment both on site and in transit, thus reducing the death rates from accidents and acute illness.

21. ___ Respite care is potentially cost effective because it helps those who need long-term care to stay at home.

22. ___ The United States government has only a limited role in the financing of health care.

23. ___ A health maintenance organization is a means of financing health care for its members but has no influence on the quality of care provided.

24. ___ Health care rationing is associated only with countries that have a national health care system.

25. ___ The fastest growing segment of the population is people over the age of 85.

26. ___ The culture of the health care system is a barrier to culturally sensitive care.

27. ___ More than 15% of the U. S. gross national product is consumed by health care.

28. ___ As a nurse you will be primarily be concerned with quality of care rather than with cost of care.

FILL-IN-THE-BLANKS

29. Improvement in general health over the last few decades can be attributed to ___health behaviors___ and ___environmental quality___.

30. ___Nurses___ are the largest group of health care professionals in the United States.

31. ___Pharmacists___ dispense medications and assist physicians in making appropriate drug choices.

32. The term ___inpatient___ describes a client who receives care in the context of at least an overnight stay in a hospital or other health care facility.

33. The predominant type of hospital today is the ___Community general hospital___

34. ___Rehabilitation___ is a long-term-care service offered to clients who need additional therapy or treatment to recover from an injury or illness.

35. ___Subacute care___ is a component of the long-term-care continuum that provides services too intensive for the average skilled nursing facility.

36. A ___physicians office___ is the primary site for the delivery of physician services.

37. ___Adult day Care___ is a daytime community-based program designed to meet the needs of functionally impaired adults through an individual plan of care and program of nursing care, rehabilitative therapy, supervision, and socialization that enables a person to remain out of institutional care.

38. The ___U.S.___ spends more money per person on health care than any other country in the developed world.

39. A ___P.P.O.___ may be organized by a group of physicians, an outside entrepreneur, an insurance company, or a company with a self-insurance plan.

40. Medicare finances health care for ___people over 65___, ___disabled people___, and ___people end stage renal disease___

41. In ___CANADA___ (country) the government finances health care, but private providers deliver health care services.

42. ___26___% of American households with children under the age of 18 include a married couple.

43. The ___Gray Panthers___ and the ___Ameri. Assoc. of Retired persons___ are political action groups that lobby Congress with the hope of influencing legislation that affects older Americans.

EXERCISING YOUR CLINICAL JUDGMENT

You are working on a cardiac unit in a community hospital. Your client is a 58-year-old male who has had a minor heart attack. You are working with this person to plan for care after discharge. The following questions address the needs you and the client have identified.

44. The client has smoked a pack of cigarettes a day for 42 years. He knows he needs to quit but has been unsuccessful despite multiple attempts. He wants to join a support group. Which source is most likely to provide access (financial support) to a support group?
    a. a preferred provider organization
    b. a health maintenance organization
    c. catastrophic health insurance
    d Medicare

45. Your client would like to try the cholesterol-reducing medication that has recently been advertised on television. You would suggest that he ask his:
    a. pharmacist.
    b. physician.
    c. respiratory therapist.
    d. managed care organization.

46. You identify several misconceptions about the low-fat diet that has been prescribed by the physician. You know that the client's insurance will pay for any of the following, so you would make a referral to:
    a. an herbalist.
    b. a physical therapist.
    c. a dietitian.
    d. a physician's assistant.

47. The physician has recommended a cardiac rehabilitation program for the next six months. You are reviewing a pamphlet about the program with the client. He asks, "What does rehabilitation mean? I thought that was for people who were paralyzed." Your best answer would be:
    a. "Rehabilitation is any long-term-care service for people who need additional therapy or treatment to recover from an illness or injury."
    b. "Using that term is a way to get your insurance to pay for the services."
    c. "Rehabilitation only refers to the exercise program that will be designed by a physical therapist."
    d. "Any service outside a hospital is rehabilitation."

TEST YOURSELF

48. A 95-year-old man is admitted to a nursing home after an episode of heart failure. Though the doctor has given him the option to have a heart valve replacement, the man has decided he prefers conservative treatment. The nursing home will monitor his medication and will help him achieve a balance of rest and activity, maintain a low-salt diet, and maintain his relationship with his family. This type of care is best labeled:
    a. illness prevention.
    b. acute care.
    c. rehabilitation.
    d. supportive care.

49. Your client is being discharged after having a growth removed from her abdomen. The doctor has assured her that the tumor was benign and that no further treatment is indicated. She says, "My neighbor uses an Ayurveda practitioner. She had cancer 15 years ago and it has never returned. What do you think?" Your most appropriate response would be:
    a. "It sounds like a good idea to me. You never know what will work."
    b. "I don't think it's safe to use alternative medicine. None of it is proven."
    c. "You should learn more about it before trying it. Let me get you a pamphlet that gives some suggestions for evaluation of alternative practices."
    d. "Ayurveda therapy won't prevent the recurrence of cancer. You need to stick with your medical doctor."

50. Your client tells you that his insurance company will allow him to see any physician he chooses, but the fees are better if he chooses a physician from a list provided by the insurance company. He is most likely describing:
    a. a health maintenance organization.
    b. a managed care organization.
    c. Medicaid coverage.
    d. a preferred provider organization.

51. If you could make a change in the delivery of health care for the growing number of Hispanic Americans, which would be most likely to result in integrating cost control and improved quality?
    a. targeting genetically transmitted diseases that only affect Hispanics
    b. increasing the number of Hispanic health providers
    c. ensuring access to health care for Hispanic people
    d. targeting the most common health problems for Hispanic people

Developing a Framework for Practice

PURPOSE

This chapter provides definitions of the terminology used in nursing theory. It describes the four components common to present nursing theories and compares and contrasts the leading nursing theories. It also examines the application of theory to practice.

LEARNING OBJECTIVES

After studying this chapter, you should be able to:

1. provide definitions of the terminology used in nursing theory.
2. describe the four components common to present nursing theories.
3. discuss the importance of theory in nursing practice.
4. compare and contrast at least five significant nursing theories.
5. describe the advantages of multiple theories.
6. discuss obstacles to implementing nursing theory in practice.
7. examine the application of three theories to practice.

MATCHING

1. ____ assumptions
2. ____ conceptual framework
3. ____ conceptual model
4. ____ hypothesis
5. ____ metaparadigm
6. ____ model
7. ____ paradigm
8. ____ phenomenon
9. ____ philosophy
10. ____ theory

a. statements that reflect the values and beliefs of a discipline

b. the incorporation of the most abstract or broad knowledge elements of a discipline; consists of more than one paradigm

c. a symbolic and physical visualization of some aspect of reality

d. refers to facts, behaviors, problems, and events that describe a reality

e. a conceptual diagram that organizes a theory

f. usually refers to a graphic explanation of theoretical relationships

g. a group of propositions used to describe, explain, or predict a phenomenon

h. beliefs about phenomena you must accept as true in order to accept a theory

(Continued on p. 22)

i. a group of related concepts that support a particular viewpoint or focus

j. a relationship statement that is to be tested

TRUE OR FALSE

11. ____ Nursing theory can be of several different types.

12. ____ Assumptions are tested and are assumed to represent reality.

13. ____ Nursing's paradigm identifies the common areas of core concern for our discipline.

14. ____ Theories are important to nurses because they help us determine the meaning of clinical experience while providing guidance for our practice.

15. ____ A nursing theory is unacceptable when the consensus of the nursing profession is that the theory provides an adequate description of reality.

16. ____ The original nursing educational system in the United States was theory-based.

17. ____ Roy believed that nursing practice should not be based on white, middle-class cultural beliefs.

FILL-IN-THE-BLANKS

18. Propositions are statements that represent the _____ view of which concepts fit together and how those concepts affect one another.

19. The concepts of _____, environment, health, and _____ are the most recognized organizing realities of nursing theory.

20. The concerns of nursing as a discipline are defined as a _____.

21. The National Center for _____ Research was established as a part of the Health Research Act of 1985.

22. It is helpful for you to know more than one nursing _____ because what you observe, document, choose as an intervention, and evaluate depends on your theoretical perspective guiding nursing practice.

23. Transcultural nursing requires that you be able to give care that is deemed _____ acceptable by the client.

24. Orem's theory focuses on the role of the _____ in helping clients meet their needs.

EXERCISING YOUR CLINICAL JUDGMENT

25. Since the half-life (i.e., half of what you learn will be outdated) of your nursing knowledge is approximately three years, you will need to do which of the following to remain knowledgeable about nursing practice?
    a. remain in one nursing specialty
    b. take college courses on nursing throughout your career
    c. remain in the clinical area and attend continuing education programs
    d. find a mentor who will help you learn about the clinical specialty

26. Your client, Mrs. Kelly, is Irish-American and has had abdominal surgery. You recognize the client's pain and her minimizing of the pain may be related to cultural ways. You stress to Mrs. Kelly that if she has adequate pain relief she will be able to tend to all of her needs. You are applying which nursing theorist's theory?
    a. Hildegarde Peplau
    b. Faye Abdellah
    c. Dorothea Orem
    d. Madeleine Leininger

27. You create a plan for meeting Mrs. Kelly's health deviation needs because she is experiencing delayed recovery from her surgery. You are applying whose nursing theory?
    a. Hildegarde Peplau
    b. Faye Abdellah
    c. Dorothea Orem
    d. Madeleine Leininger

TEST YOURSELF

28. Nursing theories do which of the following?
    a. differentiate the focus of nursing from other professions and are necessary for the continued growth and development of our profession
    b. provide a conceptual diagram of the profession
    c. are beliefs about phenomena
    d. are relationship statements that are tested

29. Which nursing leader's theory is the primary basis for psychiatric nursing?
    a. Virginia Henderson
    b. Hildegarde Peplau
    c. Faye Abdellah
    d. Dorothea Orem

30. Which of the following nursing leaders emphasized that nursing is not something a person does, but a body of abstract knowledge and a learned profession that is both science and art?
    a. Virginia Henderson
    b. Hildegarde Peplau
    c. Faye Abdellah
    d. Martha Rogers

31. According to Roy's theory, there are four ways the client can adapt. The third mode is the role function that refers to:
    a. the social expectations all people have for others.
    b. beliefs, values, and expectations for the future.
    c. activity and rest, nutrition, elimination, and self-preservation.
    d. respect, friendship, value, or love needs only being met through mutual relationships with others.

32. Which type of self-care requisite is a person's need for such things as air, water, food, activity and rest, and social interaction?
    a. partly compensatory
    b. universal
    c. developmental
    d. health deviation

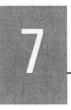

Critical Thinking and Clinical Judgment

PURPOSE

The purpose of this chapter is to help you learn to recognize the skills you use in thinking and when you are using different skills, and thus be able to improve the use of your thinking skills. It also introduces the nursing process, a patterned way of thinking used in making nursing judgments, decisions, and diagnoses. You will be able to identify how multiple thinking strategies apply to each phase of the nursing process.

LEARNING OBJECTIVES

After studying this chapter, you should be able to:

1. differentiate among critical thinking, problem solving, decision making, diagnostic reasoning, and clinical judgment.
2. describe the elements of the T.H.I.N.K. model of critical thinking.
3. discuss Benner's stages of skill proficiency in nursing practice.
4. recognize obstacles to critical thinking.
5. describe the five interwoven phases of the nursing process.
6. apply the T.H.I.N.K. model to the nursing process.

MATCHING

1. __F__ clinical judgment
2. __e__ decision making
3. __b__ nursing process
4. __C__ problem solving
5. __a__ diagnostic reasoning
6. __d__ critical thinking

a. the process of clustering related data pieces about a client situation, analyzing the cluster critically, and deriving specific nursing diagnoses for the client

b. a clinical decision-making process that includes critical thinking, diagnostic reasoning, and clinical judgment; it is composed of five inter-related parts: assessment, diagnosis, planning, intervention, and evaluation

(Continued on p. 26)

c.   a process used to arrive at an answer or a solution (There is an implied gap of information or action that needs to be provided to get to the solution, as well as the expectation that the solution be "right" according to a particular standard of measure.)

d.   purposeful self-regulatory judgment that gives reasoned and reflective consideration to evidence, contexts, conceptualizations, methods, and criteria

e.   making a choice between two or more options; may be goal directed, in which case the goal or goals will direct the outcome

f.   includes critical thinking, problem-solving, and decision–making, and is derived from the knowledge and clinical experience base of the nurse; it is holistic and partly intuitive

TRUE OR FALSE

7.   _F_   Critical thinking does not involve creative solutions to problems.

8.   _F_   The T.H.I.N.K. model is based on the idea that you use different elements of thinking in different situations. *Five modes of thinking used in combination simultaneously*

9.   _T_   Inquiry includes the quality of being curious or wondering about the meaning of information.

10. _T_   Making a judgment is a decision-making process in a situation of uncertainty.

11. _T_   Critical thinking requires an attitude of seeking the truth.

12. _T_   Critical thinking requires assessing your own thinking in specific situations.

13. _T_   Good thinking involves recognizing and considering your personal bias.

14. _F_   When you begin to recognize common patterns you have achieved competency. *advanced beginner*

15. _F_   Routines in health care facilities are antithetical to critical thinking.

16. _F_   Assessment means collecting answers to a predetermined list of questions.

FILL-IN-THE-BLANKS

17. A physical examination gathers directly observable data, otherwise known as _subjective_ data.

18. Assessment is a process of _discovering_ and _making decisions_

19. Three types of nursing diagnoses are _wellness_ diagnoses, _risk_ diagnoses, and _actual_ diagnoses.

20. In the planning phase you establish _expected outcomes_

21. Ten types of interventions include _direct care_, _teaching_, _coordination_, _collaboration_, _health promotion_, _disease prevention_, _health maintenance_, _restoration_, and _rehabilitation_.

22. An evaluation includes _data gathering_ to confirm that the problem has been resolved.

23. NANDA stands for the _North American Nursing Diagnosis Association_

24. Name six obstacles to critical thinking.
    bias
    lack of confidence
    time
    anxiety
    inadequate knowledge and
    over reliance on habits. -

25. The phases of the nursing process are _____ (interrelated or distinct).

26. Name four of the eleven attitudes of critical thinking. _____, _pg. 249_ _____, and _____.

EXERCISING YOUR CLINICAL JUDGMENT

27. You are taking an admission history. You know the medical diagnosis but the client's report of symptoms does not exactly fit the pattern of expected symptoms. Which action would be the least consistent with critical thinking?
    a.   Explore the symptoms further.
    b.   Record the symptoms as described by the client.
    c.   Record only the symptoms you believe are pertinent to the diagnosis.
    d.   Ask the client about his perception of the symptoms.

28. As a critical thinker, you attempt to make a nursing diagnosis using the NANDA list of diagnoses. You do not find a diagnosis that describes your client's symptoms. You would:
    a. pick a diagnosis anyway.
    b. conclude that nurses should not treat the problem.
    c. consider the possibility that NANDA has omitted an important diagnosis.
    d. ignore the problem.

29. You are starting a new job as a home health nurse. You must perform a procedure in the client's home. While you have done the procedure many times in the hospital, you do not have the same resources in the home. Which mode of thinking will be the most useful to you?
    a. total recall
    b. habit
    c. inquiry
    d. new ideas

30. You are working on a postsurgical unit caring for five clients. Two had surgery today. The physician's orders do not specify taking vital signs at noon on any of the clients. You know that none of the clients have had any problems with vital signs for the last eight hours, but the two who had surgery today are still in a critical postsurgical period. You decide to take vital signs on these two clients at noon. Select the response that best describes the technique you have used.
    a. decision making
    b. clinical judgment
    c. problem solving
    d. nursing diagnosis

31. A client complains of nausea. You know the physician has written an order for a medication to treat nausea if the client needs it. Using the nursing process to guide your thinking you would first:
    a. ask the client to further describe the nausea.
    b. give the anti-nausea medication.
    c. plan to cancel the client's lunch.
    d. notify the physician.

TEST YOURSELF

32. Select the response that is the least consistent with critical thinking.
    a. Select the one right answer.
    b. See a problem from multiple points of view.
    c. Make the best choice from several supportable alternatives.
    d. Consider the client's mind, body, and spirit.

33. Your client's pathology report identifies a tumor as cancerous. The client never asks his physician about the results of the report. If the physician does not give the results to the client based on the belief that this client does not want information about his illness, you would classify this belief as:
    a. a sound clinical judgment.
    b. an assumption.
    c. an act of human kindness.
    d. between the client and physician.

34. You assess your client and find sluggish skin turgor, sunken eyeballs, and a low urinary output. You know these are signs of dehydration and conclude that your client should drink more water. You have:
    a. made an interpretation of data.
    b. made an assumption.
    c. engaged in problem solving.
    d. recognized the purpose of thinking.

35. Your client has cancer. The cancer specialist believes that the client's life can be prolonged with chemotherapy and has offered to treat the cancer. The client chooses not to accept the treatment. Because the client is a mother of two small children, you are strongly opposed to the decision and tell the client your opinion. Your behavior is an example of:
    a. egocentricity.
    b. sociocentricity.
    c. humility.
    d. confidence in reasoning.

36. You are assigned to work with a staff nurse. The two of you enter a client's room and find the client slumped in bed. You assume the client is sleeping, but the staff nurse puts on the call light and picks up the phone to page for a resuscitation team. Which of Benner's stages apply to the staff nurse?
    a. advanced beginner
    b. competent
    c. proficient
    d. expert

37. You are assigned to a different nurse on the following day. A client tells you she does not need a laxative. The nurse tells you a laxative is always given after the procedure the client has had and you should insist the client take the laxative. This nurse is most likely in which stage?
    a. novice
    b. advanced beginner
    c. competent
    d. proficient

8

Assessing the Client: History Taking

PURPOSE

The purpose of this chapter is to describe the thinking skills associated with assessment and introduce a general pattern for taking a nursing history. You will add additional information about nursing history with each clinical chapter you study. By the end of the course you should be able to take a complete nursing history for a variety of clients.

LEARNING OBJECTIVES

After studying this chapter, you should be able to:

1. understand assessment as a critical thinking process.
2. make preliminary decisions to prepare for data collection.
3. identify methods to meet the assessment standard established by the American Nurses Association.
4. develop mental processes associated with effective data collection.
5. develop a systematic framework for organizing data.
6. appropriately document the assessment.

MATCHING

1. _X_ assessment
2. _r_ closed question
3. _v_ cue
4. _⧧_ demographic data
5. _o_ inference
6. _s_ database
7. _y_ data
8. _u_ cardinal signs and symptoms
9. _h_ functional health patterns
10. _e_ chief complaint
11. _w_ active listening
12. _q_ biographic data
13. _a_ working phase
14. _c_ validation
15. _n_ minimum data set
16. _m_ nursing history
17. _i_ signs
18. _d_ subjective data
19. _b_ symptoms
20. _g_ objective data

a. a phase of the interview process during which the client and the nurse work together to review the client's health history and establish potential and actual problems that will be addressed as part of the care plan

b. subjective information that is indicative of disease as perceived by the client

c. substantiating or confirming the accuracy of the information against another source or by another method

d. information that is provided by the client and cannot be directly observed

(Continued on p. 30)

21. __k__ orientation phase

22. __i__ open-ended question

23. __p__ leading question

24. __f__ interview

25. __j__ intuition

26. __z__ active processing

e. the problem that caused the person to seek health services, to call the doctor or to request a visit from the nurse; a description of what the person thinks is the problem

f. a planned series of questions designed to elicit information for a particular purpose

g. any directly observable information about the client

h. the positive and negative behaviors a person uses to interact with the environment and maintain health

i. a question designed to allow the client freedom in the manner of response

j. a process of reasoning from understanding the whole without having systematically examined the parts

k. a brief exchange to establish the purpose, the procedure, and the nurse's role as a phase of the interview process

l. objective data that are evidence of disease or dysfunction

m. a narrative of the client's past health and health practices that focuses on information needed to plan nursing care

n. the least information allowable to be collected on every client entering an institution or being admitted to a particular service within the institution

o. the process of attaching meaning to data or reaching a conclusion about data; based on a premise or proposition that supports or helps support a conclusion

p. question that suggests a possible appropriate response

q. information that identifies and describes the person, such as name, address, age, gender, religious affiliation, race, or occupation

r. question that calls for a specific response from the client

s. all of the information that has been collected about the client and recorded in the health record as a baseline for the initial plan of care

t. factual information that can be counted to describe populations of clients

u. the data of greatest significance in diagnosing a particular illness, disease, or health problem

v. a stimulus to the action of looking for related data

w. participation in a conversation with a client in which the nurse attends to what the client says and has a part in helping the client clarify, elaborate, and give additional pertinent information

x. the process of gathering data about the client's health status to identify the concerns and needs that can be treated or managed by nursing care

y. pieces of subjective or objective information about the client or the signs and symptoms of disease

z. a systematic series of mental actions to analyze and interpret the information about the client

TRUE OR FALSE

27. __T__ When prevention is the focus of care, the assessment includes risk and lifestyle factors.

28. __T__ When, how often, and how to assess a client is a nursing judgment based on individual client needs.

29. __F__ It is always appropriate to gather data from the client's family.

30. __T__ Collecting data in a systematic way is a standard of nursing practice.

31. __T__ Grouping data into meaningful patterns helps you translate the data into a meaningful statement.

32. __F__ For any client, the purpose of an admission interview is always to collect a standard set of data.

33. __F__ The termination phase of an interview is limited to the last few minutes of the interview.

34. __F__ Biographical data is collected only to help you know the client as a person.

35. __F__ The medical history is not part of the nursing history.

36. __T__ Beliefs about health and about the ability to change health are a key element of the health perception-health management pattern.

37. __T__ A functional health pattern includes both functional and dysfunctional patterns.

38. __F__ The activity-exercise pattern only includes the musculoskeletal system.

39. __F__ Only objective data is documented in the medical record.

40. __T__ It is legally advisable to document the facts that lead to a conclusion or opinion rather than your own conclusion or opinion.

FILL-IN-THE-BLANKS

41. Assessment begins with __thinking__.

42. When the goal is __restoration__, assessment focuses on the need for support of body functions and the detection and prevention of complications.

43. To decide how often to assess you need to anticipate __potential for A____, __potential for rate of A__, and __evidence of A__.

44. The seven general factors used to assess a symptom are __location, quality, chronology, setting, aggravor alleviating factors__, and __assoc. Fac.__

45. __Rapport__ is established in the orientation phase of an interview.

46. __Rapport__ implies a sense of understanding and trust between the nurse and client.

47. Questions describing the onset of symptoms, when symptoms occur, and the events surrounding symptoms are classified as __chronology__.

48. A description of a client's dietary habits is included in the __nutritional__ - __metabolic__ pattern.

49. A description of a client's tolerance for activity is included in the __activity__ - __exercise__ pattern.

50. A description of the client's perception of body image is included in the __self__ - __perception__ / __self__ - __concept__ pattern.

EXERCISING YOUR CLINICAL JUDGMENT

51. A female client who has four children, works full time, and volunteers in her church is admitted. She has peptic ulcer disease, an illness that is sometimes exacerbated by stress. In assessing the coping-stress tolerance pattern you would:
    a. assume the illness is exacerbated by stress.
    b. plan to teach the client stress reduction techniques.
    c. avoid discussion of the many stressors in the client's life.
    d. validate the client's experience of stress by eliciting information about the client's perceptions.

52. You would assess the self-concept pattern on every client by:
    a. asking a series of questions to elicit information about the self-concept.
    b. observing, listening, and being sensitive to covert messages.
    c. administering a standardized test for self concept.
    d. asking the person to rate his or her self-concept on a scale of 1–10.

53. A 55-year-old male is hospitalized for heart disease. His doctor has suggested he needs to retire. Which functional health pattern would you explore to help him through this experience?
    a. sexuality-reproductive pattern
    b. role-relationship pattern
    c. coping-stress tolerance pattern
    d. sleep-rest pattern

54. You are taking an admission history. The client tells you that he has pain in his leg. Which question is most pertinent to his safety in the hospital?
    a. "How long have you had the pain?"
    b. "Where is it located?"
    c. "Do you have any difficulty walking?"
    d. "What aggravates the pain?"

55. Your client has requested pain medication. If you could only ask one question for further assessment, which would you choose?
    a. "Did the last pain medication relieve the pain?"
    b. "How long have you had the pain?"
    c. "What brought on the pain?"
    d. "Is your pain less than yesterday's pain?"

TEST YOURSELF

56. Select the statement that is true of assessment.
    a. Assessment means collecting data.
    b. Assessment includes analyzing data to determine the need for nursing care.
    c. Assessment does not include physical examination.
    d. Assessment is a separate activity from planning and implementing care.

57. Select the response that most closely describes focused assessment. Focused assessment means:
    a. paying close attention to the client's needs.
    b. concentrating on an identified need and getting more information.
    c. identifying the client's needs.
    d. using the acronym F.O.C.U.S.

58. Select the best description of objective data. Objective data:
    a. is pertinent to an objective or goal.
    b. can be gathered through the use of one of the five senses.
    c. is elicited from the client in an objective manner.
    d. is about the objects in the client's room.

59. You are sharing information with the client's physician that the wife of your client has given you. The physician asks you if the wife is a reliable source. Select the response that is the most useful in deciding that the wife is a reliable source (all of the following information was shared with you).
    a. The couple have been arguing about the nature of his symptoms.
    b. The husband has told you to talk to his wife about his symptoms.
    c. The wife presents information factually and has kept a diary of the symptoms.
    d. The husband shows evidence of minor memory impairment.

60. *Fact:* Your client's prescription for antihypertension medication was filled 15 days ago with 60 tablets. He is supposed to take two tablets a day. He has 40 tablets left. *Premise:* There is a high incidence of failure to take blood pressure medications correctly among people with hypertension because of side effects. Select the most accurate conclusion.
    a. The client does not understand how to take the medication.
    b. The client does not want to take the medication.
    c. The client has taken the medication incorrectly.
    d. The side effects have been intolerable for the client.

Assessing the Client: Vital Signs

PURPOSE

The purpose of this chapter is to help you learn an accurate technique for measuring vital signs and to understand the physiological changes that affect vital signs. You will also begin the process of interpreting or attaching meaning to your findings.

LEARNING OBJECTIVES

After studying this chapter, you should be able to:

1. safely and accurately measure axillary, oral, rectal, and tympanic temperatures; apical and radial pulses; respirations; and blood pressure.
2. identify nursing responsibilities related to the assessment of vital signs.
3. measure vital signs in an organized, accurate manner.
4. know the normal ranges of each vital sign according to the client's age.
5. describe the normal physiology of each vital sign.
6. list factors that influence temperature, pulse, respirations, and blood pressure.
7. document and report vital sign measurements correctly.

MATCHING

1. _e_ basal metabolic rate
2. _c_ thermogenesis
3. _d_ apical pulse
4. _a_ pulse deficit
5. _b_ thermolysis

6. _l_ hypertension
7. _o_ systolic blood pressure
8. _g_ eupnea
9. _m_ hypotension
10. _p_ tachypnea
11. _k_ diastolic blood pressure
12. _n_ Korotkoff's sounds
13. _f_ pulse pressure
14. _i_ bradycardia
15. _q_ vascular resistance
16. _j_ bradypnea
17. _h_ auscultatory gap

a. the condition of the apical pulse rate exceeding the radial pulse rate

b. the processes through which heat is dispersed from the body through radiation, conduction, convection, and evaporation expressed as calories per hour per square meter of body surface

c. the generation of heat from the chemical reactions that take place in cellular activity

d. the heart rate counted at the apex of the heart on the anterior chest

e. the amount of energy needed to maintain essential basic body functions expressed as calories per hour per square meter of body surface

f. the difference between the systolic and diastolic pressure

g. normal quiet respiration

(Continued on p. 34)

h. the absence of Korotkoff II sound; sometimes present in hypertension

i. a heart rate insufficient to produce adequate tissue perfusion (when it continues over a long time), usually < 60

j. a respiratory rate insufficient to take in enough oxygen (when it continues over a long time), usually below 10

k. the pressure in the blood vessels that remains during relaxation of the ventricles

l. generally defined as a BP over 140/90

m. generally defined as a blood pressure below 100/60.

n. five distinct sounds heard as a blood pressure cuff is deflated from total occlusion of the artery to complete free flow of blood

o. the pressure in the arteries produced by the cardiac output during contraction of the ventricle

p. rapid respiration

q. hindrance to blood flow through an artery

TRUE OR FALSE

18. F The absolute value of vital signs is the basis for inferences about vital signs. Compare to baseline V/S

19. T How often you take vital signs is a nursing judgment.

20. T The body's cells work within a narrow range of normal temperature but can tolerate some changes for a brief period.

21. T High temperatures damage cells by inactivating proteins and enzymes.

22. F An oral temperature can be accurately measured by placing the thermometer anywhere in the mouth.

23. F Clean a glass thermometer by wiping from the bulb toward the end.

24. F A heart rate of 100 is always a cause for concern.

25. T Vomiting can cause bradycardia.

26. T Adrenalin increases the heart rate.

27. F Head injuries always cause the heart rate to increase. can cause bradycardia

28. F The strength of the pulse wave is only a function of the strength of myocardial contraction.

29. F The carotid artery is the most common site for counting the pulse.

30. T The most accurate pulse count is obtained at the apex of the heart.

31. T The medullary control center for respiration responds to high levels of carbon dioxide.

32. T Sighing is a protective mechanism that periodically expands unused alveoli.

FILL-IN-THE-BLANKS

33. vital signs are the signs of life.

34. The processes through which the body balances heat production and heat loss to maintain a temperature between 96.8° F and 99.4° F is called thermoregulation

35. The glass thermometer is inexpensive, accurate, and easily disinfected; however, it may be difficult to read for some clients in their homes.

36. The tympanic thermometer is accurate if the probe is directed on the eardrum.

37. Children have a slightly higher heart rate than adults do because they have a higher metabolic rate.

38. Adrenergic drugs (acting like adrenalin) will cause the heart rate to _____ (increase, decrease).

39. When the pulse wave increases during inhalation and decreases back to normal during exhalation, the phenomenon is called pulsus paradoxus

40. When blood vessels constrict, blood flow is impeded because the lumen of the vessels is smaller. The smaller diameter creates peripheral vascular resistance.

41. The systolic blood pressure is created by the _____ (contraction, relaxation) of the ventricles.

42. The diastolic blood pressure is the pressure that remains during _____ (contraction, relaxation) of the ventricles.

43. The width of the blood pressure cuff should be about two-thirds of the length of the upper arm.

EXERCISING YOUR CLINICAL JUDGMENT

44. Your client has a temperature of 103° F, respiration of 30, pulse of 50. She is cold and clammy and her blood pressure is 100/60. Which conclusion is most consistent with these findings?
    a. The temperature has caused a decrease in her pulse rate. Correcting the temperature will fix the problem.
    b. The low pulse is causing a decrease in cardiac output, thus reducing the blood pressure. It may or may not be related to the temperature.
    c. The low pulse and blood pressure is a compensatory response to decrease the metabolic rate.
    d. The high temperature is consistent with the low pulse and blood pressure.

45. The physician tells you that the client has atherosclerotic vascular disease that is increasing peripheral vascular resistance. Which vital signs would be consistent with this information?
    a. Blood pressure 140/100, pulse 90, respiration 18
    b. Blood pressure 110/60, pulse 60, respiration 18
    c. Blood pressure 160/80, pulse 56, respiration 16
    d. Blood pressure 140/84, pulse 80, respiration 20

46. Your client's blood pressure is 180/106. You administer an anti-hypertensive and come to the room to recheck the blood pressure in one hour. You find the client in the bathroom and she is pale, sweating, and feels faint. You get her back to bed and take her vital signs. Which would you expect?
    a. BP 180/106; the medication did not work.
    b. BP 120/80; the sudden drop caused the symptoms.
    c. BP 160/96; the medication is taking effect, but has made her sick.
    d. BP 120/80; the medication has been effective, and the symptoms have another cause.

47. Digitalis is a medication that slows the heart rate and strengthens the contraction. Before giving digitalis it is a common practice to check the pulse. If the client's pulse has been averaging 80 for the last three days, which pulse rate would suggest that the expected result has become a toxic effect?
    a. pulse 56
    b. pulse 66
    c. pulse 76
    d. pulse 96

48. Your client was burned on the right arm while lighting a charcoal fire. He has an IV in the left arm that was inserted with difficulty finding a vein. Which action would you take related to vital signs?
    a. Since he is awake and alert, skip taking a blood pressure.
    b. Use a smaller size cuff for the blood pressure.
    c. Take the blood pressure in the thigh.
    d. Assess the systolic pressure only by palpating the radial artery.

49. You have admitted a 16-month-old with fever of unknown origin. The child's cheeks are red and the skin feels warm to the touch. The tympanic thermometer reads 98.6° F. Select the best action.
    a. Check the temperature in the room and lower the thermostat for comfort.
    b. Ask the mother about the technique she used to take the temperature to determine if the reported fever was accurate.
    c. Straighten the ear canal and recheck the temperature. Use another method if necessary to accurately measure the temperature.
    d. Re-calibrate the thermometer and check the temperature.

TEST YOURSELF

50. You take a client's temperature at 6 a.m. It is 96.8° F. What is the most probable cause?
    a. a cold room
    b. drinking ice water
    c. circadian rhythms
    d. a faulty thermometer

51. Select the activity that is appropriate when preparing to take an axillary temperature.
    a. Dry the axilla before inserting the thermometer.
    b. Lubricate the thermometer before insertion.
    c. Position patient in the side-lying position.
    d. Shave the axilla.

52. The client's rectal temperature is 100°F. Select the comparable axillary temperature.
    a. 97° F
    b. 98°F
    c. 99°F
    d. 101°F

53. You should avoid taking a blood pressure on the same arm with an intravenous infusion. The primary reason is that:
    a. the blood pressure will be inaccurate.
    b. blood from the IV line will contaminate the blood pressure cuff.
    c. the increased venous pressure will cause blood to back up in the IV tubing.
    d. the blood pressure reading will be higher.

54. Nurses have some discretion in selecting the route to take a temperature. Which of the following represents the best judgment?
    a. taking an oral temperature in a 12-month-old child
    b. taking a rectal temperature in a confused 85-year-old man
    c. taking an axillary temperature in a newborn
    d. taking an oral temperature on a client who had oral surgery

55. Select the situation that may result in an inaccurate measurement of blood pressure.
    a. The width of cuff is 20% greater than the diameter of arm.
    b. The aneroid sphygmomanometer is viewed from the side.
    c. The meniscus of the mercury manometer is at eye level.
    d. The cuff is placed one inch above the fold of the elbow.

56. The diastolic pressure in an adult is recorded as:
    a. the first distinct beat that is heard.
    b. the change in sound from a clear, distinct tapping to a soft, muffled sound.
    c. the middle sound between the first and last beat heard.
    d. the last sound that is heard.

57. To obtain the most accurate blood pressure reading the cuff should be inflated to:
    a. 20-30 mm Hg above the palpated systolic pressure.
    b. the systolic reading last recorded on the client's chart.
    c. 50 mm Hg above last diastolic reading.
    d. 200 mm Hg in an adult client.

58. Which action might result in a falsely low systolic BP reading?
    a. allowing the client to cross legs while BP is being taken
    b. deflating the cuff too rapidly while BP is being auscultated.
    c. requiring the client to support arm isometrically while BP is being taken
    d. having the client think relaxing thoughts

59. Select the inference that is most accurate without further assessment.
    a. A right radial pulse of 88 beats/minute indicates that the person has adequate oxygenation to the right hand.
    b. Respirations of 18 per minute indicate that the person is taking in sufficient amounts of oxygen.
    c. The auscultated blood pressure of 130/88 is a normal blood pressure for this particular person.
    d. When the apical pulse is 80 and the radial pulse is 60 the client has a pulse deficit.

60. A client is admitted to the hospital with an irregular pulse of 110. Select the best method to use to further evaluate the pulse.
    a. Take an apical-radial pulse and subtract the difference.
    b. Subtract the difference between the right and left radial pulses.
    c. Count the time it takes for an apical beat to reach the radial pulses.
    d. Count the number of irregular beats to determine a pulse deficit.

61. A client has just been admitted with a lung infection. His vital signs indicate hypotension, tachycardia, and tachypnea. This information would be supported by which set of data?
    a. B/P 150/105, pulse 123, respirations 12
    b. B/P 90/40, pulse 110, respirations 28
    c. B/P 120/80, pulse 50, respirations 40
    d. B/P 115/80, pulse 100, respirations 30

62. A client had a temperature of 104° F at 10 a.m. At 1 p.m. the skin is warm and wet with perspiration. The nurse retakes the temperature. Select the finding that would be expected.
    a. A normal or near-normal temperature is found.
    b. The fever has not abated.
    c. The temperature has increased.
    d. The client is anxious.

63. Select the client for whom you would take a rectal, rather than an oral, temperature.
    a. 10-year-old girl admitted with a urinary tract infection
    b. 79-year-old man with dentures who is NPO for surgery
    c. 40-year-old male admitted for new onset confusion
    d. 80-year-old female admitted for a total hip replacement

64. A 45- year-old client has been in a motor vehicle accident (MVA). He was examined in the Emergency Department and transferred to your unit for observation. Vital signs are BP 100/60, P 94, R 22, and T 98.6° F. Select the best conclusion concerning these findings.
    a. The vital signs may indicate impending shock; notify the physician.
    b. These are normal findings for this age; routine monitoring.
    c. These may be normal findings, but there is concern about the BP; continue monitoring.
    d. He probably received pain medication in the emergency room.

Assessing the Client: Physical Examination

PURPOSE

When you finish studying this chapter you should know the basic techniques of the physical examination and be able to identify normal findings. You will also be introduced to some abnormal findings as a way to help you begin the process of comparing normal to abnormal findings.

LEARNING OBJECTIVES

After studying this chapter, you should be able to:

1. define and describe each of the four techniques used in physical examination: inspection, palpation, percussion, and auscultation.
2. identify and understand the primary instruments used in physical assessment.
3. acquire courteous nonthreatening techniques to ensure client comfort and prepare the client for each regionally focused area of a complete physical examination.
4. perform a complete physical examination on a client.
5. recognize normal physical findings.
6. recognize abnormal physical findings.
7. learn the techniques of performing certain special maneuvers used in physical assessment.
8. learn the techniques used in obtaining certain specimens routinely collected during a complete physical examination.

MATCHING

1. _b._ accommodation
2. _c._ adventitious breath sounds
3. _g_ atrial gallop
4. _y_ vesicular breath sounds
5. _k_ turgor
6. _n_ lesion
7. _s_ S_1
8. _t_ S_2
9. _v_ S_3
10. _o_ murmur
11. _l_ bruit
12. _m_ inspection
13. _e_ percussion
14. _j_ auscultation
15. _z_ apical pulse
16. _i_ broncho-vesicular breath sounds
17. _f_ respiratory excursion
18. _q_ otoscope
19. _r_ tactile fremitus

a. the abnormal accumulation of serous (edematous) fluid within the peritoneal cavity

b. adjustment of the eye for seeing objects at various distances

c. produced by a source other than the normal lungs

d. the area on the anterior chest overlying the heart and great vessels

e. the use of short, sharp strikes to the body surface to produce palpable vibrations and characteristic sounds

f. the ability of the lungs to expand as evidenced by the degree to which the chest wall expands

(Continued on p. 40)

20. __l__ ophthalmo-scope

21. __d__ precordium

22. __w__ S₄

23. __v__ point of maximum impulse (PMI)

24. __h.__ palpation

25. __a.__ ascites

26. __k__ bronchial breath sounds

g. an abnormal cardiac rhythm in which a low pitched, extra heart sound is heard late in diastole, just before the S₁, on auscultation of the heart; also called S₄

h. a form of touch or feeling with the hand; it is used to obtain information regarding temperature, moisture, texture, consistency, size, shape, position, and movement

i. normal breath sounds that occur between sounds of the bronchial tubes and those of the alveoli, or a combination of the two sounds

j. the process of listening to sounds generated within the body

k. a normal sound heard with a stethoscope over the main airways, including trachea and sternum

l. an abnormal blowing or swishing sound or murmur heard while auscultating a carotid artery, organ, or gland, such as the liver or thyroid

m. the systematic visual examination of the client

n. a wound, injury, or pathological change in the body

o. abnormal sounds that occur when there is turbulent blood flow in the heart or great vessels; they are heard as a swooshing or blowing sound when auscultated

p. an instrument used to visualize the retina, including the optic disk, macula, and retinal blood vessels through the pupil

q. an instrument used to examine the external ear, the eardrum and, through the eardrum, the ossicles of the middle ear; consists of a light, a magnifying lens, a speculum, and sometimes a device for insufflation

r. a vibration, as in the chest wall, over an area of secretions, felt on the thorax when the client is speaking

s. the first heart sound, produced by the vibration of the chest wall set in motion by the closures of the mitral and tricuspid valves

t. the second heart sound, produced by the vibration of the chest wall set in motion by the closure of the aortic and pulmonic valves

u. the third heart sound thought to be caused by vibrations of the ventricle walls when they are suddenly distended by blood from the atria; heard most clearly at the apex of the heart

v. the point where the heart comes the closest to the chest wall at the apex of the heart

w. a fourth heart sound which may be heard at the apex of the heart during expiration; caused by vibrations of the atria after contraction

x. a reflection of the skin's elasticity measured as the time it takes for the skin to return to normal after being pinched lightly between the thumb and forefinger

y. a normal sound of rustling or swishing heard with a stethoscope over the lung periphery, characteristically higher pitched during inspiration and falling rapidly during expiration

z. the heart beat heard with a stethoscope at the apex of the heart

TRUE OR FALSE

27. _F_ A good quality stethoscope has a thin wall.

28. _F_ A stethoscope amplifies sounds to enable you to hear.

29. _f_ You should always begin the physical examination with the client in the sitting position.

30. _T_ The sagittal plane divides the body into right and left halves.

31. _F_ The heart is located lateral to the midline on the right side.

32. _T_ The advantage of the balanced scale is accuracy because the scale can be balanced at zero with each use.

33. _F_ If the client can tell you that the current time of day is after lunch time, you may assume orientation to time.

34. _T_ Damage to the facial nerve (cranial nerve VII) results in lack of control of the muscles needed to close the eye.

35. _T_ Yearly eye exams are indicated for people with bleeding disorders or those on antico-agulant therapy.

36. _F_ PERRLA is checked on the unconscious client to determine visual acuity.

37. _T_ Arteries are distinguishable as brighter than veins when checking the ocular fundus.

38. _f_ You should angle the otoscope at a ninety-degree angle to the ear to visualize the ear drum. _Toward nose_

39. _f_ The thyroid gland should feel smooth and hard. _Should be soft_

40. _T_ A cervical lymph node that is less than 1 cm with definite margins, that is also mobile and nontender, is a normal finding.

41. _T_ Assessing the breast for lumps includes assessing the axilla.

42. _T_ The upper lobe of the right lung is assessed above an imaginary line from the posterior fold of the axilla to the midaxillary line at the sixth rib.

43. _T_ Decreased respiratory excursion occurs with any condition that limits the expansion of the lungs.

44. _F_ S_2 is associated with the closure of the mitral and aortic valves. _aortic + pulmonic valves_

45. _F_ An apical/radial pulse should be checked on every client with heart disease. _usually occurs c' irregular rhythms_

46. _T_ A rapid rhythm with an S_3 sound is described as a ventricular gallop.

47. _F_ A grade 6 murmur is barely audible. _loudest easily heard s stethoscope_

48. _F_ A bruit is normally heard at the carotid artery because of the vessel's large size. _never normal_

49. _T_ If you cannot feel a popliteal pulse you should confirm its absence with a Doppler.

50. _F_ Identifying hypoactive bowel sounds is a precise measurement of the volume and frequency of the sounds.

51. _T_ A gastric bubble causes a tympanic sound with percussion over the right upper quadrant.

52. _T_ The Babinski reflex should be absent in an adult.

FILL-IN-THE-BLANKS

53. Use the technique of _light palpation_ to identify and examine lesions or masses on the surface of the skin or immediately under the skin.

54. Use _percussion_ to tap on the abdomen to detect the presence of "gas" or flatus.

55. Using the technique of listening to the abdomen is called _auscultation_.

56. _Affect_ refers to the external expression of emotion attached to ideas or mental representation of ideas.

57. _Cognitive Function_ refers to patterns of thinking such as logic, relevance, organization, and coherence of thought.

58. Skin is best assessed in _natural_ light.

59. Assess superficial lesions for _size_, _consistency_, _shape_, _attachment_, _color_, and _mobility_.

60. _crepitus_ is a crackling or rubbing sound heard during movement of joints, such as the temporomandibular joint.

61. A reported result of 30/60-2 on a visual acuity test means the person is able to read with _2_ error at a distance of _30_ a line of print which a person with normal vision could read at _60_.

62. PERRLA means _pupils_ _equal_ _Round_ _reactf_ _ligh_ and _accomodation_

63. The _Rhinne_ test is a hearing test that compares air and bone conduction using a tuning fork.

64. In periodontal disease the client often has red, swollen gums indicating _gingivitis_ .

65. _Kussmaul_ respiration is the deep, rapid breathing seen in diabetic ketoacidosis.

66. If you hear an abnormal breath sound in part of the cycle of respiration (such as with inspiration and not expiration) you would describe the sound as _discontinuous_ (continuous, discontinuous).

67. _Deep_ _tendon_ reflexes are elicited by stretching a tendon by tapping with a percussion hammer.

68. A _Cystocele_ , the protrusion of the bladder into the vagina, is seen as a bulging mass arising from the anterior vaginal wall.

69. _Bartholins_ glands are located bilaterally at the base of the vaginal opening.

70. The _pap_ _smear_ is a cytology test to screen for cervical cancer.

71. The _prostate_ gland encircles the male urethra.

72. The _epididymus_ lies on top of the testes.

73. A _varicocele_ can be felt as a string of bead-like nodules or "bag of worms" in the scrotum.

EXERCISING YOUR CLINICAL JUDGMENT

74. Your client is a 90-year-old who is admitted to the hospital with a respiratory problem. She seems clean, well groomed, and well nourished, but is unsteady when walking, seems a little confused, and has pain in her chest. Select all of the elements of the physical exam that you would consider essential.
    a. assess for adventitious sounds
    b. formal mental status exam
    c. assess all pulses
    d. complete abdominal assessment
    e. rectal examination
    f. skin assessment
    g. complete musculoskeletal assessment
    h. inspection of the toenails
    i. hearing and vision screening
    j. assess the rate and rhythm of the heart
    k. listen for murmurs

75. Your client has returned from a cardiac catheterization. The catheter was threaded through the right femoral artery. You are checking for blood clots traveling from the artery to the lower leg. The dorsalis pedis pulse is strong. What would you do next?
    a. Check the popliteal pulse.
    b. Check the femoral pulse.
    c. Check the color and warmth of the toes.
    d. Conclude that the circulation is good.

76. Your client has an irregular heartbeat and the apical/radial pulse is 80/60. Select the additional findings you would expect.
    a. talkative, color pink, looking forward to visitors
    b. blood pressure low, skin pale, feels weak
    c. skin hot, face flushed, feels anxious
    d. mentally alert, BP 140/90, respiration 16

77. Which assessment data provides the nurse with the best information regarding the client's ability to perfuse distal tissues?
    a. blood pressure, Homan's sign, and breath sounds
    b. respirations, peripheral pulses, and skin turgor
    c. capillary refill, peripheral pulses, and skin color
    d. skin turgor, skin color, and quality of pulse

78. During lung auscultation, the nurse would ask the client to:
    a. breathe deeply with mouth open.
    b. cough with each inhalation.
    c. hold his or her breath.
    d. breathe quietly and normally.

79. During assessment you cannot palpate the pedal pulses bilaterally. The best nursing action to do next would be:
    a. palpate the femoral arteries.
    b. immediately call the doctor.
    c. assess color and temperature of the client's feet.
    d. ask the client to wiggle his or her toes.

80. A client's left radial pulse is assessed as irregular. The best nursing action would be to:
    a. take an apical pulse for one full minute.
    b. recount the radial pulse for two minutes to assess for regularity.
    c. have another nurse check the right radial pulse while the first nurse recounts the left pulse.
    d. record the finding without further assessment.

81. After auscultating a client's abdomen for 30 seconds, the nurse hears hypoactive bowel sounds in the RUQ and LUQ, and hears no bowel sounds in the RLQ and LLQ. The best action would be to:
    a. immediately report this information to the physician.
    b. listen one to three minutes in each of the lower quadrants.
    c. chart this information and reassess in eight hours.
    d. assess for abdominal distention.

82. When doing a physical examination of a client's lower extremities, if the nurse elicits calf pain on dorsiflexion of the client's right foot, it should be charted as:
    a. complains of cramping pain in right calf.
    b. positive Homan's sign right leg.
    c. painful right leg bruit.
    d. deep vein thrombosis.

TEST YOURSELF

83. Your client is telling you about the difficult times he has had since the death of his wife. He is smiling and periodically interrupts his story with a giggle. You most likely would describe this behavior as:
    a. flat affect.
    b. inappropriate affect.
    c. nonplus affect.
    d. timorous affect.

84. Your client's skin has a yellow cast and you observe yellow color of the conjunctiva. You would describe this finding as:
    a. cyanosis.
    b. flushing.
    c. normal.
    d. jaundice.

85. You ask the client to smile, frown, raise his eyebrows, or tightly close his eyes. Which cranial nerve are you testing?
    a. I
    b. III
    c. V
    d. VII

86. When you ask a client to read a newspaper or pamphlet, you are testing:
    a. distance vision.
    b. near vision.
    c. discrimination.
    d. accommodation.

87. To check the ocular fundus, begin with the ophthalmoscope about _____ inches from the eye.
    a. 5
    b. 10
    c. 15
    d. 20

88. When you palpate the sinuses you are primarily looking for:
    a. changes in temperature.
    b. changes in color.
    c. tenderness.
    d. nodules.

89. Assessing the oropharynx includes examination of the tonsils. You would expect to see:
    a. tonsils somewhat darker that the rest of the oropharynx.
    b. an irregular tonsillar surface.
    c. tonsils that do not protrude beyond the tonsillar pillar.
    d. tonsils that protrude between the pillars and the uvula.

90. To palpate cervical lymph nodes you feel on both sides of the neck at the same time. The reason for this technique is:
    a. to save time.
    b. for bilateral comparison.
    c. to prevent distortion.
    d. to compress the neck.

91. When you are assessing for breast symmetry you would expect:
    a. both breasts to have perfectly equal symmetry.
    b. the right breast to be larger in right-handed people.
    c. the breasts to have the same general shape, with some minor variation.
    d. the breasts to be of equal size.

92. To detect excess mucus in the bifurcation of the bronchi you would listen:
    a. at the third intercostal space on the right.
    b. over the sternum at the angle of Louis.
    c. over the sternum at the level of the fourth rib.
    d. at the sternal angle.

93. To assess the bases of the lungs you would listen posteriorly:
    a. over the 12th intercostal space.
    b. over the 10th intercostal space.
    c. over the 8th intercostal space.
    d. over the 6th intercostal space.

94. The physician's physical examination report identifies a grade 3 holosystolic murmur. You would expect to hear:
    a. a moderately loud muffled or non-distinct sound throughout S$_1$.
    b. a moderately loud muffled or non-distinct sound throughout S$_2$.
    c. a barely audible S$_1$ and S$_2$.
    d. a barely audible muffled or non-distinct sound throughout S$_2$.

95. Even if the client has liver disease, the liver is not assessed every shift or even daily. The rationale for this action is that:
    a. nurses can't legally perform liver assessment.
    b. it involves deep palpation causing unnecessary discomfort.
    c. there are other better signs of liver enlargement.
    d. liver enlargement is a normal finding in many people.

96. Observing your client from the posterior, you notice an S-shaped curve to the spine. Select the medical term you would use to describe this finding.
    a. ankylosing spondylitis
    b. lordosis
    c. scoliosis
    d. kyphosis

97. Screening for sexual abuse includes external inspection of the genitalia. In a three-year-old female, you would be less suspicious of sexual abuse if you find that the:
    a. hymen is edematous.
    b. hymen is intact.
    c. hymen is absent.
    d. hymen is torn.

98. A finding associated with scrotal edema is:
    a. slightly darker pigmentation than the rest of the body.
    b. absence of rugae.
    c. the left testicle is lower than the right.
    d. presence of a varicocele.

Making a Nursing Diagnosis

PURPOSE

This chapter provides information about the process of making a nursing diagnosis. It also discusses nursing diagnosis classification systems, diagnostic reasoning, and preventing nursing diagnostic errors.

LEARNING OBJECTIVES

After studying this chapter, you should be able to:

1. discuss the classification of nursing diagnoses.
2. describe the five components of a NANDA nursing diagnosis.
3. compare and contrast four types of nursing diagnoses.
4. describe the process of diagnostic reasoning.
5. discuss several sources of diagnostic error and how to avoid them.

MATCHING

1. _g_ clinical judgment
2. _I_ collaborative problem
3. _h_ cue
4. _i_ defining characteristics
5. _b_ diagnostic label
6. _d_ diagnostic reasoning
7. _M_ differential diagnosis

8. _l_ nursing diagnosis
9. _n_ qualifier
10. _e_ related factors
11. _c_ risk factors
12. _f_ "risk for" nursing diagnosis
13. _a_ taxonomy
14. _k_ wellness nursing diagnosis

a. a system of identification, naming, and classification of phenomena

b. the name of the nursing diagnosis

c. internal or external environmental factors that increase the vulnerability of a person, family, or community to an unhealthful event

d. a process of logical, flexible thinking to solve problems and plan nursing care that accounts for individual client needs and uses the individual strengths of the client and nurse to the fullest

e. those factors that appear to show some type of patterned relationship with the nursing diagnosis

f. describes human responses that may develop in a vulnerable person, family, or community

g. a conclusion or an opinion that a problem or situation requires nursing care and that determines the cause of the problem, distinguishes between similar problems, or discriminates among two or more courses of action

(Continued on p. 46)

h. an indicator of the presence or existence of a problem or condition that represents a client's underlying health status

i. descriptors of a client's behavior that determine whether a nursing diagnosis is present and whether a particular diagnosis is appropriate or accurate

j. a clinical problem that cannot be solved by the nursing staff alone, but requires medications or treatments that nurses are not licensed to order

k. describes human responses to levels of wellness in an individual, family, or community with a potential for growth and/or enhancement to a higher state

l. a clinical judgment about individual, family, or community responses to actual or potential health problems or life processes

m. the process of deciding among several possible diagnoses to most accurately describe the client's problem

n. a word, such as *impaired, altered, decreased, ineffective, acute,* or *chronic,* that gives the nursing diagnosis greater specificity

TRUE OR FALSE

15. __T__ A nursing diagnosis is a problem for which nurses are accountable and can diagnose and treat independently.

16. __T__ Nursing diagnosis is part of the nursing process.
N A N A A
17. __F__ The American Nurses Association is the group that develops, refines, and promotes a taxonomy of nursing diagnoses.

18. __T__ A benefit of nursing diagnosis is that it contributes to the autonomy and self-regulatory capacity of nursing.

19. __F__ "Experiencing" is one of the nine NANDA patterns of response.

20. __T__ A nursing diagnosis staged as Level 1 incorporates a diagnosis from the time it is recommended with a label until it is placed on the taxonomy list for study.

21. __T__ A limitation of the current NANDA diagnosis group is that it does not adequately include wellness diagnoses, community health nursing diagnoses, or psychiatric diagnoses.

22. __F__ A diagnostic label gives a nursing diagnosis greater specificity. qualifier

23. __T__ The process of making a nursing diagnosis involves several interrelated steps.

24. __F__ Nursing diagnoses should never be discussed with the client.

FILL-IN-THE-BLANKS

25. Nursing diagnosis is the ___Second___ step of the nursing process.

26. A nursing diagnosis that has been refined or revised is classified as Level ___Four___.

27. The ___Omaha___ System has developed from 15 years of research and includes nursing diagnoses that reflect the home and community health setting.

28. The first part of a nursing diagnostic statement is the ___diagnostic label___.

29. *Family coping: potential for growth* is an example of a ___wellness___ nursing diagnosis.

30. After gathering nursing assessment data, the nurse ___clusters___ it to gain insight into the client's condition.

31. The nurse who is engaged in the nursing diagnosis step of ___differentiating___ among possible diagnoses is narrowing the number of possible nursing diagnoses to identify the most appropriate one.

32. A ___defining characteristic___ is a descriptor of a client's behavior that determines whether a nursing diagnosis is present and appropriate or accurate.

33. The nursing diagnosis *Ineffective infant feeding pattern related to negligent mothering and maternal selfishness* written in a client's chart could be viewed as ___libel___ in a court of law.

34. Trying to include every possible nursing diagnosis that could ever apply to a client would be considered to be the nursing diagnosis error of ___overdiagnosing___.

EXERCISING YOUR CLINICAL JUDGMENT

Mrs. Marcus had her gallbladder removed in surgery earlier in the day, and has an incision in the right upper abdomen near the diaphragm. Her temperature is 98.8° F., pulse is 92, respirations 22/minute and shallow. Blood pressure is stable at 128/78 mm Hg. Mrs. Marcus has an intravenous line for fluid replacement and has an indwelling Foley catheter to drain urine from the bladder. She complains that it hurts to take a deep breath and exhibits guarding of the incision area. She says she feels "achy" from being immobilized on the operating room table. The last dose of a prn narcotic analgesic was given three hours ago and is now due. The nurse who admitted Mrs. Marcus from the postanesthesia care unit must formulate a list of nursing diagnoses and develop a plan of care.

35. Which of the following nursing diagnoses represents the most well-constructed nursing diagnostic statement about this client's pain?
    a. Pain related to right upper abdominal incision and operative positioning
    b. Risk for pain related to frequency of ordered narcotic analgesic
    c. Pain related to insufficient pain medication frequency
    d. Risk for pain related to overall surgical experience

36. If the nurse is considering the nursing diagnosis *Risk for urinary retention*, it should be instituted when:
    a. the nurse writes the initial care plan.
    b. the Foley catheter is discontinued.
    c. the client's urine output falls below 30 mL/hour with the catheter in place.
    d. the client is ready for discharge to home.

37. The most appropriate nursing diagnosis for the client's respiratory status would be:
    a. Risk for impaired gas exchange due to increased secretions.
    b. Risk for ineffective breathing pattern related to subdiaphragmatic incision and guarding.
    c. Ineffective airway clearance related to weak cough and shallow respirations.
    d. Impaired gas exchange due to anesthesia and abnormal respiratory rate.

38. If the nurse considers the possibility that the client could develop an infection in the wound or because of invasive lines, the nursing diagnosis would be written as a(n):
    a. actual diagnosis.
    b. wellness diagnosis.
    c. medical diagnosis.
    d. "Risk for" diagnosis.

TEST YOURSELF

39. One of the limitations of the current NANDA system for classifying nursing diagnoses is that it:
    a. is specific to only a few nursing specialties.
    b. is not well accepted in nursing education.
    c. is endorsed by the American Nurses Association.
    d. contains diagnoses at different levels of abstraction.

40. The part of the nursing diagnostic statement that contains a qualifier is called:
    a. a diagnostic label.
    b. a definition.
    c. the defining characteristics.
    d. the etiologic factors.

41. The broadest and highest level type of thinking that may be required for clinical nursing practice is:
    a. ordinary, logical thinking.
    b. clinical judgment.
    c. critical thinking.
    d. diagnostic reasoning.

42. A nurse working in a community health setting would choose which of the following nursing diagnoses as the most realistic after taking into consideration the care setting?
    a. Impaired home maintenance management
    b. Decreased cardiac output
    c. Ineffective thermoregulation
    d. Decreased adaptive capacity: intracranial

43. The nursing diagnosis *Ineffective airway clearance related to infrequent suctioning* is most inappropriate because it:
    a. is judgmental.
    b. is derogatory.
    c. suggests negligence.
    d. suggests poor opinion of colleagues.

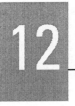

Planning for Intervention

PURPOSE

The purpose of this chapter is to introduce you to the planning process. While the chapter focuses on the individual, you will also consider planning for groups of clients who have a common set of needs. Planning is an inherent part of designing services to meet the needs of a client population. Individual planning considers the specific needs of a client within the population.

LEARNING OBJECTIVES

After studying this chapter, you should be able to:

1. describe types of planning for individual clients and client groups.
2. identify priorities for planning client care.
3. describe the process of establishing client expected outcomes.
4. discuss the essential skills needed to implement client care.
5. describe the intervention process.
6. describe types and components of interventions to individualize care for each client.
7. describe the criteria for developing a nursing care plan.

MATCHING

1. _c_ consultation
2. _m_ clinical pathway
3. _d_ computerized care plan
4. _a_ care plan conference

5. _f_ individualized care plan
6. _g_ indirect care intervention
7. _e_ implementation
8. _i_ physician-initiated intervention
9. _j_ nursing intervention
10. _h_ nurse-initiated intervention
11. _l_ discharge planning
12. _k_ direct care intervention
13. _b_ collaboration

a. the action of a group conferring or consulting together to plan care for the client

b. the act of two or more health care professionals performing work cooperatively to achieve a common goal

c. the act of two or more health care professionals deliberating for the purpose of making decisions; the primary caregiver generally retains the authority for the decision

d. a standardized care plan that is set up by software vendors

e. the action phase of the nursing process; this phase is where the nurse provides actual care to clients

(Continued on p. 50)

f. written separately for each client who enters a health care facility; allows for the nurse to identify the unique problems of each client to decide on the outcomes to be achieved and to identify which nursing interventions will be appropriate to achieve those outcomes

g. a treatment performed away from the patient but on behalf of a patient or group of patients

h. within the independent scope of nursing practice and prescribed by the nurse independent of the physician

i. within the scope of nursing practice but requiring a physician's order for the nurse to implement

j. any treatment, based upon clinical judgment and knowledge, that a nurse performs to enhance patient/client outcomes

k. a treatment performed through interaction with the client(s)

l. addresses the needs of the client that will continue when the present services are no longer needed

m. a multidisciplinary plan that projects the expected course of the client's progress over the hospital stay

TRUE OR FALSE

14. _F_ Planning occurs only at the beginning of the nurse-client relationship. ongoing

15. _F_ Planning is a distinct step in the nursing process. interelated c other steps

16. _F_ A nursing care plan for clients who are undergoing a hysterectomy is sufficient for all hysterectomy clients.

17. _F_ The nursing care plan does not include interventions performed by other team members, such as the dietitian.

18. _T_ Planning includes projecting the desired outcomes of the care.

19. _F_ The term *nursing care planning* only applies to the written or documented plan.

20. _T_ Staffing should be planned based on the level of care needs of the clients on the unit.

21. _F_ Priorities are always based on physiological needs first.

22. _T_ Because needs are often interrelated, several problems may be grouped together as a priority.

23. _T_ To use the Nursing Outcomes Classification system, the nurse must choose which measurement parameters are needed in a given client situation.

24. _T_ Nursing interventions are clarified by indicating who, what, when, how, and why.

25. _T_ Nursing interventions include all acts of nurses on the client's behalf.

26. _T_ Nursing interventions include technical care and the therapeutic use of self.

FILL-IN-THE-BLANKS

27. Discharge planning begins with the _first client contact_

28. The frequency of planning during a client's span of care depends on how often the client's condition _A's_.

29. Basic survival needs take first priority when your client has a threat to _physiological integrity_.

30. Verbs for the goal of adaptation of a psychomotor skill include _adapts_, _alters_, _changes_, _rearranges_ _reorganizes_ _revises_, and _varies_.

31. Assessment data is documented in the health care record in _admiss._ _history_, _daily_ _assess_ _rec_, and _nurs_ _progr_ _notes_.

32. Nursing diagnoses are documented in the health care record in the _nursing_ care plan or the _multidisiplinary_ care plan.

33. Interventions are documented in the _graphic checklist_ or _nurse progress notes_.

34. Evaluation data is documented in _nursing_ _prog_ _notes_ or _daily_ _assess_ _rec_.

35. Through the development of expected outcomes nurses can be held _accountable_ for the results of nursing care.

36. In planning nursing care you should choose outcomes that are _Sensitive_ to nursing care.

37. The Nursing Outcomes Classification system uses a _Likert_- or _5_-point scale to measure outcomes, thus allowing for variable client outcomes.

38. The six domains of the Nursing Outcome Classification System are

    _____,

    _____ _____, _____

    _____, _____,

    _____ _____, and

    _____, _____ _____, and

    _____ _____.

39. List nine skills of intervention: _____,

    _____, _____, _____,

    _____, _____, _____,

    _____, and _____.

40. A standardized language provides a common language for _communication_

EXERCISING YOUR CLINICAL JUDGMENT

41. All of the following interventions are missing some of the five elements of who, what, when, how, and why. Select the one you think would be the most consistently carried out across all three shifts.
    a. turn q2h
    b. turn on even hours, side to back to side
    c. turn as needed to prevent decubiti
    d. nursing assistant to turn client

42. You refer a client to AIDS Services (a local volunteer agency) for assistance in obtaining his medication. Which domain of interventions (NIC) have you used?
    a. physiological
    b. behavioral
    c. safety
    d. health systems

43. Your client needs to learn to give an injection to himself on a weekly basis. Select the most measurable outcome. The client:
    a. understands the mechanics of the injection technique.
    b. demonstrates the correct injection technique before discharge.
    c. develops a procedure for injection suitable to his lifestyle.
    d. knows how to give his own injection.

44. A client has a fractured ankle. He is learning to walk on crutches. Select the outcome that best reflects the client's long-term goal. The client:
    a. safely demonstrates stair climbing with crutches.
    b. can walk the length of the corridor correctly using a three-point gait.
    c. can use crutches independently at discharge.
    d. bears weight on ankle without pain.

45. Select the activity that most clearly reflects a nurse-initiated intervention. The nurse:
    a. safely administers intravenous Gentamycin.
    b. establishes schedule for the administration of medication.
    c. observes for side effects of medication.
    d. teaches client to self-administer medication after discharge.

TEST YOURSELF

46. The most significant disadvantage of a computerized nursing care plan is:
    a. difficult care plan development and revision.
    b. low rating for readability.
    c. lack of individualization.
    d. lack of clarity of the terms used in planning.

47. Select the statement that reflects an advantage to the NIC system for documentation of interventions.
    a. Each intervention is specific for a NANDA diagnosis.
    b. Provides ease of documentation of individualized care.
    c. Provides the specific details of the activities used for each client.
    d. Provides a short notation that implies the same set of activities to all nurses using the system.

48. Select the statement that best exemplifies the purpose of case management. Seeks to:
    a. ensure quality care in a health care system focused on cost control.
    b. expand the hospital's control beyond the acute care experience.
    c. increase the number of roles for professional nurses in acute care.
    d. ensure that clients get access to all possible services.

49. Select the statement that best describes a clinical pathway.

    a.   describes the specifics of nursing care in measurable terms

    b.   is a multidisciplinary plan with criteria for daily progress of a client with a particular diagnosis

    c.   is a plan of care for an individual client

    d.   predicts the course of a client's illness based on the identification of that client's individual risk factors

50. There are multiple methods of documenting a nursing care plan (NCP). Which of the following is essential?

    a.   using a form developed for the agency for documentation of the NCP

    b.   using columns for expected outcomes, interventions, and resolution of the problem

    c.   documenting the elements of diagnosis, expected outcomes, and interventions

    d.   having the plan on a separate form from the documentation of care

Evaluating Care

PURPOSE

This chapter explores the process of evaluating nursing care. It discusses evaluation as it relates to measuring expected client outcomes and determining the degree to which an institution's external and internal standards are met.

LEARNING OBJECTIVES

After studying this chapter, you should be able to:

1. describe the purposes and process of establishing expected outcomes.
2. discuss the process of evaluating care you provided.
3. evaluate yourself regarding factors affecting outcome attainment.
4. evaluate yourself regarding the compliance with standards established by the American Nurses Association.
5. describe the evaluating process of the Joint Commission on Accreditation of Healthcare Organizations (JCAHO) regarding an organization's quality of care.
6. discuss the purposes and types of internal standards established by health care organizations.
7. discuss the methods that an organization uses to evaluate compliance with internal standards.

MATCHING

1. _J_ case management
2. _h_ concurrent audit
3. _e_ continuous quality improvement
4. _n_ evaluation
5. _K_ peer review
6. _O_ performance appraisal
7. _M_ policy
8. _b_ procedure
9. _d_ protocol
10. _f_ quality assurance
11. _i_ retrospective audit
12. _a_ standards of care
13. _g_ standards of client care
14. _p_ standards of practice
15. _l_ standards of professional performance
16. _v_ variance

a. authoritative statements that describe a competent level of clinical nursing practice demonstrated through assessment, diagnosis, outcome identification, planning, implementation, and evaluation

b. a detailed description of a specific method of performing nursing care

c. any deviance from a clinical pathway

d. contains detailed guidelines for nursing care for clients with specific conditions

e. a systematic approach to control and improve quality from both professionals' and clients' perspectives

(Continued on p. 54)

f. a process of evaluating the outcome of care measured against predetermined standards and implementing methods of improvement

g. the essential elements of nursing care prescribed for specific client populations

h. an evaluation method to inspect the nursing staff's compliance with predetermined standards and criteria while the nurses are providing care

i. an evaluation method to inspect the medical record for documentation of compliance with the standards

j. a care delivery system that focuses on the management of client care across an episode of illness

k. the evaluation of the performance of one staff member by another staff member to judge the quality of care provided

l. authoritative statements that describe a competent level of behavior in the professional role, including activities related to quality of care, performance appraisal, education, collegiality, ethics, collaboration, research, and resource utilization

m. a set of rules and regulations that govern nursing practice and nursing care

n. a systematic and ongoing process of examining whether expected outcomes have been achieved and whether nursing care has been effective

o. a systematic and standardized evaluation of an employee's work contribution, quality of work, and potential for advancement, made by the employee's supervisor

p. what the nursing staff should assess, plan, implement, and evaluate during daily and ongoing care for specific client populations

TRUE OR FALSE

17. __T__ Nursing practice that consistently upholds standards of care is important in achieving positive client outcomes.

18. __F__ If client outcomes are not achieved, only the nursing interventions are revised.

19. __F__ Nurses can often determine a client's level of satisfaction with care by asking the opinions of other nurses assigned to that client.

20. __T__ Formulating measurable and realistic client outcomes is a factor that facilitates attainment of those outcomes.

21. __T__ Inadequate information about a client's disease, treatment, or care is a barrier that impedes attainment of expected outcomes.

22. __F__ The ANA standards of care include a statement that nurses should contribute to the professional development of peers, colleagues, and others. *standards of professional performance*

23. __T__ An institution must be accredited by the JCAHO to be certified or licensed, or to receive reimbursement for services.

24. __F__ A nurse who is verifying information for properly submitting a vacation request form would consult the nursing procedure manual. *policy*

25. __T__ A nurse using a clinical pathway in the care of an assigned client would document the reasons for any variances in the client's medical record.

26. __T__ A nurse measuring nurses' compliance with documentation of intravenous site assessments would most likely use the retrospective audit method.

FILL-IN-THE-BLANKS

27. A nurse orientee who requests that the designated mentor nurse observe her while she performs a wound irrigation is engaged in the __Concurrent__ audit method.

28. An assumption of a continuous quality improvement program is that quality can always be __improved__.

29. If a client has begun to achieve expected outcomes, but has not yet fully met them, the nurse would consider that the goals for this client have been ___partially___ met.

30. A nurse whose evaluation shows that a client has fully met the expected outcomes for a nursing diagnosis would determine that the nursing diagnosis should be ___resolved___.

31. A factor that impedes the ability of a client to meet an expected outcome is considered to be a ___barrier___.

32. A health care organization's standards are often influenced by ___external___ standards, such as those from federal, state, and regulatory agencies.

33. Criteria used to measure competent practice of the ANA standards of care are called ___indicators___.

34. A health care organization that has demonstrated exemplary performance in meeting JCAHO standards receives accreditation with ___commendation___.

35. The nursing care of a client who is at risk for skin breakdown may be outlined in a ___protocol___.

36. A ___performance appraisal___ is often used to determine promotion, selection, termination, or pay raise for an individual nurse.

EXERCISING YOUR CLINICAL JUDGMENT

Mr. Stanley, the man identified in the chapter case study, has an ongoing care plan for pain management following total knee replacement (TKR). At the time we last read about him, he was receiving adequate doses of morphine (a narcotic analgesic) through a patient-controlled analgesia (PCA) pump. Yesterday Mr. Stanley was weaned from PCA and his pain was being managed with oral narcotic analgesics. The nurse in turn modified and wrote additional client outcomes for the nursing diagnosis of Pain based on the newly prescribed regimen. The nurse expanded the outcome of "verbalizes that pain is reduced or controlled" to "verbalizes that pain is reduced or controlled with oral analgesics." Other outcome criteria currently include "verbalizes proper use of oral analgesics prior to discharge" and "identifies and uses noninvasive adjunct pain relief measures effectively." You have just come onto the clinical nursing unit and have been assigned to the care of Mr. Stanley.

37. Which of the following evaluative questions would you ask Mr. Stanley to best determine the extent of pain relief obtained with oral medication?
a. "Are you just as comfortable now as you were before?"
b. "Can you rate your pain using a 0–10 scale now that 30 minutes has passed since your last dose?"
c. "Which type of medication works better, the old or the new?"
d. "What do you think about this new pain medication?"

38. Mr. Stanley tells you that he finds music soothing, and that it helps him to relax and feel less pain. You notice that Mr. Stanley fell asleep and took a 90-minute nap after he put on earphones to listen to a portable CD player. You would evaluate that the outcome "identifies and uses noninvasive adjunct pain relief measures effectively" is:
a. being met.
b. being partially met.
c. not being met.
d. irrelevant to the care of this client.

39. You notice as you sign out a narcotic analgesic for Mr. Stanley that a record is kept of how many tablets are used and how many remain in the locked storage area. You realize that this recordkeeping provides a means for doing which of the following types of evaluation?
a. peer review
b. retrospective audit
c. performance appraisal
d. quality improvement

40. You are assigned to present in clinical conference an overview of the health care facility's regulations for obtaining, monitoring, and dispensing controlled substances, such as narcotic analgesics, on the clinical unit. You describe to the group that these regulations are based on:
a. internal standards only.
b. external standards only.
c. both internal and external standards.
d. neither internal nor external standards.

TEST YOURSELF

41. A client expresses satisfaction with the nursing care received on the clinical unit, and completes a patient satisfaction survey describing it as caring, thoughtful, and respectful. The nurse manager documents this anecdote from the client, knowing that this information is an example of which of the following?
    a. quality indicator
    b. internal standard
    c. external standard
    d. compliance with federal regulation

42. A nurse who is facilitating a client's attainment of expected outcomes would:
    a. have a vague idea of the client's plan of care.
    b. assess the client thoroughly and accurately.
    c. not be overly concerned with revising the plan of care.
    d. consult with the family, but not the client, about expected outcomes.

43. The nurse who is practicing nursing within the standards of a specialty nursing organization knows that these standards most often are derived from those of the:
    a. employer.
    b. Joint Commission on Accreditation of Healthcare Organizations.
    c. Department of Health and Human Services.
    d. American Nurses Association.

44. A nurse working on the cardiac telemetry unit has a set of standing physician's orders for treating chest pain. The nurse implementing these orders is working with a:
    a. policy.
    b. procedure.
    c. protocol.
    d. parameter.

45. The nurse would determine that a case management approach was effective for a particular client if that client:
    a. was approved by the insurance company to remain in the hospital an extra day or two.
    b. achieved a satisfactory clinical outcome and did not require rehospitalization.
    c. received every type of service available.
    d. incurred the least cost even if the outcome was not satisfactory.

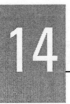

Documenting Care

PURPOSE

This chapter explains the purpose, principles, and methods of documenting client care. It differentiates among the various charting formats and describes the usefulness of various types of flow sheets.

LEARNING OBJECTIVES

After studying this chapter, you should be able to:

1. explain the purpose of documentation.
2. state the purpose of using appropriate medical terminology and standard abbreviations when documenting care.
3. discuss the importance of recording information legibly, concisely, completely, and sequentially.
4. identify significant data that should be documented in clients' records.
5. explain the value of recording complete data entries using clear and objective terms.
6. relate the need for variation in documenting for special populations and facilities.
7. differentiate among various charting formats.
8. describe the usefulness of various types of flow sheets.

MATCHING

1. _d_ admit note
2. _f_ APIE charting
3. _k_ charting by exception
4. _a_ discharge note
5. _l_ documentation

6. _J_ flow sheet
7. _b_ focus charting
8. _l_ interval or progress note
9. _C_ narrative charting
10. _g_ PIE charting
11. _h_ problem-oriented medical records
12. _n_ SOAP charting
13. _e_ source-oriented medical records
14. _m_ transfer note

b. a method of charting that addresses client problems or needs and includes a column that summarizes the focus of the entry

c. a method of charting that provides information in the form of statements that describe events surrounding client care

d. the opening nurse's note acknowledging the arrival of a new client

e. a type of medical record with separate divisions according to health discipline (e.g., medicine, nursing, laboratory, respiratory care)

f. the acronym that stands for assessment, problem identification, interventions, and evaluation

a. nursing note that reflects the circumstances surrounding the release of a client from a facility

(Continued on p. 58)

g. the acronym that stands for problem identification, interventions, and evaluation

h. a form of documentation originally designed to reorganize information according to identified client problems, with all members of the health team documenting information sequentially

i. recording of information relevant to data collection, planning, implementation, and client response to care given

j. forms used to document data that can be more easily followed in graphic or tabular form

k. provides documentation in progress notes only if data are significant or abnormal

l. nursing notes entered at various times during a shift that reflect any aspect of change in client condition, or anything affecting the client such as tests, STAT or prn medications, and procedures

m. nursing note that reflects the movement of a client from one location to another, either within the agency or to another agency

n. a method of charting used to record progress notes with problem-oriented medical records; it includes subjective data, objective data, assessment, and plan

19. ___T___ You are responsible for charting how your client responds to your teaching, and whether the client and/or family can return-demonstrate a skill such as wound care or explain the instructions in their own words.

20. ___T___ Narrative charting is unstructured, providing you with flexibility in determining how information is recorded.

21. ___T___ The use of computer systems for documentation has raised concerns over security of client information in order to protect client rights.

FILL-IN-THE-BLANKS

22. Accurate _documentation_ of information is essential in order to communicate information to all members of the health team, to ensure _nursing_ accountability, and to demonstrate effective use of the _nursing_ _process_ and appropriate _standards_ of care.

23. Quality assurance focuses on providing care according to established _standards_.

24. _Black_ is the choice of color for charting, unless an agency has a different policy.

25. When you chart you do not include the _client's_ name or the word client or patient.

26. Copying a chart usually requires written consent by the _client_ or responsible party.

27. Upon admission to a facility, most health care agencies require a health _Hx_ to be completed followed by a current _needs_ assessment.

28. Nursing notes should state _observations_ rather than opinion.

TRUE OR FALSE

15. ___T___ Client outcomes serve as the measure of quality and are monitored through complete and accurate documentation.

16. ___F___ Agencies do not chart errors in client's charts to avoid being sued.

17. ___F___ Medical abbreviations are used consistently throughout the medical/nursing community.

18. ___T___ Charting should be done in complete sentences, using as much description of the situation as possible.

EXERCISING YOUR CLINICAL JUDGMENT

29. You admitted Ms. Peters, the client mentioned at the beginning of the textbook chapter, to your hospital unit. You charted: *68-yr-old female admitted to room 268A via stretcher from ER with dx FX L h P 92, BP142/89, T 98. C/o pain to L hip from mid-thigh to greater trochanter area, marked bruising noted in same area.* The agency where you work is using which type of charting format?
    a. narrative
    b. focus
    c. APIE
    d. charting by exception

30. You charted the following nursing note in black ink: *12:00 ate lunch; 7:30am prn medication given for pain; 1:00 transferred to X-ray via a stretcher, accompanied by aide.* What is incorrect about this entry?
    a. The prn medication should not have been recorded.
    b. The recording of the information is not done sequentially.
    c. Black ink is not the ink of choice for most institutions.
    d. The charting should have included the client's name.

31. Ms. Peters, the elderly client from the chapter's case study, has been on your unit for several days. You chart the following: *Dr. Warren visited c̄ orders to d/c current meds. Neighbor notified and on the way. Home Health Nurse S. Beil, notified of discharge and arrangement for first visit made. PT visited concerning walker and reinforced proper use.* This is an example of which type of nursing note?
    a. progress
    b. interval
    c. discharge
    d. assessment

TEST YOURSELF

32. Your client has his dressing changed every four hours. You forgot to chart the morning dressing change. You remembered the omission when you began to document your client's afternoon dressing change. The client's morning dressing had no drainage on it and the wound was healing without any problems. How would you handle this situation?
    a. chart the morning results with your afternoon charting.
    b. call the physician and report you did not chart the dressing change the client's chart
    c. add the information as an addendum to the afternoon charting
    d. do nothing; since the dressing is changed frequently, it is not necessary to add the morning dressing change to the client's chart

33. You are about to chart and notice that the previous charting was not signed. How should you chart?
    a. sign previous nurse's charting and then do your charting and sign it
    b. have the head nurse sign the previous nurse's charting and then do your own
    c. no is action necessary; do only your own charting
    d. do not sign for the previous nurse; report it to the head nurse and chart and sign your own charting

34. You charted the following nursing note regarding your client's current condition: *Awake, alert and oriented x3. Skin warm and dry. IV D₅W infusing in R lower arm at 100cc/h with 450 TBA. Site without redness or edema. Reports pain in L hip. States pain is 8 on scale of 1-10. Tylox tabs ii given PO.* Which type of nursing note is this?
    a. admit note
    b. change-of-shift note
    c. assessment note
    d. interval note

35. You chart a progress note on your client's condition using the same problem list as the client's other health care providers used. What type of medical record is your facility using?
    a. source-oriented
    b. problem-oriented
    c. critical pathways
    d. narrative

36. Which type of charting addresses client problems or needs and includes a column that summarizes the focus of the entry?
    a. focus
    b. SOAP
    c. narrative
    d. PIE

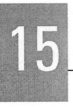

The Nurse-Client Relationship

PURPOSE

This chapter will orient you to beginning theories, principles, and techniques of therapeutic communication related to the nurse-client interaction.

LEARNING OBJECTIVES

After studying this chapter, you should be able to:

1. identify the tasks associated with each of the three phases of the therapeutic relationship.
2. list and describe the six elements of the communication process.
3. identify how Peplau, Travelbee, Satir, and Watzlawick contributed to an understanding of the nurse, the client, and communication.
4. compare and contrast the two main forms of verbal communication.
5. identify the elements of body language and paralanguage.
6. describe the nursing attitudes and action-oriented characteristics that facilitate effective therapeutic techniques.
7. identify some techniques that impair therapeutic communication.
8. list and give examples of seven techniques that enhance therapeutic communication.
9. identify a variety of characteristics of effective communication techniques.

MATCHING

1. __c__ acting-out behaviors
2. __p__ attending behaviors
3. __m__ body language
4. __h__ context
5. __g__ decoder (receiver)
6. __r__ empathy
7. __d__ encoder (sender)
8. __i__ feedback
9. __k__ language
10. __e__ message
11. __l__ nonverbal communication
12. __n__ paralanguage
13. __o__ personal space
14. __s__ positive listening
15. __f__ sensory channel
16. __b__ therapeutic rapport
17. __a__ therapeutic relationship

a. a helping relationship

b. a special bond that exists between a nurse and a client who have established a sense of trust and a mutual understanding of what will occur in their relationship

c. inappropriate or unexpected client behaviors that communicate about the client's true or subconscious feelings and concerns

d. person who initiates a transaction to exchange information, convey thoughts and feelings, or engage another person

e. the content a sender wishes to transmit to another person (the receiver) in the process of communication

(Continued on p. 62)

18. _q_ unconditional positive regard

19. _j_ verbal communication

f. a means by which a message is sent

g. a person to whom a message is aimed

h. a condition under which a communication occurs

i. the process by which effectiveness of communication is determined

j. involves the use of words to convey messages

k. a set of words that have meanings that are comprehensible within a group

l. a set of behaviors that conveys messages either without words or by supplementing verbal communication

m. refers to nonverbal communication behaviors that are accomplished by the movement of our bodies or body parts, by the presentation of ourselves to the world, and by the use of our personal space

n. refers to nonverbal components of spoken language

o. a private zone or "bubble" around our body that we believe is an extension of oneself and that belongs to us

p. shows that you are paying attention and listening to what the client is saying

q. term coined by psychologist Carl Rogers; describes respect for the client that is not dependent on the client's behavior

r. the accurate perception of the client's feelings

s. understanding the auditory messages sent by a sender

TRUE OR FALSE

20. _T_ A therapeutic relationship is personal, client-focused, and aimed at realizing mutually-determined goals.

21. _F_ Peplau, a nurse theorist, believed that the
Travelbee nurse is a human being who is vulnerable to stereotypes, labels, and generalizations.

22. _T_ Nonverbal communication includes body posture. For example, when your client stands with an erect posture, this usually signifies a feeling of fitness and confidence.

23. _F_ Generally speaking, a person's personal space is similar for most cultures.

24. _T_ A rule of thumb is to ask permission before touching a client.

25. _T_ According to Tannen's theories, women speak to connect and men speak to preserve status and independence.

26. _F_ _ask client to concider what to do_
To encourage a formulation of a plan of action, you consider what might be the best thing to do in a future situation.

27. _T_ Summarizing can help bring closure in the termination phase of a therapeutic relationship.

FILL-IN-THE-BLANKS

28. Confidentiality is an _ethical_ obligation to share health care information about a person only with other persons who have a _profession_ need to know the person's health status.

29. _Positive_ feedback affirms your efforts to communicate by rewarding and reinforcing successful communication.

30. Personal appearance, conscious and unconscious changes in facial expressions, body posture and gestures, and the distances maintained from others are examples of _body language_.

31. You can help the client to be ___Concrete___ by role-modeling concreteness and by asking the client to remain in the "here-and-now" during discussions.

32. If you are using therapeutic techniques correctly, your client will be doing most of the ___talking___ as you listen and guide the interaction.

33. Many people (nurses and clients) are uncomfortable with ___silence___ and will talk continuously about nothing in particular just to avoid it.

34. ___Active___ listening is a means of "being with" the client and indicating acceptance and agreement by using verbal and nonverbal cues.

EXERCISING YOUR CLINICAL JUDGMENT

35. You say to your client who is five years old, "Why don't you stop crying?" This is an example of which type of nontherapeutic technique?
    a. requesting an explanation
    b. probing
    c. challenging
    d. testing

36. You say to your adolescent client, "Maybe you would explain more about what you mean so I can be more helpful." You are using which therapeutic communication technique?
    a. offering self
    b. focusing
    c. asking for clarification
    d. reflecting

37. You say to your adult client, "I haven't really known of anyone getting direct messages from God." This is an example of which therapeutic communication technique?
    a. presenting reality
    b. voicing doubt
    c. summarizing
    d. reflecting

TEST YOURSELF

38. "I don't know the right answer right now. But I will find out and let you know in an about hour." This is an example of being honest with the client, which is an essential step in:
    a. developing a trusting relationship with the client.
    b. developing a friendship with the client.
    c. helping the client with termination issues.
    d. believing that you are a competent nurse.

39. During which phase of the nurse-client relationship do you complete nursing interventions that address expected nursing outcomes?
    a. working phase
    b. termination phase
    c. orientation phase
    d. therapeutic phase

40. "Hmm, I believe you are right," is an example of which type of paralanguage?
    a. rate
    b. pitch
    c. quality
    d. pause

41. You say to your adult client, "I have 30 minutes available to talk with you at 10 a.m. today." This is an example of which therapeutic communication technique?
    a. offering self
    b. presenting reality
    c. focusing
    d. testing

42. You say to your client who is three years old, "Do you want your Baby Lisa? Is she your doll?" Which therapeutic communication techniques are you using?
    a. focusing
    b. placing events in sequence
    c. providing broad openings
    d. seeking consensual validation

Client Teaching

PURPOSE

This chapter introduces you to the key concepts that you must understand to provide effective client teaching. It introduces teaching-learning theory and processes, and guides you to use the nursing process effectively in meeting clients' learning needs.

LEARNING OBJECTIVES

After studying this chapter, you should be able to:

1. discuss the rationale for client teaching, including its benefits and purpose.
2. describe the teaching and learning process, including domains of learning and principles of effective teaching.
3. summarize the client characteristics to consider when assessing teaching needs.
4. compare and contrast factors that facilitate learning and those that are barriers to learning.
5. discuss the nursing diagnosis Knowledge deficit and compare it to a related diagnosis.
6. develop a teaching plan for a client.
7. discuss strategies for effectively implementing client teaching.
8. write sample documentation for teaching and learning processes.
9. discuss methods for evaluating, teaching, and learning.

MATCHING

1. _g_ learning objective
2. _h_ teaching plan
3. _a_ psychomotor learning domain
4. _d_ teaching
5. _i_ learning
6. _c_ cognitive learning domain
7. _f_ perceptual learning domain
8. _b_ learning contract
9. _e_ affective learning domain

a. the learning domain concerned with physical and motor skills, such as giving injections

b. much like any business contract; each party, nurse and client, agrees to contribute certain things to the agreement

c. the learning domain which encompasses knowledge, comprehension, and critical thinking skills

d. a set of planned activities performed to impact knowledge, behavior, or skill

e. the learning domain that relates to ethics or principles that guide moral behavior and to reasoning that determines right behavior

(Continued on p. 66)

f.   being able to perceive (see, hear, understand, and respond) written and spoken words, and pictures or symbols.

g.   describes the intended results of learning rather than the process of instruction

h.   an organized, individualized, written presentation of what the client must learn and how the instructions and information needed will be provided

i.   a process that involves perceiving and acquiring new knowledge, information, and skills, and subsequently changing one's behavior

TRUE OR FALSE

10. ___T___ JCAHO supports the client's right to education specific to his or her health care needs throughout a hospital stay.

11. ___T___ Client education is a factor in quality control in that it ensures that clients have the knowledge they need to provide self-care.

12. ___F___ The client must reach the synthesis level of learning about his of her health care problem to be successful.

13. ___F___ In the United States, literacy is not a concern for those who provide client education.

14. ___T___ A child's imagination may create greater fear than the truth, told directly and simply.

15. ___T___ For the adult learner you should assume that the learner has some knowledge you can use to build on to enhance education.

16. ___F___ In a hospital setting, the best method of teaching is verbally providing information in a one-on-one situation with the client.
      written supplementals

17. ___F___ It is safe to assume all clients want to learn about their health problems.

18. ___F___ Knowledge deficit is the only nursing diagnosis used for client learning needs.

19. ___T___ Teaching from the simple to the complex is a principle of teaching.

20. ___T___ Writing specific measurable objectives helps to clarify your teaching plans.

FILL-IN-THE-BLANKS

21. The advantage of __individual__ instruction is pacing and customizing to meet an individual client's needs.

22. The advantage of __group__ instruction is economy of teaching time and sharing of experiences.

23. The advantage of __written__ instruction is learning at an individualized pace and readily available reinforcement.

24. Repetition is used to __reinforce learning__

25. Discussion allows the learner to be an __active participant__ in learning.

26. Evaluation has two types of goals. Assessing the client's ability to repeat the information is a __short__ - __term__ goal.

27. Assessing for a change in lifestyle at a three-month follow-up is a __long__ - __term__ goal.

EXERCISING YOUR CLINICAL JUDGMENT

28. Your client has just been admitted with an asthma attack. This is the third admission in six months and the client is highly anxious. You suspect the client does not fully understand the preventive measures recommended by the physician. You would:
    a.   review the measures while the client is waiting for the medications to take effect.
    b.   gather limited information at this time; postpone teaching.
    c.   give the client written information to be read later.
    d.   use the opportunity to emphasize the importance of prevention.

29. The physician has recommended that your client follow a low-fat diet and wants you to introduce the topic to the client. Knowing you should teach from the simple to the complex you would start with the topic of:
    a.   a general list of foods to avoid.
    b.   pathophysiology of the formation of fatty plaque in arteries.
    c.   planning menus.
    d.   maintaining a diet that is less than 30% fat based on grams of fat in common foods.

30. Your client is going to go home on a new medication to lower blood pressure (anti-hypertensive medication). Based on the axiom that adult learners learn best when there is a need to know, which of the following would you emphasize?
    a. how the medication works in the body
    b. the need to memorize all side effects
    c. the importance of maintaining the pre-scribed dose schedule
    d. the possible complications of high blood pressure

31. Your client is having surgery and expects to be in the hospital for four days. The postoperative care will involve complex wound care after discharge. The best time to start the teaching is:
    a. preoperatively.
    b. on the first day after surgery.
    c. on the day of discharge.
    d. after the client is at home.

32. Select the client who would most likely need repetition to ensure learning.
    a. a 90-year-old using insulin injections for the first time
    b. a 20-year-old who needs to take a pre-scription for 10 days for a urinary tract infection
    c. a person with long-standing asthma who has a prescription for a different inhaler
    d. a surgical client being discharged; wound is healing without complications and the sutures have been removed

TEST YOURSELF

33. Early discharge for hospitalized clients has changed client teaching by:
    a. increasing the client's need for information.
    b. shifting the responsibility for teaching from the hospital nurse to the home health nurse.
    c. reducing the need for teaching because complications are reduced.
    d. allowing hospital nurses to focus only on acute physical needs.

34. Quality care is improved when:
    a. the client and family are active partici-pants in restoring health.
    b. clients do what they are told without asking questions.
    c. the physician is in control of all decision making.
    d. clients have absolute faith in health care providers.

35. A client has 20/200 vision. You are planning to teach the care of a new colostomy (colon opens on the abdomen and the client must wear a pouch). Which domain of learning would you address first?
    a. perceptual
    b. cognitive
    c. affective
    d. psychomotor

36. Which behavior represents the complex overt response level of psychomotor learning?
    a. performs the skill precisely following the steps as taught
    b. performs the skill correctly while visiting with a friend
    c. modifies the skill to meet lifestyle needs
    d. creates a new way of performing the skill

37. Your client is a shy seven-year-old. She is learning to use an asthma inhaler. Her asthma attacks occur no more frequently than once a week. Her mother has received permission from the school for the child to have the inhaler with her in the classroom, but the child says she cannot use it in front of her friends. Which teaching activity would you select?
    a. telling her that her friends won't care
    b. role play asking the teacher if she can be excused from the room to use her inhaler
    c. getting the prescription changed to a tablet taken four times a day
    d. telling her mother that she has to do it whether she likes it or not

38. Which of the following is most likely true of an adult learner?
    a. prefers the nurse to identify what knowl-edge is needed
    b. is bored with being shown how to per-form a skill
    c. likes to know why knowledge is needed
    d. likes role playing as a method of learning

39. The client who exhibits the greatest motivation to learn:
    a. asks questions about planning a low-fat diet.
    b. thanks the nurse and says he will read the information provided.
    c. talks about the difficulties of managing a low-fat diet.
    d. tells the nurse to talk to his wife about the diet.

40. You have planned to do a client's wound care at 10 a.m. Your schedule is busy and you know the client will probably be discharged tomorrow. When you enter the room you find that the client's son has just arrived from out of state. You would:
    a. know that psychosocial needs are important and delay the wound care.
    b. ask the son to leave the room and hurriedly do the wound care without teaching.
    c. ask the client if the son can stay and include him in the teaching.
    d. tell the son he will have to come back later.

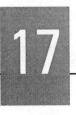

Nursing Management

PURPOSE

This chapter introduces you to nursing management and the roles of a nurse manager at different levels in an organization. It describes how these roles involve managing quality, budgets, people, change, and risk.

LEARNING OBJECTIVES

After studying this chapter, you should be able to:

1. discuss theories and types of management.
2. describe the characteristics and roles of managers.
3. explain the role of the nurse manager in ensuring quality client care.
4. discuss the nurse manager's role in financial management.
5. discuss leadership styles, communication patterns, and organizational methods nurse managers use to work with people.
6. describe the change process and strategies for managing resistance to change.
7. explain the nurse manager's role in managing risk.
8. compare and contrast the roles of nurse managers and nursing leaders as participants in multidisciplinary health care teams.

MATCHING

1. ____ accountability
2. ____ authority
3. ____ delegation
4. ____ leadership
5. ____ management
6. ____ nurse manager
7. ____ quality assurance
8. ____ responsibility
9. ____ risk management

a. being held answerable for personal actions or the actions of others

b. the obligation to provide an accounting or rationale for personal actions or the actions of others

c. a nurse responsible for managing the operation and expenses of a health care organization that employs nurses as the means to produce health

d. the process of identifying, evaluating, and reducing or financing the cost of predictable losses

e. the ability or legitimate power to make decisions, implement strategies, and elicit work from others

f. involves assigning responsibility for certain tasks to other people, thereby allowing the manager to concentrate on organizational goals and productivity

(Continued on p. 70)

g. involves showing others the way, directing others in a course of action, going before others, or going with and inspiring others.

h. the implementation of strategies that promote effective and efficient use of resources to achieve organizational goals

i. refers to the process of achieving an optimal degree of excellence in the services rendered to every client

TRUE OR FALSE

10. ____ Theory Y proposes that workers are negatively motivated.

11. ____ Nurse managers have become consensus builders who facilitate client care rather than acting as control systems.

12. ____ A middle-level nurse manager is called a nurse executive.

13. ____ Only middle-level managers can hire and fire staff.

14. ____ A front-line manager typically works as a charge nurse, team leader, or client care coordinator.

15. ____ A nurse manager who wanted to hire a new nurse could use information gained as part of fiscal management to justify the need.

16. ____ The overall definition of the business of health care for each institution is written in the form of a policy.

17. ____ A mission statement is used to identify institutional goals.

18. ____ Organizational goals are translated into specific objectives to guide the day-to-day operation of work units.

19. ____ Cost containment remains a major goal in health care today and affects all health care practitioners.

FILL-IN-THE-BLANKS

20. Theory X proposes that workers are _____ motivated.

21. Based on Theory Z, organizational structures in health care have become more _____.

22. Regardless of whether the setting is a home care agency or a hospital, the goal of a nurse manager is to promote _____.

23. Because the position of a nurse manager involves inspiring others to work, all nurse managers should be _____.

24. An _____ is defined as a social system deliberately established to carry out some defining purpose.

25. Most organizations create a diagram called an _____ _____ that depicts the hierarchical arrangement of its managers.

26. Managing _____ means accentuating positive outcomes as well as avoiding negative outcomes.

27. Nurse managers evaluate how well policies and procedures facilitate the attainment of goals by measuring _____.

28. _____ and _____ are rules and outlined processes that define the steps taken to meet objectives.

29. Nurse managers strive to ensure the highest quality care at the lowest possible _____.

EXERCISING YOUR CLINICAL JUDGMENT

Kristen Williams is a middle-level nurse manager on a 40-bed surgical unit in a local hospital. She arrived at work at 7 a.m. and is developing her plan for the day after reviewing her scheduled appointments and meetings. She must attend a 9 a.m. meeting of the Policy and Procedure Committee, followed by a budget meeting at 10 a.m. In the afternoon she has a staff meeting planned to explore with staff how they can achieve more timely client discharges on the unit before new admissions arrive from the post-anesthesia care unit. As she gathers the materials needed for the morning meetings, she realizes that in her role today she will be managing quality, people, budget, and change. She glances at her watch and determines that she has plenty of time to talk to the first-line nurse manager and nursing staff about concerns on the unit before her planned schedule begins.

30. As Kristen enters the nurses' station, the first-line manager reports that there has been a sick call already for the evening shift. Which of the following actions would represent the best use of Kristen's time and skills and those of other staff?
    a. Delegate to the front-line manager the responsibility for calling part-time off-duty nurses to see if they can work.
    b. Call the nurse executive to complain about how short-staffed the unit always is.
    c. Make a mental note to bring this problem up at the budget meeting and try to use it to demand more staff.
    d. Tell the staff at 3 p.m. that they will have to work short and "make do."

31. At the Policy and Procedure Committee meeting, the first item on the agenda is a review of the effectiveness of a new policy and procedure for blood transfusion intended to reduce turn-around time from receipt of an order in the blood bank to the start time for infusion into the client. The committee determines that based on data available, 20 minutes have been eliminated in the process. The new policy and procedure are determined to be effective in improving:
    a. communication.
    b. quality.
    c. cost.
    d. goals.

32. At the budget meeting, Kristen must determine projected revenue from her nursing unit for the coming year. She would use concepts related to which of the following in order to complete this work?
    a. negotiation
    b. lobbying
    c. forecasting
    d. staffing

33. At the staff meeting later that day, a group of nurses express an interest in beginning to use a self-scheduling process to determine their work schedules. Kristen asks for an interested group of nurses to get wider input from nurses on the unit, determine feasibility, and report back to the group in a month. In this instance, Kristen is using which of the following management styles?
    a. Theory Q
    b. Theory X
    c. Theory Y
    d. Theory Z

TEST YOURSELF

34. Which of the following members of the hospital staff would not be part of a multidisciplinary team working with a client?
    a. social worker
    b. billing clerk
    c. pastoral care provider
    d. client's family

35. Which of the following activities undertaken as part of a planned change correlates with the analysis phase of the nursing process?
    a. identify the need for change
    b. identify potential action plans
    c. identify the potential cause of a problem
    d. incorporate new behaviors into structures or processes

36. Which of the following time management tips would be least useful and productive for a nurse manager?
    a. write down identified tasks, obligations, and activities
    b. work on the most important task first
    c. do not accept assignments that you are not capable of completing
    d. adopt a strategy of needing to be perfect

37. A new first-line manager tends to be autocratic and authoritarian in nature, and does not seem to trust that the staff will complete their assignments unless they are monitored frequently during the day. This new manager is exhibiting which of the following management styles?
    a. aggressive
    b. assertive
    c. passive
    d. passive-aggressive

38. The nurse managers of an institution are meeting to determine how well they are complying with regulations of the Joint Commission for Accreditation of Health Care Organizations. The group is motivated to be in compliance because this is necessary for:
    a. praise from the chief executive officer.
    b. national recognition.
    c. accreditation.
    d. high profit margins.

Nursing Research

PURPOSE

The purpose of this chapter is to provide introductory information about nursing research methodology to assist you in reading research studies.

LEARNING OBJECTIVES

After studying this chapter, you should be able to:

1. describe the importance of nursing research.
2. identify the influence of ethical dilemmas in nursing research and the mechanisms for the protection of human subjects.
3. describe the personnel involved in research studies, types of studies, and the parts of a typical research study.
4. identify and discuss the steps of the research process.
5. identify ways of implementing nursing research findings in your nursing practice.

MATCHING

1. _h_ data
2. _c_ experimental research
3. _g_ dependent variable
4. _i_ nonexperimental research
5. _f_ instruments
6. _i_ institutional review board

7. _a_ abstract
8. _b_ data collection
9. _d_ hypothesis
10. _o_ operational definition
11. _n_ quantitative research
12. _m_ informed consent
13. _e_ independent variable
14. _k_ quasi-experimental research
15. _j_ qualitative research
16. _r_ research problem
17. _s_ theoretical framework
18. _q_ sampling
19. _p_ research design

a. a short summary that contains brief information about the purpose of the study, the number of subjects, methodology used to select subjects, the type of study being conducted, and the major results from the study

b. the process by which the researcher acquires subjects and collects the information necessary to answer the research question

c. a type of research study in which the researcher manipulates a treatment or intervention, randomly assigns subjects to either a control or experimental group, and has control over the research situation

d. a tentative prediction of the relationship between two or more variables being studied

e. the variable in a research design that may show variation, but the variation is expected to remain constant in the study, although it influences or even causes change in another variable.

(Continued on p. 74)

f. the tools a re-searcher uses to conduct a study

g. the variable in a research design that is hypothesized to change with the treatment (i.e., have been caused by an independent variable)

h. used to designate the information the researcher is interested in collecting

i. a type of study in which the re-searcher collects data without the introduction of a treatment or intervention

j. a type of study that uses ideas that are analyzed as words

k. a type of study in which the re-searcher manipu-lates a treatment or intervention, but is unable to random-ize subjects into groups or lacks a control group

l. a committee whose duties include insuring that the proposed research meets the federal requirements for ethical research; the federal govern-ment mandates the committee if the institution is receiving federal funds for research

m. means that the subjects have been provided with sufficient informa-tion regarding the research to enable them to consent voluntarily to participate or decline to partici-pate.

n. a type of study that uses variables that are analyzed as numbers

o. the meaning of the concept precisely as it is being used in the study, defined in a manner that specifies how the concepts will be measured

p. a researcher's strategy for testing a hypothesis

q. the process of collecting data from a portion of the group being studied

r. an observation, situation, occur-rence, or even a hunch which an investigator chooses to research

s. a logical but abstract structure that suggests the relationship among the variables for a research study

TRUE OR FALSE

20. ____ One of the ANA priorities for nursing research is to analyze home health care services and data on elders at home and in long-term care facilities.

21. ____ One of the priorities for the National Center for Nursing Research is to test interventions for coping with chronic illness.

22. ____ Informed consent for research includes a clear statement that the subject is free to discontinue participation at any time the subject wishes.

23. ____ In the absence of a requirement for institu-tional review, researchers are free to skip some ethical guidelines.

24. ____ Research should not be performed on human subjects unless there is a clear possibility of benefit to society or individu-als.

25. ____ When a research study shows a good correlation between two variables, causa-tion can be inferred.

26. ____ Reading an abstract is sufficient to evaluate a study.

27. ____ The results of a study are a factual presenta-tion of what is found.

28. ____ In the discussion that follows the results, the researcher tells what the findings mean in his or her opinion.

29. ____ Not all problems are amenable to research methods.

30. ____ The Index Medicus does not contain nursing journals.

31. ____ As a user of research, the operational definition can help you know if the infor-mation applies in a specific client situation.

32. ____ A research study is not worthwhile unless it proves the hypothesis.

33. ____ Research begins with a problem or a question that arises in the clinical practice setting.

34. ____ When you are reading a research study, always ask yourself, "What else could have caused this effect?"

35. ____ The goal of using research findings is to improve the quality of care in the clinical setting.

FILL-IN-THE-BLANKS

36. _Nursing   research_ is the method used to develop or search for knowledge about issues important to nurses and nursing practice.

37. _Florence Nightingale_ was the first nurse researcher.

38. Because nursing research often involves _human   subjects_, ethical standards are especially important.

39. A _case   study_ is a type of research that involves the detailed investigation of an individual, group, or institution to understand which variables are important to the subjects—history, care, or development.

40. The concepts under investigation in a study are called _variables_.

41. In _____ (random, nonrandom) sample each member of the population has an equal chance of being selected as part of the sample.

42. In qualitative research the data is analyzed by _reduction_ of large volumes of narrative data into categories that can be identified as the concepts present in the situation.

43. Controlling _extraneous_ variables controls research bias.

44. When you ask if the passage of time has affected the results, you are asking a question about the validity classification of _maturation_.

45. _Transferability_ refers to whether it makes good sense to attempt an innovation in your practice situation.

EXERCISING YOUR CLINICAL JUDGMENT

46. Select the statement that is true about the case study method of research.
    a. Case studies increase knowledge of clients with similar conditions.
    b. Case studies are not a valid method of research.
    c. Case studies focus on the psychosocial needs of clients.
    d. Case studies rule out the need to consider multiple variables.

47. Before you use the findings of a research study to make decisions in the clinical setting, you should ask:
    a. if the elements of the situation are precisely like those of the study.
    b. if you have the qualifications to make decisions using research.
    c. if your hospital is a research hospital.
    d. if the elements of the situation are sufficiently similar to the conditions of study to make it likely that the intervention will work in this situation.

48. Select the phrase that would be consistent with one of the ANA priorities for nursing research.
    a. finding a cure for AIDS
    b. testing lifestyle management strategies for preventing AIDS
    c. developing a vaccine against AIDS
    d. describing the mutation mechanisms of the HIV virus

TEST YOURSELF

49. Select the most important criteria for deciding if a problem is worth studying.
    a. The solution can be expected to improve the quality of life for a number of clients.
    b. The solution to the problem will make the researcher famous.
    c. The problem is unusual and therefore interesting to study.
    d. Enough is known about the problem to make a solution feasible.

50. A nurse wants to study a technique for reducing infection rates in premature infants. Select the behavior that would be within ethical guidelines for research.
    a. not informing the parents of the control group because nothing will change for their child
    b. not informing the parents of the experimental group because their participation is not necessary
    c. selecting the babies with greater weights for the experimental group to prevent causing harm
    d. fully informing and seeking consent from parents of all infants

51. The review of a research protocol by an institutional review board is required:
    a. when federal support is sought to conduct the study.
    b. only when invasive procedures are used in the study.
    c. only when the subject is of a sensitive nature.
    d. only when the methods are known to cause harm.

52. When considering the issue of informed consent for research, a vulnerable population is one that is:
    a. unable to give informed consent.
    b. more likely to be harmed by the intervention.
    c. at greater risk for complications.
    d. unlikely to want to participate in the study.

53. The population being studied refers to:
    a. both the research subjects and the control group.
    b. the group with the characteristics of the people who are selected as subjects.
    c. the clients on the nursing unit where the study is being conducted.
    d. everybody living in a given geographical area.

The Well Newborn, Infant, and Toddler

PURPOSE

This chapter explores concepts of growth and development and factors that affect them. It introduces you to the use of the nursing process in caring for the well newborn, infant, and toddler.

LEARNING OBJECTIVES

After studying this chapter, you should be able to:

1. compare and contrast three significant theories of growth and development.
2. identify developmental milestones in the newborn, infant, and toddler.
3. describe environmental, socioeconomic, nutritional, and physiological factors affecting growth and development.
4. describe the assessment of growth and development in the newborn, infant, and toddler.
5. discuss the conditions related to altered growth and development in the child from birth to age 3.
6. discuss assessment strategies to detect altered growth and development.
7. identify situations that could result in problems of health maintenance.
8. select an appropriate nursing diagnosis for a newborn, infant, or toddler with problems in growth and development.
9. plan interventions to promote healthy growth and development.
10. plan interventions to promote maintenance of a newborn's, infant's, or toddler's health.
11. evaluate outcomes for a newborn, infant, or toddler with Altered health maintenance.

MATCHING

1. ____ accommodation
2. ____ adaptation
3. ____ assimilation
4. ____ attachment
5. ____ bonding
6. ____ cephalocaudal
7. ____ cognitive development
8. ____ critical periods
9. ____ development
10. ____ developmental milestones
11. ____ developmental task
12. ____ differentiated development
13. ____ growth
14. ____ infant
15. ____ newborn
16. ____ object permanence
17. ____ proximodistal
18. ____ psychosocial development

a. the physiological development of a living being and is the quantitative change seen in the body

b. a child from the age of 1 month to the end of 12 months

c. development that starts with a generalized response and progresses to a skilled specific response

d. an important activity that arises at a certain period in life

e. a progression of behavioral changes that involve the acquisition of appropriate cognitive, linguistic, and psychosocial skills

f. a child aged 1–3 years

g. a child born within the last 28 days

(Continued on p. 78)

19. _____ sensory stimulation

20. _____ teratogen

21. _____ toddler

h. a process of changing, or modifying old ways of thinking to fit new situations.

i. the awareness that unseen objects do not disappear; evidenced by the infant searching for an object that has been moved out of sight

j. a progression of mental abilities from illogical thinking to logical thinking, from simple to complex problem solving, and from understanding concrete ideas to understanding abstract ideas

k. periods of time when a person has an increased vulnerability to physical, chemical, psychological, or environmental influences

l. an agent or influence that causes physical defects in the developing fetus

m. a pattern of neuromuscular growth and development that starts at the head and moves toward the feet

n. a pattern of skill development that starts at the midline of the body and moves outward

o. the development of strong ties of affection by an infant with a significant other

p. the development of subjective feelings and interpersonal relationships

q. a change that occurs as a result of assimilation and accommodation, also called coping behavior

r. the process of learning from new experiences

s. predictable patterns of normal development according to age

t. the process of forming an attachment between parent and newborn

u. the activation and exhilaration of the senses

TRUE OR FALSE

22. _____ Each stage of development depends on adequate completion of the previous one and forms the foundation for development of new skills.

23. _____ Stages of physical growth rarely correspond to certain developmental changes.

24. _____ Jean Piaget described cognitive development as involving the increasing ability to think and reason in a logical manner.

25. _____ The list of developmental tasks is the same for all cultures.

26. _____ A newborn can smell at birth once the nose is cleared of mucus and other fluids.

27. _____ Crying is the secondary means by which newborns make their needs and wants known.

28. _____ During parallel play, toddlers play beside, but not with, their friends.

29. _____ Socioeconomic factors, such as income, educational level, and single parenthood, influence the growth and development of children.

30. _____ The cerebral palsies can involve either a single limb or can produce total disability.

FILL-IN-THE-BLANKS

31. A newborn's length is measured from _____ to _____.

32. The development of a newborn's ability to move and to control the body is called _____ development.

33. Eyes begin to focus and fixate at _____ months.

34. An infant who cries when separated from parents or approached by strangers is having _____ _____.

35. The ability to _____ is an important developmental milestone for toddlers.

36. Temper tantrums usually make their appearance at about age _____.

37. Human milk is the most desirable form of milk for the first _____ months of life.

38. _____ is a genetic disorder of amino acid metabolism in which phenylalanine cannot be converted to tyrosine.

39. More than 75% of children have at least one episode of _____ _____, an infection and inflammation of the middle ear.

EXERCISING YOUR CLINICAL JUDGMENT

Yung Hi, the 33-month-old Korean girl who was introduced in the chapter case study, has undergone orthopedic surgery to reduce a fractured femur and is in skeletal traction. She has a nursing diagnosis of *Altered growth and development related to prescribed dependence (traction) and separation from parents at night.* You are assigned to work with Yung on the evening shift, and are thus able to work with her while her mother is present, and on a one-on-one basis after the parents have gone home for the evening.

40. Which of the following age-appropriate toys would you recommend be brought to the hospital for Yung to play with during her recuperation?
    a. mobile
    b. rattle
    c. toys that float in water
    d. non-toxic crayons

41. You are trying to encourage continued physical growth during the period of recuperation. Which of the following strategies would be most useful?
    a. Try to have Yung eat the same amount of food every day.
    b. Keep foods separated from each other on the tray, and use her favorite cup at each meal.
    c. Use food as a reward for good behavior.
    d. Encourage Yung to eat every bit of food on her plate.

42. Which of the following tools would you use to assess the amount of pain that Yung is experiencing due to surgery and traction?
    a. pain scale using words as descriptors
    b. pain scale using numbers as descriptors
    c. pain scale using facial expressions as descriptors
    d. a word board listing words associated with pain in Korean

43. You would plan age-appropriate care by allowing time for Yung to have a 1-2 hour nap each day at:
    a. 9 a.m.
    b. 10 a.m.
    c. 1 p.m.
    d. 4 p.m.

TEST YOURSELF

44. Bringing toys and games to the bedside of an immobilized child would be primarily useful interventions for which of the following nursing diagnoses?
    a. Altered health maintenance
    b. Altered growth and development
    c. Diversional activity deficit
    d. Health-seeking behaviors

45. The nurse would bring rattles that make noise and vinyl or cloth books to the bedside of a client who is how old?
    a. 1–2 months
    b. 2–3 months
    c. 4–8 months
    d. 1–2 years

46. The nurse providing immunizations to children would teach the parents to report to the health care provider which of the following adverse effects of an immunization?
    a. high fever
    b. mild discomfort at the site
    c. rash at the site
    d. soreness in the area

47. The home health nurse would provide parent education after noting which of the following behaviors when visiting the home of a pediatric client?
    a. all crib rails raised
    b. mother left toddler in tub to answer door
    c. safety handles on all cabinet doors
    d. gate positioned at the head of the stairs

48. The nurse would avoid giving toys with small removable parts to a client under the age of:
    a. 1.
    b. 2.
    c. 3.
    d. 4.

20

The Well Child

PURPOSE

This chapter focuses on the principles of child growth and development. It identifies factors affecting growth and development of the preschool and school-age child. It also discusses assessment of growth, development, and health maintenance for the preschool and school-age child. In addition, it gives nursing interventions that may be used to give parents anticipatory guidance.

LEARNING OBJECTIVES

After studying this chapter, you should be able to:

1. describe the normal growth and development of the preschool and school-age child.
2. identify factors affecting growth and development of the preschool and school-age child.
3. discuss assessment of growth, development and health maintenance for the preschool and school-age child.
4. plan nursing care that demonstrates knowledge of normal growth and development of the preschool and school-age child.
5. identify areas in which the parents of preschool and school-age children can benefit from the nurse's anticipatory guidance.
6. describe evaluation of expected outcomes for the preschool and school-age child experiencing Altered growth and development or Altered health maintenance.

MATCHING

1. ____ attention-deficit/hyper-activity disorder
2. ____ concrete operations
3. ____ conservation
4. ____ decentering accommodation
5. ____ latchkey children
6. ____ learning disability
7. ____ preschooler
8. ____ school-age child
9. ____ sibling rivalry
10. ____ symbolic play

a. a child between the age of 3 and 5 years

b. pretend or imaginative play that enables preschool children to recreate experiences and to try out roles

c. a child in the developmental stage between 6 and 11 years old

d. the stage of cognitive development at which children begin to project the self into other people's situations and realize that their own way of thinking isn't the only way

e. a child's ability to adapt thought processes to perceive more than one reason for a person's actions

f. a child's ability to understand that changing the shape of a substance does not change its volume

(Continued on p. 82)

g. refers to the competition of brothers and sisters for the attention, approval, and affection of the parents

h. a neuropsychological disorder associated with disturbances in attention, impulsivity, and hyperactivity.

i. lifelong disorder that affects the manner in which people of normal or above-average intelligence select, retain, and express information

j. describes children in elementary school who spend some part of their time before or after school without adult supervision

21. _____ _____ is the child's ability to adapt thought processes to perceive more than one reason for a person's actions.

22. Optimum childhood _____, _____, and _____ of illness are the objectives of pediatric health supervision.

23. Deaths from bicycling injuries usually result from _____ injuries and almost always are the result of _____ between bicycles and motor vehicles.

24. Children under the age of _____ should not use skateboards or in-line skates because they are not developmentally prepared to protect themselves from injury.

TRUE OR FALSE

11. _____ The preschool years are a time of rapid weight gain for a toddler.

12. _____ All 20 deciduous teeth generally erupt during the preschool period.

13. _____ It is normal for preschool children to create imaginary companions that they talk to and play with, and who become a regular part of their daily routines.

14. _____ Children between the ages of 6 and 11 have few fears, such as fear of darkness, animals, and high places.

15. _____ Attention-deficit/hyperactivity disorder is more prevalent in boys than girls.

16. _____ Children cannot be trusted to handle a gun safely, even though they have the mechanical skill and strength to fire one.

17. _____ Latchkey children are often afraid and lonely while at home alone.

FILL-IN-THE-BLANKS

18. During the preschool years, a toddler's future body type becomes apparent. Body types include _____ (lanky build), mesomorphic (medium muscular build) and _____ (large build).

19. Preschoolers experience tremendous improvement in large and fine _____ coordination.

20. The vivid imagination of the _____-_____ child can turn a stuffed toy by day into a threatening monster in the dark.

EXERCISING YOUR CLINICAL JUDGMENT

25. Timmy, the child referred to in the chapter's case study, is a four-year-old who was injured in a water-skiing accident. His parents had unrealistic expectations about Timmy's athletic abilities. They thought that if he just had more practice he would become skilled at water skiing. What nursing diagnosis would be most appropriate?
    a. Altered growth and development
    b. Altered health maintenance
    c. Altered childhood achievement
    d. Altered family processes

26. During your interview with Timmy, he confides in you that his parents beat him. Which of the following nursing diagnoses would be most appropriate for this situation?
    a. Altered parenting
    b. Altered growth and development
    c. Altered health maintenance
    d. Altered childhood achievement

27. Timmy discusses how he is a good skateboarder. Knowing that it is not recommended that children under age 5 use skateboards, the most appropriate nursing diagnosis is:
    a. Altered parenting
    b. Altered growth and development
    c. Altered health maintenance
    d. Risk for injury

TEST YOURSELF

28. Your client is upset because his mother left the room. She told him that she was returning in two hours. Fear of abandonment is a common concern for which of the following age groups?
    a. four- to six-year-olds
    b. teenagers
    c. school-age children
    d. preschoolers

29. Establishing guidelines for behavior is which of the following?
    a. developing morality
    b. discipline
    c. limit-setting
    d. parenting skills

30. The recommended screening for tuberculosis (TB) during childhood is at which of the following times?
    a. twice during childhood
    b. four times during childhood: 1, 4, 8, and 12 years old
    c. three times during childhood: 12–15 months, before entering kindergarten, and at 14–17 years of age
    d. at the entrance of school, unless otherwise indicated

31. Children may use symptoms such as vomiting, headaches, or abdominal pain as an excuse to say home from school because they have a fear of school. This is an example of:
    a. a phobia.
    b. school avoidance.
    c. acting-out behavior.
    d. a defense mechanism.

32. Advice you can give working parents of latchkey children is to:
    a. not leave their children unsupervised.
    b. use the community resources available to latchkey children (provide a list).
    c. encourage them have their children remain at school until they can pick them up.
    d. consider working in jobs that allow them to be at home when their children are home.

The Well Adolescent

PURPOSE

This chapter discusses the principles of adolescent growth and development. It describes general assessment of adolescent growth and development and factors affecting it. It also gives nursing interventions to maintain wellness and reduce risk factors for adolescents.

LEARNING OBJECTIVES

After studying this chapter, you should be able to:

1. describe the normal growth and development of an adolescent.
2. discuss factors that affect adolescent growth and development, including environmental, socioeconomic, lifestyle, psychosocial, and physiological factors.
3. describe the general assessment of adolescents for normal function and risk factors.
4. compare and contrast at least three nursing diagnoses that may be especially appropriate for use with adolescents.
5. plan nursing interventions to maintain wellness and reduce risk factors for adolescents.
6. discuss interventions to improve adolescents' access to health care.
7. evaluate nursing care using outcome criteria.

MATCHING

1. ____ adolescence
2. ____ anorexia nervosa
3. ____ bulimia nervosa
4. ____ constitutional delay of puberty
5. ____ egocentrism
6. ____ familial short stature
7. ____ formal operations
8. ____ gynecomastia
9. ____ menarche
10. ____ nocturnal emission
11. ____ obesity
12. ____ puberty
13. ____ scoliosis

a. the period of transition between childhood and adulthood

b. the time of the first menstrual period

c. the sequence of physiological events that cause the reproductive organs to mature, making conception and childbirth possible

d. the ability to reason abstractly

e. refers to the tendency to spend so much time thinking about and focusing on your own thoughts and changes in your own body that you come to believe that others are focused on them as well

f. an absence of early signs of puberty

g. term used to describe a height below the third percentile on the growth chart

(Continued on p. 86)

h. body weight or body fat percentage that exceeds a chosen reference point

i. a benign increase in breast tissue associated with puberty

j. a complex disorder characterized by self-induced weight loss driven by a morbid fear of becoming fat

k. a disorder characterized by binge eating coupled with purging via emetics, laxatives, or self-induced vomiting

l. a structural lateral curvature of the spine

m. a discharge of semen during sleep

23. Adolescents who live in poverty typically have poor nutrition, substandard housing, and limited access to _____ _____.

24. A common complaint of _____ _____ is gynecomastia, which is a benign increase in breast tissue associated with puberty.

25. The primary causes of adolescent morbidity and mortality are _____ health-risk _____.

26. An important goal of care for hospitalized adolescents is to avoid disruption of their _____ development.

27. Adolescents with a chronic illness may engage in risk taking by failing to _____ with their treatment program.

TRUE OR FALSE

14. ____ Children grow and develop at different rates, so any definition of adolescence should be flexible at both ends.

15. ____ Adolescents who are abused and neglected are at high risk for Altered growth and development.

16. ____ Girls are affected by a constitutional delay of puberty more often than boys are.

17. ____ Most of the cases of short stature result from underlying disease.

18. ____ The number of adolescents living with chronic illness has increased, not because the incidence of disease has changed but because more children with chronic conditions are surviving.

19. ____ Alcohol is a cofactor in the most common causes of deaths and injuries among adolescents.

20. ____ You should be cautious when asking adolescents questions about illegal, unsafe, or otherwise undesirable behavior.

FILL-IN-THE-BLANKS

21. The hallmark of adolescence is a physical process known as _____.

22. The chief developmental task of adolescence is the development of _____ versus _____ diffusion.

EXERCISING YOUR CLINICAL JUDGMENT

28. Malik, an 18-year-old senior, referred to in this chapter's case study, has been sexually active for the past two years with multiple partners. He refuses to use condoms since he believes it is unmanly to use them. Which of the following nursing diagnoses would be most appropriate?
    a. Altered health maintenance
    b. Ineffective individual coping
    c. Self-esteem disturbance
    d. Altered growth and development

29. One of Malik's girlfriends, a 16-year-old, seeks your advice because she is afraid of getting a STD from him if she continues to have unprotected sex with him. Which of the following nursing diagnoses would be most appropriate?
    a. Altered health maintenance
    b. Ineffective individual coping
    c. Risk for infection
    d. Altered growth and development

30. Malik is about to graduate from high school. He admits he is stressed about graduation. He has increased his drinking with friends on weekends, but he is unsure why. Which of the following nursing diagnoses would be most appropriate?
    a. Altered health maintenance
    b. Ineffective individual coping
    c. Risk for infection
    d. Altered growth and development

TEST YOURSELF

31. You are discussing preventive health issues with an adolescent client. The response you get is, "Other people may have to worry about that, but I don't have to worry about it." This is an example of which hallmark of adolescent cognitive development?
    a. egocentrism
    b. elitism
    c. fantasy world
    d. concrete thinking

32. Which of the following statements is true for constitutional delay of puberty?
    a. It affects more girls than boys, and is more likely to arise in a family in which the pubertal development of the same-sex parent was delayed.
    b. It is more likely to arise in a family in which the pubertal development of the same-sex parent was delayed.
    c. It affects more boys than girls, and is more likely to arise in a family in which the pubertal development of the same-sex parent was delayed.
    d. It affects males and females equally and is related to heredity.

33. Your adolescent client was involved in a homicide. Which of the following statements is the most accurate?
    a. Homicide is a serious public health problem in the United States, and a leading cause of deaths among young adults.
    b. Homicide-related deaths are among the top three causes of death among adolescents.
    c. Homicide deaths occur among adolescents, but are not among the primary causes of deaths among adolescents.
    d. Homicide is a serious problem because of alcohol abuse among teenagers.

34. One of the most effective ways for parents to help prevent their teenagers from becoming pregnant is to:
    a. use the just say "no" approach.
    b. buy them condoms.
    c. condone their adolescents' behaviors, so they feel comfortable coming to their parents when they want advice.
    d. talk with their teenagers about sex in a nonjudgmental and informative manner.

35. Your client, a high school student, earns straight As and is very active in school activities. She is thin and appears underdeveloped for her age. Her weight is 98 lbs. and height is 5'8". She confides in you that she feels fat. Which of the following nursing diagnoses would be most appropriate?
    a. Altered health maintenance
    b. Ineffective individual coping
    c. Body image disturbance
    d. Altered growth and development

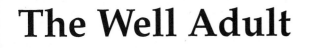

The Well Adult

PURPOSE

This chapter discusses key concepts related to the developmental tasks of young and middle-aged adults. It identifies the various factors that affect adult development. It also differentiates among the variety of diagnoses appropriate for the adult seeking knowledge or health care related to growth and development and discusses nursing interventions to maintain health and reduce risk factors.

LEARNING OBJECTIVES

After studying this chapter, you should be able to:

1. discuss the developmental tasks a young adult must complete.
2. describe the developmental tasks of the middle years.
3. identify a variety of factors affecting adult development.
4. describe the assessment of a well adult for normal function and risk factors.
5. differentiate among the variety of nursing diagnoses appropriate for the middle-aged adults seeking knowledge or health care related to growth and development.
6. plan nursing interventions to maintain wellness and reduce risk factors as appropriate to the adult's developmental level.
7. evaluate nursing care using outcome criteria.

MATCHING

1. _d_ alcohol abuse
2. _h_ evaluation
3. _b_ fetal alcohol syndrome
4. _g_ health history
5. ___ menopause
6. _e_ middle adulthood
7. _f_ midlife crisis
8. _i_ poverty
9. _c_ sandwich generation
10. _a_ young adulthood

a. refers to the period from ages 20 to 35

b. a distinct cluster of physical and mental impairments caused by prenatal exposure to alcohol

c. caught between the needs of adjacent generations; caring for ill or frail parents while handling the competing demands of children and employment

d. may cause cirrhosis of the liver, inflammation of the pancreas, damage to the brain and heart, and malnutrition

e. the period from ages 35 to 64

(Continued on p. 90)

f. a stressful life period during middle adulthood, precipitated by the review and reevaluation of one's past, including goals, priorities, and life accomplishments, during which the person experiences inner turmoil, self-doubt, and major restructuring of personality

g. includes the client's biographical data, past health history, chief complaint, and present health status

h. a systematic, ongoing process in evaluating the client's progress toward the attainment of goals

i. associated with limited access to heath care, poor nutrition, substandard housing, and inadequate prenatal care

j. the second stage in the female climacteric, during which hormone production is reduced, the ovaries stop producing eggs, and menstruation ceases

TRUE OR FALSE

11. __T__ Always, a person's growth and development represent the interaction of genetic makeup and environment.

12. __T__ Traditionally, biologists have divided the life span into three phases. The last phase is a decline of physical abilities after age 45.

13. __F__ Erickson's theory of psychosocial development identifies the young adult stage as generativity versus stagnation. *intamacy vs. isolation*

14. __F__ The Centers for Disease Control and Prevention (CDC) report that approximately 1 in 100 deaths is related to cigarette smoking. *1 in 5 deaths*

15. __T__ Stress is the most common cause of illness in our society, probably underlying as much as 70% of all visits to primary care providers.

16. __T__ Homicide is the third leading cause of fatal injury for male workers and it is the leading cause of injury and death for women in the workplace.

17. __F__ Changing a client's high-risk behavior involves giving the client appropriate health information. *health education + counceling*

FILL-IN-THE-BLANKS

18. __Growth__ refers to the quantitative change a person undergoes and __development__ refers to the progressive increase in skill and capacity to function.

19. Erickson's seventh stage of psychosocial development, __generativity__ versus __stagnation__ is reached during middle adulthood.

20. Levinson conceived of development as a sequence of qualitatively distinct eras or __seasons__, each of which has its own time and brings certain psychological challenges to the forefront of a person's life.

21. Chronic drug users are particularly susceptible to __infectious diseases__ and are considered high-risk transmitters.

22. Clients who are __depressed__ experience a great deal of functional impairment, resulting in lost work time, decreased job performance, and decreased family and social functioning.

23. __Poverty__ is associated with limited access to health care, poor nutrition, substandard housing, and inadequate prenatal care.

24. Nearly half of all worker-compensation costs reported to the Bureau of Labor Statistics each year represent __ergonomic__-related disorders.

25. Each plan of care must be __individualized__ to a client's needs, age, and culture.

EXERCISING YOUR CLINICAL JUDGMENT

26. Mr. Biaggio, the 42-year-old client from the chapter's case study, is struggling with balancing his roles as a husband, parent, and new employee. His children are in high school and plan to attend college in another state. He has become self-absorbed and distant from his family. Mr. Biaggio may be experiencing which psychosocial stage of development?
    a. intimacy versus isolation
    b. industry versus inferiority
    c. integrity versus despair
    d. generativity versus stagnation

27. Mr. Biaggio has been reviewing and re-evaluating his life including his life accomplishments. He has been experiencing inner turmoil and self-doubt. He is most likely experiencing:
    a. poor job performance.
    b. a situational crisis.
    c. a midlife crisis.
    d. poor family relationships.

28. To help persuade Mr. Biaggio to change his high-risk behaviors, you will need to:
    a. give Mr. Biaggio both oral and written health education material.
    b. have Mr. Biaggio join a support group made up of men his age.
    c. identify Mr. Biaggio's beliefs relevant to his high-risk behaviors and provide him information based on this foundation.
    d. give Mr. Biaggio your recommendations regarding his most serious high-risk behavior so he may begin working on modifying it.

TEST YOURSELF

29. Middle adulthood is the period from ages 35–64 when mature adults are concerned with:
    a. developing philosophies of life and personal lifestyles.
    b. balancing a career with raising small children.
    c. establishing a significant relationship with a partner.
    d. establishing and guiding the next generation in their roles as parents, teachers, mentors, guardians of the culture, etc.

30. Your client has a child in high school and is caring for his elderly parent. As a group, clients in this situation are often commonly called the:
    a. mid-level generation.
    b. x-generation.
    c. sandwich generation.
    d. midlife transition generation.

31. You are admitting a client to your health care facility. What is the most important thing you need to do to ensure that you obtain a thorough and accurate history of the client's problems?
    a. read the client's admission record prior to your assessment
    b. develop trusting relationship with the client
    c. obtain biographical data, history, chief complaint
    d. obtain family history, chief complaint

32. You should do which of the following diagnostic screening tests with your young adult clients?
    a. TB, vision, Papanicolaou smear, breast exam
    b. TB, prostate-specific antigen test, cholesterol
    c. BP, breast exam, prostate-specific antigen test
    d. TB, sigmoidoscopy, vision

33. Your assessment of your client, who is 20 years old, reveals that she is suicidal, has had several unwanted pregnancies, and abuses alcohol. Which nursing diagnosis would be appropriate?
    a. Altered health maintenance
    b. Knowledge deficit
    c. Ineffective management of therapeutic regimen
    d. Altered growth and development

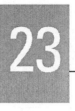
The Well Older Adult

PURPOSE

This chapter introduces you to the older adult in terms of stages of life, demographics, and factors affecting health. It provides you with information on how to use the nursing process to assist the older adult to maintain his or her health status.

LEARNING OBJECTIVES

After studying this chapter, you should be able to:

1. describe the older adult by stages of life and demographics.
2. discuss factors affecting health in older adults.
3. describe modifications of the health history and physical examination for the older adult.
4. discuss nursing diagnoses relevant to health maintenance for the older adult.
5. plan for goal-directed interventions for health maintenance of the older adult.
6. evaluate the outcomes that describe progress toward the goals of health maintenance.

MATCHING

1. __b__ ageism
2. __d__ older adult
3. __a__ polypharmacy
4. __c__ retirement

a. the use of more drugs than is clinically indicated

b. a stereotype, prejudice, or discrimination against people based on their age

c. the permanent withdrawal from one's job

d. any person 65 years of age or older

TRUE OR FALSE

5. __T__ The majority of people in the 65-and-older age group are female.

6. __F__ Almost all Americans who are older adults are not concerned about an inadequate supply of food.

7. __T__ Regular exercise is important for the older adult to promote appetite, mental health and balance, and to reduce stress.

8. __F__ Alcohol abuse in the older adult is often very easy to determine.

9. __T__ Older adults generally require 5–7 hours of sleep each night, and may need rest periods during the day.

10. __T__ The rate of motor vehicle accidents increases with older adults who have visual changes and increased arthritis.

11. __T__ Older adults can learn new skills, but sometimes at a slower rate.

12. __F__ The normal aging process necessarily limits mobility.

13. __F__ Older adults only rarely participate in ageist thinking.

14. __T__ An older adult's values and culture-specific needs are embedded in his or her coping strategies.

FILL-IN-THE-BLANKS

15. Physical changes associated with aging begin as early as the decade of the __forties__.

16. Chair-bound older adults can benefit from __range-of-motion__ exercises.

17. Regular replacement of smoke detector batteries will support __home safety__ for the older adult.

18. Older adults who drink __alcohol__ should not drive.

19. Most older adults have at least __one__ chronic disease(s).

20. Glaucoma can lead to __optic__ nerve damage if left untreated in the older adult.

21. An older adult who is able should be encouraged to walk 3–4 times a week for __twenty__ minutes at a time.

22. __Falls__ are the primary cause of femoral neck fractures in the older adult.

23. An important age-related change that can affect bones is the decreased amount of __calcium__ absorption.

24. Urinary __incontinence__ is not a normal age-related change in the older adult.

EXERCISING YOUR CLINICAL JUDGMENT

Betty Ellerton, the 81-year-old African-American woman identified in the chapter case study, has a nursing diagnosis of *Altered health maintenance*. She is living in her daughter's home after falling and fracturing the tibial head in one leg. Mrs. Ellerton was widowed six months earlier, and has reduced mobility and psychosocial well-being. She has very recently withdrawn further and become more immobile after suffering another fall at her daughter's house, so that she now does not want to get out of bed or ambulate in the home.

You have been assigned to fill in for the home health nurse following Mrs. Ellerton while that nurse is on vacation.

25. As you begin to consider what you will do to provide culture-specific care to Mrs. Ellerton, you should recall that which of the following is often valued by older African-American women?
    a. religion
    b. distance from family
    c. independence with all aspects of self-care
    d. warmth and trust when working with new health care providers

26. Because Mrs. Ellerton is at risk for falls, you should do which of the following to promote home safety?
    a. tell the client not to get out of bed at night, since it is dark
    b. tell the client to leave the overhead light on in the bedroom at night
    c. instruct the client to wear shoes with non-skid soles
    d. place loose throw rugs along paths where the client walks

27. While you are gathering routine health screening information, you determine that Mrs. Ellerton does not perform breast self-examination (BSE). After discussing the importance and rationale, you teach the client that this self-screening measure should be done by an older adult:
    a. once a week.
    b. once a month.
    c. once every six months.
    d. once a year.

28. Mrs. Ellerton states that her appetite is decreased and that she is eating less than she has in the past. Which of the following strategies would you recommend knowing she needs adequate nutrition for healing and repair of the leg?
    a. make sure almost all calories come from milk-based products
    b. decrease empty calorie intake and select foods high in nutritional value
    c. increase intake of foods containing protein
    d. increase intake of foods containing fat

29. You note during one visit that Mrs. Ellerton has reduced her fluid intake because it will reduce the number of trips she must make to the bathroom. You teach her the importance of fluid intake, stressing that she should drink how many glasses of fluid each day?
    a. 1–2
    b. 2–4
    c. 4–6
    d. 6–8

TEST YOURSELF

30. An otherwise healthy older adult client who lives alone has decreased mobility. The nurse places highest priority on assessing whether this client is able to do which of the following to meet his own nutritional needs?
    a. chew thoroughly
    b. swallow liquids
    c. shop for food
    d. wash dishes

31. The nurse interviewing an older adult inquires about the frequency of alcohol use. The nurse includes this information in planning care knowing that which of the following occurs in older adults who abuse alcohol?
    a. there is a higher ratio of body water to solid tissue
    b. there is greater production of protective mucus in the stomach
    c. there is faster excretion time for alcohol
    d. there is slower metabolism of alcohol

32. In discussing the ability of an older adult to drive, the nurse understands that the primary issue is one of:
    a. confusion.
    b. independence.
    c. cost.
    d. illness.

33. An older adult client tells the nurse that presbyopia has been diagnosed. When discussing the health problem with the client, the nurse explains that this will likely result in:
    a. cataract formation.
    b. the need to wear glasses.
    c. other signs of glaucoma.
    d. eventual blindness.

34. The nurse would be most careful to assess for signs of depression as a medication side effect in an older adult client taking medication for:
    a. high blood pressure.
    b. asthma.
    c. urinary tract infection.
    d. arthritis.

35. An older adult using diet as a complementary therapy to control cardiovascular disease should focus on which of the following?
    a. reduced potassium intake and increased protein intake
    b. increased carbohydrate and protein intake
    c. reduced caloric and salt intake
    d. reduced water and salt intake

CHAPTER 24

Health Perception

PURPOSE

This chapter discusses key concepts that relate to the nursing diagnosis Health-seeking behaviors. It provides you with definitions of health and describes the perception of health for individuals, families, and communities. In addition, this chapter identifies health goals and expected outcomes when planning care for individuals, families, and communities. It also discusses factors affecting health and interventions you can use to promote health.

LEARNING OBJECTIVES

After studying this chapter, you should be able to:

1. describe the perception of health for individuals, families, and communities.
2. list factors that affect health.
3. understand the focus of assessment of health in individuals, families, and communities.
4. identify health goals and expected outcomes when planning for individuals, families, and communities.
5. discuss the use of the nursing diagnosis Health-seeking behaviors.
6. identify methodologies of intervention for improving the health of individuals, families, and communities.
7. evaluate health outcomes in individuals, families, and communities.

MATCHING

1. _g_ disease
2. _j_ etiology
3. _i_ health goals
4. _k_ health-illness continuum
5. _a_ health perception
6. _d_ health promotion
7. _c_ health within illness
8. _b_ illness
9. _n_ longevity statistics
10. _o_ morbidity statistics
11. _p_ mortality statistics
12. _f_ population health
13. _s_ preventive health care
14. _m_ primary health care
15. _h_ primary prevention

a. knowledge and experience of one's state of wellness and well-being

b. personal experience of feeling unhealthy, caused by changes in a person's state of well-being and social function

c. an event that can expand human potential by providing an opportunity for personal growth and well-being despite having an illness

d. the advancement of health through the encouragement of activities that enhance the wellness of individuals, families, and communities

(Continued on p. 98)

16. ___ secondary prevention

17. ___ tertiary prevention

18. ___ well-being

19. ___ wellness

e. a subjective perception of a good and satisfactory existence in which the individual has a positive experience of personal abilities, harmony, and vitality

f. considers health problems encountered as a result of being a part of a group and focuses intervention on the population rather than on the individual

g. a specific disorder characterized by a recognizable set of signs and symptoms and attributable to heredity, infection, diet, or environment

h. consists of actions that are considered true prevention because they precede disease or dysfunction and are applied to clients considered physically and emotionally healthy to protect them from health problems

i. outlines broadly what needs to be done to achieve health for individuals, families, and communities

j. the cause of the disease

k. ranges from high-level wellness—an optimal state of mental and physical well-being—to premature death

l. consists of actions that focus on the early diagnosis and prompt treatment of people with health problems or illnesses and who are at risk for developing complications or worsening conditions

m. all care necessary to people's lives and health, including health education, nutrition, sanitation, maternal and child health care, immunizations, and prevention and control of endemic disease

n. life expectancy

o. illness rate

p. death rate

q. involves minimizing the effects of a permanent, irreversible disease or disability through interventions directed at preventing complication and deterioration

r. a state of optimal health or optimal physical and social functioning

s. the recognition of the risk for disease and actions taken to reduce that risk

TRUE OR FALSE

20. ___ Health perception is the knowledge and experience of one's state of wellness and well-being.

21. ___ Countries around the world are seeking to establish and attain health goals for their citizens.

22. ___ The World Health Organization (WHO) has declared that it is unrealistic to believe that health is a fundamental right of all people.

23. ___ All diseases can be cured by removing their etiology.

24. ___ Every person exists at some point on the health-illness continuum and may move back and forth between the two extremes.

25. ___ Population health perspective excludes consideration of individual needs and responsibility.

26. ___ The key element of Health-seeking behaviors is choice.

27. ___I___ Society at large is responsible for the health of its members.

FILL-IN-THE-BLANKS

28. The _World Heath Organ_ has defined health as a state of complete physical, mental, and social well-being, and not merely the absence of illness.

29. The three broad goals of *Healthy People 2000: National Health Promotion and Disease Prevention Objectives* are to increase the span of life, reduce health disparities among Americans, and achieve _preventativ_ services for all Americans.

30. The overarching goal of *Healthy People 2010* is increasing the _quality_ and _years_ of healthy life.

31. Health care is the _diagnosis_ and treatment of disease based on a specific disorder and its etiology.

32. The _health - illness continuum_ recognizes that more than one factor is necessary to determine a person's state of health.

33. Factors known to influence population health include living and _working_ conditions, economic well-being, and a personal sense of control over and skills for coping with the challenges and stresses of everyday living.

34. A statement of health goals flows from the _perception_ of health

35. Primary _medical_ care refers to care provided at the point at which a client first enters the health care system.

EXERCISING YOUR CLINICAL JUDGMENT

36. You are organizing a public forum to identify health goals for the local teen center. Your plan is to have teens actively seek ways to alter detrimental personal health habits so they can move toward a higher level of health. You are doing your health care planning based on the goals of *Healthy People 2010*. The enabling goals of *Healthy People 2010* include which of the following?
    a. to increase healthy behaviors, protect health, and strengthen community prevention
    b. Essential health services must be available to all persons without regard to age, risk category, present health status, or ability to pay.
    c. Essential services should be planned, funded, and supervised on a nonprofit basis by public authorities.
    d. Essential health services should be available to those eligible when they are away from home.

37. When planning your assessment of the teen center, which broad social issues might you consider assessing?
    a. whether it is a safe environment, and whether they offer cost-effective health services
    b. whether individual teens have good relationships with their peers
    c. whether the teens have good coping skills
    d. whether individual teens have the capacity to make healthy lifestyle decisions

38. You are concerned about the high levels of depression in the teen population. You organize and screen the teens for depression. This type of prevention is:
    a. primary.
    b. secondary.
    c. tertiary.
    d. evaluation.

TEST YOURSELF

39. The World Health Organization (WHO) has defined health as:
    a. the absence of disease.
    b. a state of complete physical, mental, and social well-being.
    c. knowledge and experience of one's state of wellness and well-being.
    d.  a state of complete physical, mental, and social well-being, and not merely the absence of disease.

40. In the United States, health care planning is commonly based on the two overarching goals of *Healthy People 2010*. These goals are:
    a. to provide essential health services to those eligible when they are away from home and to include a wide range of services, including health promotion and disease prevention.
    b. to ensure access to quality health care and strengthen community prevention.
    c. to increase the span of healthy life and eliminate health disparities among different populations.
    d. to promote healthy behaviors and protect health.

41. Your client has a family history of diabetes. The methods of managing this client's genetically transmitted disease include:
    a. case-finding and treating the manifestations of the illness.
    b. assessing the client's living conditions.
    c. ensuring the client has access to nursing and social services.
    d. encouraging a supportive environment.

42. When assessing community health, your nursing care plan may include which of the following broad social issues of community health?
    a. positive, supportive interpersonal family relationships, safety and security issues, affordable housing
    b. community design, joint action for minority and cultural health, social services, and public policy
    c. a safe environment, preventive health services, and consequences of lower-status occupations
    d. access to and appropriate use of health care services, affordable housing, and a safe environment

43. Immunization programs are an example of which level of preventive care?
    a. primary prevention
    b. secondary prevention
    c. tertiary prevention
    d. disease prevention

Health Maintenance: Lifestyle Management

PURPOSE

This chapter introduces you to world views of health, health care, and behavior change that affect one's decisions about lifestyle changes as part of a therapeutic regimen. It helps you to use the nursing process in working with clients seeking to make these lifestyle changes to enhance health and well-being.

LEARNING OBJECTIVES

After studying this chapter, you should be able to:

1. describe world views of health and health care and models of behavioral change that underlie decision making about lifestyle changes to manage a therapeutic regimen.
2. describe factors affecting behavioral change.
3. assess a client who is experiencing problems in maintaining health when a therapeutic regimen requires alterations in lifestyle.
4. write diagnoses for clients who need to manage a therapeutic regimen to maintain health.
5. plan nursing interventions that would assist a client to effectively manage the lifestyle changes needed to implement a therapeutic regimen.
6. evaluate the behavioral outcomes of lifestyle changes made to maintain health through a therapeutic regimen.

MATCHING

1. __d__ action stage
2. __f__ contemplation stage
3. __o__ counseling

4. __i__ emic dimension
5. __m__ etic dimension
6. __k__ lifestyle
7. __h__ maintenance stage
8. __w__ perceived barriers
9. __p__ perceived benefits
10. __e__ perceived severity
11. __a__ perceived susceptibility
12. __b__ precontemplation stage
13. __g__ preparation stage
14. __l__ referral
15. __g__ self-efficacy
16. __j__ social support
17. __n__ termination stage

a. a person's subjective perception of the risk of contracting a health condition

b. a behavioral stage in which the person does not intend to change a high risk behavior in the foreseeable future, primarily because of lack of awareness of the long-term consequences of the behavior

c. perceived negative aspects of a health action or the perceived impediments to undertaking the recommended behaviors

d. a behavioral stage in which the person changes risky behaviors and the context of the behavior (environment, experience) and makes significant efforts to reach goals

e. the perceived seriousness of contracting an illness or leaving it untreated

(Continued on p. 102)

f.   a behavioral stage in which the person intends to change within the next six months.

g.   the conviction that one can successfully execute the behavior required to produce the outcomes

h.   a behavioral stage that takes place during the six months after the person changes the high-risk behavior

i.   refers to an individual's or social group's subjective perceptions and experiences related to health

j.   the client's social network that may be of assistance to the client

k.   a behavior or group of behaviors, chosen by the person, which may have a positive or a negative influence on health

l.   a process designed to provide the client with access to health care and supportive services that are not available form the sending institution

m.   refers to the objective interpretation of health by a scientifically trained practitioner

n.   a behavioral stage in which the person is no longer tempted to engage in an old behavior

o.   a method of communication that actively involves the client in the recognition of personal risk factors and management of necessary behavior changes

p.   the person's perceptions and beliefs about the effectiveness of the recommended actions in preventing the health threat

q.   a behavioral stage in which the person intends to take action in the very near future, usually within the next month

TRUE OR FALSE

18. ___T___ To effectively help others, health care professionals must first understand the impact of their own beliefs about health on the health practices of their clients.

19. ___T___ According to the health belief model, clients will take action to control ill health if the anticipated barriers to taking the action are outweighed by the benefits.

20. ___F___ Impaired verbal skills or language differences do not interfere with the ability of a client to effectively express health needs to health care professionals.

21. ___T___ Clients with health insurance are more likely to seek health care at the onset of symptoms than those who do not have insurance.

22. ___F___ A client's spiritual values and beliefs always coincide with recommended interventions to promote, maintain, or restore health.

23. ___T___ The nursing diagnosis Noncompliance is used when a client has adequate knowledge and ability to improve health but makes an informed decision not to adhere to the treatment plan.

24. ___T___ Counseling is different from education in that counseling involves guiding the client through decision making rather than merely providing the information needed to make a decision.

25. ___T___ A nurse should anticipate problems in managing the therapeutic regimen if the client has poor eyesight, decreased mobility, or reduced manual dexterity.

26. ___F___ The nurse is solely responsible for the discharge planning process.

27. ___T___ If no noticeable change occurs in unhealthy behaviors within a reasonable time, the client should be reassessed to determine what prevented progress.

FILL-IN-THE-BLANKS

28. The theory of __reasoned__ __action__ is a human behavior framework designed to explain a person's intention to perform a behavior.

29. Health practices and behaviors that have potential negative effects on health are known as __risk factors__.

30. A health-risk appraisal provides clients with essential information about threats to health to which they may be __vulnerable__.

31. The client with a nursing diagnosis of Health-seeking behaviors does not necessarily have a __medical__ diagnosis.

32. A nurse who provides specific information to a client about a health problem in order to motivate health behavior is striving to increase the client's __knowledge__ level.

33. __values clarification__ is a self-discovery process that may be helpful in assisting a client to make health-related choices when faced with one or more alternatives.

34. Building rewards into effective management of the health care regimen is a method of providing __reinforcing__ or __motivating__ factors.

35. A client who is in __denial__ is not likely to see the need for or benefit of health care services that are provided through referral.

36. __Discharge__ planning begins at the time of admission, but should be finalized with a specific plan before the client leaves an institution.

37. The assistance of family and friends in facilitating health-related behavioral change is considered to be a type of __social__ support.

EXERCISING YOUR CLINICAL JUDGMENT

Mr. Kitchener, the African-American man identified in the chapter case study, has a nursing diagnosis of *Ineffective management of therapeutic regimen*. His identified health problem is heart failure and he was prescribed digoxin (a cardiac glycoside), Hygroton (a thiazide diuretic), and Lasix (a loop diuretic) at his first clinic visit. Mr. Kitchener did not return to the clinic when he was scheduled for a follow-up appointment, but came today after experiencing a return of shortness of breath. He had stopped taking his medication because he felt better, and also because he disliked having to go to the bathroom so frequently because of medication therapy. Recall that he is a widower with no family nearby, and he does not carefully plan meals or attend to his health. He also is a smoker who is not motivated as yet to stop smoking. You have been asked by the clinic nurse to provide teaching to Mr. Kitchener to enhance his ability to manage his health problems at home.

38. If Mr. Kitchener does not yet perceive that there are health benefits from smoking cessation, you would determine that he is in which of the following stages in the transtheoretical model of behavior change?
    a. precontemplation
    b. contemplation
    c. preparation
    d. action

39. Which of the following factors is most likely to be responsible for Mr. Kitchener's lack of adherence to the medical regimen?
    a. complexity of the therapeutic regimen
    b. side effects of therapy
    c. financial cost of the regimen
    d. complexity of the health care delivery system

40. The most effective strategy to use when providing information to Mr. Kitchener about his health problem would be to:
    a. explain that he will have a steady downhill course if he does not adhere to the treatment plan.
    b. share with him the results of research studies that show the cost of treating other noncompliant clients who have similar health problems.
    c. increase his awareness that unhealthy lifestyle habits are related to the development of his symptoms.
    d. encourage him to hire a companion to cook his meals and make sure he takes his medication.

41. You realize that Mr. Kitchener needs supportive care in order to achieve and maintain lifestyle changes. Given this client's particular situation, you would select which of the following as the most important intervention for this client?
    a. Make referrals to all available services that are provided within the clinic setting.
    b. Contact other outside agencies to give follow-up care.
    c. Ask him to renew his relationships with family that lives out of town.
    d. Establish a trusting therapeutic relationship with him.

TEST YOURSELF

42. To improve overall health, the nurse would place highest priority on assisting the client to make lifestyle changes for which of the following habits ?
    a. drinking a six-pack of beer each day
    b. eating an occasional chocolate bar
    c. exercising twice a week
    d. using relaxation exercises to deal with stress

43. A nurse who is assessing the health-related physical fitness of a client as part of a health assessment would focus on which of the following aspects of the assessment?
    a. agility
    b. speed
    c. body composition
    d. power

44. A nurse would interpret that which of the following clients is most likely to have a reduced ability to acquire knowledge about a newly prescribed diet and medication regimen due to cognitive perceptual impairment?
    a. one who has a slight decrease in hearing acuity
    b. one who has chronic confusion
    c. one who wears corrective lenses
    d. one who is 48 years old

45. A client with a newly diagnosed health problem has the choice of using either of two acceptable treatments for the problem. If the client has difficulty choosing between the two, the nurse would consider which of the following nursing diagnoses as most appropriate?
    a. Health-seeking behaviors
    b. Knowledge deficit
    c. Altered health maintenance
    d. Decisional conflict

46. A nurse is trying to motivate a client toward more effective management of a therapeutic regimen. Which of the following actions by the nurse is most likely to be effective in increasing the client's motivation?
    a. Determine whether the client has any family or friends living nearby.
    b. Develop a lengthy discharge plan and review it carefully with the client.
    c. Teach the client about the disorder at the client's level of understanding.
    d. Make a referral to an area agency for client follow-up.

Health Maintenance: Medication Management

PURPOSE

This chapter describes concepts of medication management and a wide variety of factors that can influence the effectiveness of medication therapy. It provides specific guidelines and nursing process information about how to effectively deliver medication therapy to clients.

LEARNING OBJECTIVES

After studying this chapter, you should be able to:

1. discuss important concepts related to safe and effective medication management.
2. describe a variety of factors that influence drug actions in individual clients.
3. explain how to assess a client who is receiving medication therapy.
4. formulate appropriate nursing diagnosis statements for a client receiving medications.
5. plan appropriate expected outcomes for a client taking medications.
6. incorporate safe and effective nursing interventions for a client receiving medications.
7. evaluate the effectiveness of medication therapy on goals formulated to improve a client's health.

MATCHING

1. _d_ adverse effect
2. _l_ anaphylaxis
3. _p_ antagonistic effect
4. _y_ biotransformation
5. _a_ chemical name
6. _o_ controlled substance
7. _i_ generic name
8. _b_ hypersensitivity reaction
9. _k_ idiosyncratic response
10. _u_ intradermal route
11. _m_ intramuscular route
12. _e_ intravenous route
13. _g_ loading dose
14. _t_ official name
15. _x_ parenteral route
16. _g_ pharmacokinetics

a. precisely describes the chemical and molecular structure of a medication; is of special interest to pharmacists

b. a mild allergic reaction to a drug

c. involves injection into the subcutaneous tissue just under the dermis

d. a medication side effect that is potentially harmful to a client

e. involves injection of a medication into a vein

f. the likelihood that a medication will harm a developing fetus

g. refers to a drug's activity from the time it enters the body until it leaves

h. a serious adverse effect of a medication that may even threaten life

(Continued on p. 106)

17. __V__ prescription

18. __n__ side effect

19. __c__ subcutaneous route

20. __i__ synergistic effect

21. __j__ target organ

22. __k__ teratogenic potential

23. __r__ therapeutic effect

24. __s__ topical route

25. __h__ toxic effect

26. __w__ trade name

i. an effect that occurs when one drug enhances or increases the effect of another drug

j. a body tissue or organ that is specifically affected by a drug

k. an unexplained and unpredictable response to a medication

l. the name assigned to a drug when it is first manufactured; also known as the nonproprietary name

m. involves injection into muscle tissue, specifically the body of a muscle

n. an effect of a medication that is not intended or planned but may occur as a result of use

o. drug that affects the mind or behavior, may be habit forming, and has a high potential for abuse

p. an effect that occurs when one drug reduces or negates the effect of another

q. an initial medication dose that exceeds the maintenance or therapeutic dose

r. the intended effect or action of a medication

s. used to deliver medication directly into a body site, such as skin, eyes, or ears

t. the name assigned by the FDA after it approves a drug; often the same name as the generic name

u. involves injection into the dermis

v. an order for a medication that contains the client's name, medication name, dose, route, frequency, amount of medication to be dispensed, and the number of refills allowed

w. a copyrighted name given by a specific manufacturer to a medication; also known as the brand name or proprietary name

x. a drug route that is outside the GI tract

y. the process of inactivating and breaking down a medication

z. a life-threatening allergic reaction to a drug that requires immediate intervention to prevent possible death

TRUE OR FALSE

27. __T__ In some states, revised Nurse Practice Acts have allowed selected groups of advanced practice nurses to write prescriptions.

28. __T__ The blood-brain barrier permits transport of lipid-bound medications while preventing transport of many water-soluble drugs.

29. __F__ No drug reaches the liver until it has passed through all body tissues.

30. __T__ The peak serum concentration of a medication usually occurs just as the last bit of the most recently administered dose is being absorbed.

31. __F__ There is a national standard recognized throughout all states that regulates how and when telephone and verbal medication orders should be given.

32. __T__ The most common medication system in use today is the unit-dose system.

33. __T__ A client's overall nutritional status can either positively or negatively affect medication actions in the body.

34. __F__ Dehydration has no effect on drug transport because the dosage is unchanged.

35. __T__ A client who subscribes to Western beliefs about health and illness typically expects to receive medication as part of the treatment plan.

FILL-IN-THE-BLANKS

36. In the U.S., the _Drug Enforcement_ Agency is empowered to enforce narcotic laws.

37. _Drug tolerance_ refers to the diminishing therapeutic effect of the same dosage of a drug over time, requiring increased dosing to achieve the same therapeutic effect.

38. _Enteric - Coated_ drugs are coated to prevent them from dissolving until they reach the alkaline environment of the small intestine.

39. A drug that should be avoided during pregnancy because the risks outweigh any benefits is labeled as belonging to FDA Pregnancy Risk Category _X_.

40. Drug dosages for infants and children are calculated according to either body surface area or _body weight_.

41. Nursing diagnoses that could apply due to the gastrointestinal side effects of medications include _Constipation_ and _Diarrhea_.

42. A client who develops signs such as oral lesions, diarrhea, or vaginal itching while taking antibiotic therapy could be developing _Superinfection_.

43. A medication should be administered within _30_ minutes before or after its scheduled time.

EXERCISING YOUR CLINICAL JUDGMENT

Mr. Connell, the 62-year-old Irish-American introduced in the chapter case study, has high blood pressure, but stopped taking prescribed medications because he "felt better." He has been treated in the local hospital emergency department for chest pain and is now diagnosed with angina pectoris. You must teach Mr. Connell about the medications that are being resumed.

44. Which of the following items would you include in a discussion with Mr. Connell about general principles of medication self-administration?
   a. If the prescription runs out, use that of a relative or friend until it can be refilled.
   b. Change brand names depending on cost to motivate compliance with therapy.
   c. Develop and use a reminder system if forgetting medications is a problem.
   d. Put all types of medications into a single large container to make storage easier.

45. You are teaching Mr. Connell strategies to prevent dizziness, a common side effect of anti-hypertensive medications. Which of the following would you recommend?
   a. Use alcohol at will since it adds to the anti-hypertensive effect.
   b. Sit or stand up slowly when getting out of a bed or chair.
   c. Go out for long walks in hot weather for additive medication effects.
   d. Take the medication upon arising in the morning if dizziness is a chronic problem.

46. Which of the following directions would you give Mr. Connell about taking the nitroglycerin since it is a sublingual medication?
   a. chew the tablet thoroughly
   b. swallow it whole
   c. place it between the cheek and the gum
   d. let it dissolve under the tongue

47. You would be careful to teach Mr. Connell about adverse medication effects knowing that he has an increased likelihood of experiencing these because of his:
   a. age.
   b. work history.
   c. medical diagnosis.
   d. cultural background.

TEST YOURSELF

48. A client is exhibiting a toxic effect from a medication. Which of the following actions by the nurse is most appropriate?
   a. withhold the dose and report the signs and symptoms to the prescriber
   b. administer half the dose for the next three days
   c. withhold the dose for twenty fours, then resume
   d. administer the next dose, but keep an antidote nearby

49. A client has an order for an intramuscular injection. The nurse selects an appropriate size syringe with a needle that is:
   a. 1/2–5/8 inch long.
   b. 5/8–1 inch long.
   c. 1–1 1/2 inches long.
   d. 1 1/2–2 inches long.

50. A client has a new order for a transdermal patch. Which of the following would the nurse teach the client about maintaining safety with this type of medication?
    a. apply the patch on a hairy site to prolong absorption
    b. use firm pressure, especially around the edges to ensure good skin contact
    c. if a patch falls off, leave it off until the next day
    d. trim the patch so it fits under clothing without being visible

51. A client is due for a dose of a scheduled eye drop. Which of the following would the nurse do to safely administer this medication?
    a. have the client lower the chin
    b. ask the client to look down at the floor
    c. tell the client to squint or squeeze the eye shut after administration
    d. pull downward on the bony orbit to expose the lower conjunctival sac.

52. A client has an order to take 5 ml of a medication at each dose. The home health nurse tells the client that this amount is equal to:
    a. 1/2 teaspoon.
    b. 1 teaspoon.
    c. 2 teaspoons.
    d. 1 tablespoon.

Health Protection: Risk for Infection

PURPOSE

This chapter introduces you to the important problem of infection and infection control as it relates to nursing practice. It uses the nursing process as a framework in describing how to assess, diagnose, plan, implement, and evaluate strategies used either to prevent or treat infection.

LEARNING OBJECTIVES

After studying this chapter, you should be able to:

1. discuss the course of an infection, physiological defenses against infection, and chain of infection as they relate to infection control.
2. describe the assessment of a client's risk for infection, actual infection, and responses to infection.
3. identify appropriate nursing diagnoses for a client with either an active infection or an increased risk for infection.
4. plan for goal-directed interventions to prevent or correct the infectious process.
5. identify specific interventions needed to prevent transmission of infection, manage a client with a compromised immune system, and reduce the personal risk of infection.
6. evaluate the outcomes that describe progress toward the goals of health protection nursing care.

MATCHING

1. _i_ antibiotic
2. _h_ antibody
3. _e_ antimicrobial
4. _a_ bacterium
5. _k_ differential cell count
6. _n_ gram stain
7. _f_ immunization
8. _g_ immunosup-pression
9. _b_ infection
10. _m_ inflammatory response
11. _o_ isolation
12. _d_ medical asepsis
13. _j_ nosocomial infection
14. _l_ pathogen
15. _g_ septicemia
16. _c_ standard precautions
17. _f_ virus

a. a small, single-celled organism that can reproduce outside of cells

b. a clinical syndrome caused by the invasion and multiplication of a pathogen

c. a set of actions, including hand-washing and the use of barriers, designed to reduce transmission of infectious organisms

d. consists of practices designed to reduce the numbers of pathogenic micro-organisms in the client's environment

e. having the ability to limit the spread of microorganisms

(Continued on p. 110)

f. a tiny microorganism, much smaller than a bacterium, that can only replicate inside the cell of a host such as a human

g. infection in the bloodstream

h. a circulating protein that recognizes and destroys foreign invaders or immunoglobulins

i. a drug that kills bacteria

j. an infection acquired from a reservoir in the hospital that may also be resistant to several antibiotics

k. breaks down the number of white blood cells into their types

l. a disease-producing microorganism

m. a localized reaction to injury that is activated when there is tissue damage

n. a specific microscopic test used to obtain rapid results on a culture sent to the laboratory

o. identification of a client who has an infection and implementation of precautions to prevent the spread of that infection

p. a medication administered to activate an immune response before exposure to the disease agent

q. suppression of the body's immune system

TRUE OR FALSE

18. __T__ The incubation period of an infection extends from the time of a client's first exposure to the organism to the appearance of the first symptoms.

19. __T__ Virulence is a measure of the aggressiveness of an organism in causing a disease.

20. __F__ Measles is an example of an infection that is carried by a vector. airborne

21. __T__ An individual's level of immunity is age-related.

22. __T__ People with dementia are at increased risk of infection due to impaired protective responses.

23. __F__ The presence of an increased number of immature neutrophils, which can indicate infection, is sometimes called a right shift. left

24. __T__ A gram stain tests the nature of bacterial cell walls by determining whether they take up a stain.

25. __F__ A person's state of anxiety has no effect on one's protection against infection.

26. __T__ Contact precautions involve use of standard precautions plus the use of barrier items such as gloves and gowns.

27. __T__ Minor cuts and bruises should be washed with mild soap and water and patted dry.

FILL-IN-THE-BLANKS

28. The period of ___Convalescence___ is the time following the height of the acute symptoms to the time the person experiences a return to normal health.

29. A place where an infectious agent can survive and, possibly, multiply until it can invade a susceptible host is called a ___reservoir___.

30. ___Opportunistic___ infections are those that result from organisms that do not ordinarily cause disease.

31. An ___environmental___ factor that contributes to increased risk of infection is overcrowded living conditions.

32. Redness, swelling, pain, and heat are signs that accompany a ___localized___ infection.

33. The sink and bathroom of a hospital room are generally considered to be ___dirty___ areas.

34. Gloves should never be used as a substitute for good ___handwashing___.

35. The ___steam___ sterilization method kills microorganisms that are sensitive to heat and moisture.

36. Enteric precautions are designed to prevent disease transmission through direct or indirect contact with ___feces___.

37. ___Droplet___ precautions refer to precautions used for organisms that can be spread through the air but are unable to remain in the air for distances greater than three feet.

EXERCISING YOUR CLINICAL JUDGMENT

Luisa Martinez, a 6-month old Mexican-American infant, is admitted with dehydration and possible sepsis following upper respiratory infection. Luisa lives with her two parents, two older siblings, and her uncle and his entire family. Her father speaks and understands English, but her mother does not. You are assigned to care for Luisa while she is hospitalized.

38. You would expect to note which of the following signs of systemic infection while caring for Luisa?
   a. malaise
   b. redness
   c. swelling
   d. pain

39. When considering what to teach Luisa's parents about reducing the risk of further infection, you would begin with which of the following health practices?
   a. food storage
   b. food preparation
   c. hand-washing
   d. bathing

40. If Luisa had been found to have a viral infection, such as influenza, as the basis for her symptoms, which of the following types of isolation would be important to implement in her care?
   a. airborne
   b. droplet
   c. contact
   d. strict

41. Luisa is started on antibiotic therapy to treat her infection. If she still had general malaise and fever after seven days of therapy, the nurse would evaluate that which of the following would be the most likely follow-up?
   a. increase her fluid intake
   b. change the antibiotic to an antiviral agent
   c. send her home since hospitalization didn't help
   d. reculture her throat and blood

TEST YOURSELF

42. A nurse who is reviewing the medical record of a client would expect that the client has some type of infection if the results of the white blood cell count differential showed:
   a. increased immature neutrophils.
   b. decreased monocytes.
   c. increased eosinophils.
   d. decreased basophils.

43. The nurse is performing hand-washing as part of medical asepsis. Which of the following nursing actions for rinsing the hands represents correct practice?
   a. hands lower than elbows, water washing down hands to fingertips
   b. hands lower than elbows, water washing from fingertips to wrists
   c. hands higher than elbows, water washing down hands to fingertips
   d. hands higher than elbows, water washing from fingertips to wrists

44. A client admitted with tuberculosis should be placed in isolation in which of the following rooms on the nursing unit?
   a. a two-bed room
   b. a four-bed room
   c. a private room with windows that open
   d. a private room with negative pressure

45. A home health nurse would provide client teaching about how to prevent infection in the home after noting which of the following?
   a. sink and bathroom are clean
   b. leftover cooked food is stored on countertop
   c. individuals wash hands before touching food
   d. individuals use tissues when sneezing

46. A nurse has an order to change a dressing using sterile technique. After opening a package of sterile gloves, the nurse would do which of the following first to put them on correctly?
   a. grasp the glove from the inside edge
   b. grasp the glove from the outside edge
   c. grasp the folded edge of the cuff
   d. grasp it anywhere desired

Health Protection: Risk for Injury

PURPOSE

This chapter introduces you to concepts of injury and internal and external factors that are associated with increased risk. It uses nursing process as a framework to help you identify nursing actions that can help prevent injury and those that can minimize risk of further injury.

LEARNING OBJECTIVES

After studying this chapter, you should be able to:

1. discuss the epidemiology of common injuries from falls, suffocation, and poisoning.
2. discuss the epidemiology of trauma from burns, electricity, motor vehicle accidents, and radiation.
3. identify the behavioral, environmental, socioeconomic, developmental, cognitive, and physiological factors that affect safety.
4. assess the client's risk of injury.
5. distinguish among related nursing diagnoses for the client at risk for injury.
6. Plan interventions to prevent injury and promote safety in the acute care setting, the client's home, and the community.
7. evaluate client outcomes and nursing interventions used to help the client reduce the risk of injury.

MATCHING

1. _f_ aspiration
2. _e_ burns
3. _a_ choking
4. _h_ injury
5. _i_ poisoning
6. _g_ restraint
7. _d_ strangulation
8. _b_ suffocation
9. _c_ trauma

a. an internal obstruction of the airway by food or a foreign body

b. a lack of oxygen caused either by airway obstruction or by oxygen starvation from insufficient atmospheric oxygen

c. a physical injury or wound caused by a forceful, disruptive, or violent action

d. constriction of the airway from an external cause

e. any injuries caused by excessive exposure to electricity, chemicals, gases, radioactivity, or thermal agents

f. the inspiration of foreign material into the airway

g. a device intended for medical purposes that limits movement to the extent necessary for treatment, examination, or protection of the client

h. trauma or damage to some part of the body

i. an adverse condition or physical state resulting from the administration of a toxic substance

TRUE OR FALSE

10. __T__ Injury can result from physical, mechanical, biological, or chemical agents.

11. __T__ The biggest concern when an older adult falls is the threat of a hip fracture.

12. __F__ Faulty electrical equipment is the leading cause of fatal residential fires.

13. __T__ A scalding type of burn injury is very distressing due to the considerable pain it causes, the need for prolonged treatment, and the possibility of permanent scarring.

14. __F__ A single, stressful lifting event is the cause of most back injuries.

15. __T__ A person's lifestyle can raise the risk of injury.

16. __T__ Potential hazards in the home are inadequate lighting, missing or broken steps or handrails, or the presence of throw rugs.

17. __T__ A person's cognitive and perceptual abilities are crucial to promoting safety.

18. __F__ All child car seats on the market are safe.

19. __T__ A client who engages in high-risk behaviors such as using drugs or alcohol while driving may require referral for a more in-depth assessment of methods needed to change the behavior.

FILL-IN-THE-BLANKS

20. Accidents that most commonly result in death include motor vehicle accidents and _falls_

21. Clients who are unconscious from drugs or alcohol, or who have a cerebrovascular accident or cardiac arrest are most at risk for _aspiration_

22. _Poisons_ can enter the body through ingestion, inhalation, injection, application, or absorption of the noxious material.

23. Motor vehicle accidents are the leading cause of _accidental_ deaths in the United States.

24. Potential _occupational_ hazards to safety may result from noise, dust, air pollution, working with dangerous machinery, or being exposed to toxic substances.

25. A frequently cited reason for ignoring safety is a lack of _money_.

26. Clients at the developmental levels of _infancy_ and _toddler_ are particularly vulnerable to accidents and injuries because of their limited awareness of potential dangers.

27. When planning care for a client with an increased risk for injury, the nurse should focus primarily on _prevention_

28. The nurse can help prevent electrical shocks by using equipment that is electrically _grounded_

29. The acronym RACE used in fire safety stands for _rescue_, _alarm/confine_, and _ext.inguish_

EXERCISING YOUR CLINICAL JUDGMENT

Juanita Soto, a 75-year-old widow with rheumatoid arthritis who lives alone, is being followed by a home health nurse due to declining mobility and partial loss of vision. She recently fell and required a brief hospitalization.

30. Which of the following factors in Mrs. Soto's physical environment places her at risk for further falls?
    a. intact stairs with treads
    b. throw rugs on tile floors
    c. night light in hallway
    d. grab bars in bathroom

31. The home health nurse would reinforce to Mrs. Soto that she should do which of the following to prevent becoming burned in the home setting?
    a. Leave electrical outlets uncovered for ease of use.
    b. Keep pot handles facing the back of the stove.
    c. Use an open-flame heater for added warmth in cold weather.
    d. Use extension cords to be able to maximize ability to use electric plugs.

32. The nurse assesses Mrs. Soto for physiological risk factors for falls. The nurse would conclude that she is at no further risk if which of the following were discovered?
    a. history of dizziness
    b. need for wheelchair due to reduced mobility
    c. weakness and fatigue noted when climbing stairs
    d. intact recent and remote memory

33. The nurse notes that Mrs. Soto has no fire extinguisher in the home. Which of the following types of fire extinguishers should be recommended?
    a. water pump extinguisher (type A)
    b. foam extinguisher (type B)
    c. multipurpose extinguisher (type A, B, C)
    d. dry powder extinguisher (type D)

TEST YOURSELF

34. The nurse working with older adults keeps in mind that falls are most likely to happen to older adults that are:
    a. in their 80s.
    b. living at home.
    c. hospitalized.
    d. living on only social security income.

35. The nurse working with a population of clients of all ages would interpret that which of the following clients has the least risk of poisoning?
    a. toddlers
    b. young children
    c. older adults with sensory impairment
    d. young adults

36. The home health nurse would recommend that a client keep a portable heater at least how many inches from anything that might be flammable?
    a. 12
    b. 18
    c. 36
    d. 60

37. A client has been diagnosed with radiation dermatitis. The nurse would assess for which of the following skin manifestations of this type of burn?
    a. blistering and skin sloughing
    b. diaphoresis
    c. poor capillary refill
    d. pale, cool skin

38. After calling the poison control center, an ambulatory care nurse prepares to induce vomiting in a client being seen with overdose. The nurse should select which of the following as the agent of choice?
    a. activated charcoal
    b. syrup of ipecac
    c. hypertonic saline
    d. any solution containing phosphate

29

Nutrition

PURPOSE

This chapter discusses key concepts that relate to normal nutrition. It provides an overview of how you will use the nursing process to assist clients in maintaining and/or improving nutritional health.

LEARNING OBJECTIVES

After studying this chapter, you should be able to:

1. describe the elements of a nutritious diet and how nutrients are used by the body.
2. distinguish among various guidelines for normal nutrition.
3. discuss the impact of factors affecting nutritional status, including lifestyle, culture, economics, developmental stage, pregnancy and lactation, and psychological and physiological state.
4. describe assessment of a client to determine optimal nutritional status.
5. identify nursing diagnoses applicable to the client with normal nutritional balance.
6. plan for goal-directed interventions to promote optimum nutrition and reduce nutritional risk factors.
7. describe specific interventions and strategies to promote optimum nutrition and reduce nutritional risk factors throughout the lifespan.
8. evaluate the outcomes of nutritional interventions.

MATCHING

1. _g_ fiber
2. _M_ metabolism
3. _e_ nutrient
4. _c_ glycogen
5. _o_ polysaccharide
6. _p_ starch
7. _a_ anthropometric measurements
8. _s_ nutritional status
9. _d_ basal metabolic rate
10. _b_ carbohydrates
11. _J_ recommended dietary allowance (RDA)
12. _K_ vitamins
13. _i_ amino acids
14. _l_ triglycerides
15. _n_ minerals
16. _s_ disaccharides
17. _h_ proteins
18. _t_ calorie
19. _f_ nutrition
20. _g_ monosaccharides

a. measurements of physical characteristics of the body (such as height and weight), as well as the amount of muscle tissue or fat tissue in the body

b. simple or complex compounds composed of carbon, oxygen, and hydrogen

c. the form in which carbohydrates are stored in humans and in meat

d. the minimal energy expended for the maintenance of respiration, circulation, peristalsis, muscle tonus, body temperature, glandular activity, and the other vegetative functions of the body

e. a biochemical substance utilized by the body for growth, maintenance, and repair

(Continued on p. 118)

f. the condition of the body resulting from the use of essential nutrients available to it

g. sub-units of carbo-hydrates that are six-carbon sugars (glucose, fructose, and galactose are examples)

h. compounds con-taining polymers of amino acids, linked together in a chain to form polypeptide bonds.

i. compounds com-posed of carbon, hydrogen, oxygen, and an amino group that are classified as essential or nones-sential, depending on whether the body can manufac-ture them from other sources

j. the level of a nutrient that is adequate to meet the needs of almost all healthy people, as determined by the Food and Nutrition Board of the National Research Council

k. organic substances found in food which serve as coenzymes in enzymatic reactions

l. composed of three fatty acids and a glycol unit; the chief form of fat in the diet and the main form of fat trans-port in the blood

m. the process by which energy from nutrients can be used by the cells or stored for later use

n. inorganic elements that are present in small amounts in virtually all body fluids and tissues

o. a group of monosaccharides joined together in a chain; they can be converted back to monosaccharides through a process called acid hydroly-sis

p. the form in which plants store glucose

q. the structure of which plants are composed; includes cellulose, hemicel-lulose, pectins, gums, and muci-lages

r. the science of food and nutrients, and the processes by which an organism takes them in and uses them for energy to grow, maintain function, and renew itself

s. molecules that form when two monosaccharides condense and join together to form a double sugar

t. a measure of the energy content of food

TRUE OR FALSE

21. __T__ A woman who is pregnant has an increased need for iron, calcium, and other vitamins.

22. __F__ Most enzymatic digestion and virtually all absorption occur in the large intestine. *Small intestine*

23. __T__ The chemical energy from food is converted by the body to electrical, thermal, or mechanical energy, depending on the needs of the body.

24. __F__ A diet high in fiber contains foods such as cereals, meats, and poultry. *raw fruit, veg*

25. __F__ When the body is storing protein, negative nitrogen balance and catabolism occur. *positive   anabolism*

26. __T__ When taking medications, it is important to note whether there are foods that can cause drug-nutrient reactions.

27. __T__ During pregnancy, the need for both calorie and fluid intake increases.

28. __F__ Taking in the RDA of a nutrient will meet the body's needs for that nutrient regard-less of whether the client is well or ill.

29. __T__ Body composition can be determined by measuring the triceps fat fold and midarm muscle circumference.

30. __T__ Eating a diet high in calories and fat or eating late at night are likely characteristics of a client with the nursing diagnosis Altered nutrition: more than body require-ments.

FILL-IN-THE-BLANKS

31. ___Digestion___ is the process by which the body changes food into elemental nutrients that can be absorbed.

32. Cellulose, pectins, gums, and mucilages are examples of ___fibers___.

33. As energy sources, both protein and carbohy-drates provide __4__ calories per gram.

34. ___Vitamins___ are organic substances found in food that serve as coen-zymes in enzymatic reactions.

35. Zinc, iron, copper, and selenium are examples of ___minerals___.

36. Analysis of the type and amount of food eaten by a client is done by taking a ___food hx___.

37. Teaching clients about the type and number of food servings to eat each day can be done using the _Food_ _guide_ _pyramid_

38. Albumin and prealbumin levels are indicators of _protein_ intake.

39. As a health promotion measure, nurses should teach clients to read the _Nutritional fact_ _Food_ _label_ that must appear on all manufactured food products.

40. The second level of the Food Guide Pyramid includes _fruits_ and _vegetables_.

EXERCISING YOUR CLINICAL JUDGMENT

Mr. Crane is a 76-year-old man living alone in his own home. He has a son and daughter-in-law who live in the area. During a routine health visit, he tells the nurse in the physician's office that he has not been very interested in food following the death of his wife (who did most of the cooking) two months ago. The nurse notes that Mr. Crane has lost 7 pounds since his last visit three months ago, and has a current weight of 149 pounds (at the low end of the normal range for a man of his size). He can drive to the grocery store, but has limited income to spend on food. He has dentures that seem to fit well, but has a history of arthritis in the hands and knees.

41. The nurse would determine that which of the following factors is a positive one, which does not negatively influence Mr. Crane's nutritional status?
    a. difficulty in using the hands
    b. financial concerns
    c. ability to chew and swallow
    d. decreased appetite secondary to grief

42. The nurse interprets that Mr. Crane's arthritis of the hands would be which of the following types of barriers to adequate nutrition?
    a. psychological
    b. physical
    c. cultural
    d. financial

43. If Mr. Crane indicates an interest in obtaining help with shopping and/or food preparation, the nurse should first investigate which of the following resources?
    a. ability of the son and daughter-in-law to help
    b. private housekeeper
    c. Meals-on-Wheels delivery service
    d. ability to use a microwave oven

44. In providing teaching to Mr. Crane about the elements of a healthy diet, the nurse would find which of the following to be the most helpful resource to use during the information session?
    a. Recommended Dietary Allowances chart
    b. nutrition book
    c. textbook on aging
    d. Food Guide Pyramid chart

TEST YOURSELF

45. A nurse who is teaching clients about lowering risk of hypertension (high blood pressure) would emphasize limiting which of the following types of substances in the daily diet?
    a. salt
    b. sugar
    c. fiber
    d. seeds and nuts

46. While fats should be used sparingly in the diet, the nurse would encourage the use of which of the following types of fats when fat is needed during food preparation?
    a. monounsaturated
    b. polyunsaturated
    c. hydrogenated
    d. saturated

47. A prepubescent child has an increased need for calcium in the diet. The school nurse would teach children of this age group to increase intake of which of the following types of foods to obtain this nutrient?
    a. meats
    b. fish
    c. raw fruits
    d. dairy products

48. The nurse would encourage a client who is pregnant to take which of the following dietary supplements that cannot be met sufficiently with proper daily diet?
    a. vitamin C and the B vitamins
    b. vitamins A and D
    c. ferrous iron and folacin
    d. iron and magnesium

49. The nurse teaching clients about intake of high-fiber foods to protect against colorectal cancer would encourage the use of which of the following types of foods in the meal plan?
    a. cooked fruits
    b. cruciferous vegetables
    c. lean meats
    d. products made with refined flour

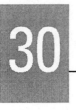
Nutritional Deficiency

PURPOSE

This chapter introduces you to nutritional deficits such as malnutrition and starvation, and the factors that aid in their development. It guides you in the use of the nursing process to facilitate optimum nutrition for clients with a nutritional deficit.

LEARNING OBJECTIVES

After studying this chapter, you should be able to:

1. describe the physiology of malnutrition and starvation.
2. discuss factors affecting nutritional deficits.
3. assess clients experiencing severe nutritional deficits.
4. formulate nursing diagnoses for nutritional deficits.
5. plan for goal-directed interventions for clients with nutritional deficits.
6. employ a variety of interventions to facilitate optimal nutrition for clients.
7. evaluate the achievement of measurable outcomes for clients with nutritional deficits.

MATCHING

1. _d_ anorexia
2. _e_ catabolism
3. _a_ deglutition
4. _f_ dysphagia
5. _g_ enteral nutrition
6. _b_ malnutrition
7. _c_ parenteral nutrition

a. the reflex passage of food, fluids, or both from the mouth to the stomach

b. any disorder of nutrition caused by unbalanced, insufficient, or excessive diet or from impaired absorption or metabolism of nutrients

c. the provision of total nutrition through a central or peripheral intravenous catheter

d. loss of appetite

e. the breakdown of muscle and lean body mass when nutrient intake fails to meet energy expenditure

f. difficulty in swallowing

g. any form of nutrition delivered to the gastrointestinal tract, although commonly used to refer to tube feedings

TRUE OR FALSE

8. __T__ Nutritional deprivation can occur with problems that raise energy needs, such as infection, trauma, stress, or surgery.

9. __F__ If a client has been starving for a period of time, the urine will be negative for ketones and nitrogen balance will be positive. *Ketones + nit. bal neg*

10. __T__ Kwashiorkor is a condition of starvation caused by decreased protein intake, and usually occurs in young children after weaning.

11. __F__ Marasmus is a condition of starvation that results from deficient caloric intake over a very short period of time. *long period of X*

12. __T__ Bleeding tendencies can be associated with a deficiency of vitamin K.

13. __T__ Approximately half of clients aged 65 and older wear dentures, which can affect nutritional intake.

14. __T__ Changes in appetite include anorexia, early satiety, lack of interest in food, and loss of taste.

15. __F__ A weight gain program is generally considered successful if the client gains at least 5 pounds per month. *2 lbs a month*

16. __T__ Food intake can be enhanced by serving meals in an attractive manner and making the environment as pleasant as possible.

17. __F__ A client who is diabetic should be allowed small amounts of concentrated sweets.

FILL-IN-THE-BLANKS

18. Involuntary control of swallowing is coordinated in the lower pons and the __medulla__ of the brain.

19. Pernicious anemia results from a deficiency of vitamin __B12__.

20. Anemia is most commonly associated with reduced intake of __iron__.

21. Premature infants may require tube feedings because the suck-swallow reflex does not develop until __34__ weeks of gestation.

22. Serum studies are often ordered to evaluate a client who has unintentionally lost __10__% of his or her weight during the last 6 months.

23. The first phase of swallowing that is evaluated when the client has impaired swallowing is the __pharyngeal__ phase.

24. A one-liter bag of 5% Dextrose in Water IV solution contains only __170__ kilocalories.

25. Ginger ale, apple juice, and gelatin are considered to be part of a __clear__ liquid diet.

26. A __2__-gram sodium diet is common for clients with hypertension.

27. If a client has severe kidney disease, such as renal failure, protein is generally __limited__ in the diet.

EXERCISING YOUR CLINICAL JUDGMENT

Mrs. Goldman, the 54-year-old Russian woman introduced in the chapter case study, is receiving chemotherapy following surgery for breast cancer. She has a nursing diagnosis of *Altered nutrition: less than body requirements related to adverse effects of chemotherapy.* Specifically, she has early satiety and anorexia and says that food does not have much taste. You are working with Mrs. Goldman in the clinic setting to increase her nutritional intake with a Kosher diet, especially during the three remaining months of chemotherapy.

28. To increase Mrs. Goldman's sense of taste, you would recommend that she take supplemental doses of which of the following minerals?
    a. magnesium
    b. calcium
    c. zinc
    d. iodine

29. You would encourage Mrs. Goldman to increase intake at which of the following times, when intake is usually best?
    a. breakfast
    b. lunch
    c. dinner
    d. bedtime

30. To reduce the discomfort of mouth sores (xerostomia) that can accompany chemotherapy, you would advise Mrs. Goldman to avoid foods that are:
    a. low in fat.
    b. spicy or acidic.
    c. high in carbohydrates.
    d. high in liquid content.

31. To determine whether Mrs. Goldman has effectively increased the amount of iron in her diet, you would review the results of which of the following laboratory studies drawn at the next clinic visit?
    a. blood urea nitrogen (BUN)
    b. total protein
    c. albumin
    d. hemoglobin

TEST YOURSELF

32. The nurse giving enteral nutrition and medications through a feeding tube uses which of the following methods to prevent the tube from becoming occluded?
    a. adequate flushing with water
    b. instillation of meat tenderizer
    c. flushing with cola
    d. flushing with cranberry juice

33. The nurse measures and documents gastric residual for a client receiving enteral nutrition every:
    a. hour.
    b. two hours.
    c. four hours.
    d. day.

34. A client is receiving parenteral nutrition via a central venous catheter. The nurse monitors this client for fluid overload from hyperosmolar fluids most effectively by:
    a. monitoring temperature.
    b. listening to lung sounds.
    c. checking results of serum osmolarity.
    d. watching the color of the urine.

35. The nurse would interpret that a client has had a mild reaction to lipid emulsion infusion if the client experiences which of the following?
    a. fever and chills
    b. vomiting
    c. pain in the back or chest
    d. itchy skin rash

36. The nurse would best promote effective swallowing in a client at risk for aspiration by having the client sit:
    a. on the right side with the head elevated to 45 degrees.
    b. upright with the neck flexed at 45 degrees.
    c. supine and on the left side.
    d. in a comfortable chair that promotes relaxation.

Fluid and Electrolyte Balance

PURPOSE

The purpose of this chapter is to introduce the concepts of fluid balance and its relationship to electrolytes in the body. You will learn introductory skills in providing intravenous therapy under a physician's directive.

LEARNING OBJECTIVES

After studying this chapter, you should be able to:

1. describe the normal physiology of fluid balance, including fluid compartments, functions of body fluids, and types of electrolytes.
2. identify 10 mechanisms that contribute to the regulation of fluid and electrolyte balance.
3. discuss five common problems related to fluid balance.
4. discuss the factors affecting fluid balance, including physiological problems and medical and nursing therapies.
5. describe the general assessment of a client's fluid balance.
6. describe the focused assessment of clients at risk for fluid problems, the manifestations of actual fluid problems, and client responses to fluid problems.
7. diagnose the problems of clients with fluid imbalances that are within the domain of nursing.
8. plan and carry out goal-directed interventions to prevent or correct fluid and electrolyte imbalances.
9. evaluate outcomes in terms of progress or lack of progress toward the goals of fluid balance with revision of the care plan as appropriate.

MATCHING

1. _Z_ anion
2. _f_ cation
3. _a_ absorption
4. _g_ filtration
5. _d_ fluid shifting
6. _h_ electrolyte
7. _C_ colloid
8. _e_ colloid osmotic (oncotic) pressure
9. _g_ hypotonic
10. _t_ hypertonic
11. _O_ insensible fluid loss
12. _n_ homeostasis
13. _s_ isotonic
14. _r_ milliequivalent
15. _I_ hydrostatic pressure
16. _✓_ secretion
17. _i_ osmolarity
18. _M_ osmolality
19. _K_ nonelectrolyte
20. _P_ milliosmole

a. the passage of liquids or other substances from one tissue into another (e.g., medication movement from the buccal cavity, dermal, subcutaneous, or muscle tissue into the blood stream; movement of end products of digestion from different parts of the GI system into the blood)

b. minimum amount of any substance that is needed in resting state to provide desired function of that substance

c. macromolecules that are too large to pass though a cell membrane and do not readily dissolve into a solution (e.g., protein)

d. movement of fluid from one compartment to another

(Continued on p. 126)

21. __Y__ plasma

22. __l__ third spacing

23. __U__ serum

24. __W__ sensible fluid loss

25. __X__ reabsorption

26. __b·__ basal requirement

e. osmotic pressure exerted by the protein molecules

f. positively charged ion (e.g., sodium, potassium, calcium, magnesium, hydrogen)

g. the passage of water and certain smaller particles through a semipermeable membrane, assisted by hydrostatic or capillary pressure

h. substance that, when placed in a solvent such as water, breaks up into positively charged particles called ions; will conduct electricity

i. the number of milliosmoles per liter of solution

j. pressure exerted by the fluid within a compartment that results from the weight of the fluid; for practical purposes it can be thought of as the portion of the pressure exerted by the fluid itself

k. substance that does not ionize, thus does not carry an electrical charge (e.g., glucose)

l. the movement of fluid into an area in which the fluid is physiologically unavailable to the body (e.g., peritoneal space—ascites; pericardial space—pericardial effusion; pleural space—pleural effusion; vesicles—burn)

m. the number of milliosmoles per kilogram of water

n. the maintenance of constant or static conditions within the body; a relatively constant balance in the internal environment maintained through adaptive mechanisms that interact within and in response to changes within the internal and external environment

o. the fluid that is lost that is not perceptible to the senses (e.g., the fluid lost through breathing and the skin in the absence of hyperventilation and diaphoresis)

p. the unit of force from the dissolved particles in a solution

q. having an osmotic pressure less than that of the solution with which it is being compared

r. one thousandth of a chemical equivalent; the measurement used to express the chemical activity or combining power of an ion

s. having an osmotic pressure equal to that of the solution with which it is being compared

t. having an osmotic pressure greater than that of the solution with which it is being compared

u. plasma in which fibrinogen has been separated by the process of clotting

v. to expel substances from cellular processes into the blood or into other compartments within the body (e.g., secretion of excess products such as hydrogen into distal and collecting renal tubule for excretion as waste products; secretion of hormones from endocrine glands into blood stream)

w. fluid loss that can be perceived by the senses (e.g., fluid lost with diaphoresis or hyperventilation)

x. the process of absorbing again (e.g., the absorption of glucose, proteins, and electrolytes from the renal tubules back into the blood)

y. the fluid portion of the blood

z. negatively charged ion (e.g., chloride, bicarbonate, phosphate, sulfate, proteinate)

TRUE OR FALSE

27. __T__ Clients with hyponatremia should be observed for low urinary output.

28. __T__ Clients with hypernatremia should be observed for fluid retention.

29. __T__ The most characteristic manifestations of hypokalemia are muscle flaccidity and EKG changes.

30. __F__ Hyperkalemia occurs in the presence of high volume urinary output.

31. ____ The client with hypocalcemia should be observed for seizures.

32. __T__ Hypercalcemia is associated with kidney stones.

33. __F__ Insensible water loss should be measured as part of intake and output.

34. __T__ Cardiac failure is associated with retention of potassium and water.

35. __T__ Tube feedings are hypertonic, thus the client may be at risk for fluid volume deficit unless water is given as a supplement.

36. __F__ 5% Dextrose in water is given primarily for its glucose content. given for fluid replacement

37. __F__ 5% Dextrose in 1/2 normal saline (a 25% solution) given at 3000 cc per day does not add sodium to the body. has sodium in it

38. __T__ Hyponatremia can result from administration of excess D_5W.

39. __T__ Plasma is used as a volume expander when a client is bleeding and there is not time to type and cross match blood.

40. __T__ Caution should be used with IV therapy to prevent air from entering a client's veins.

FILL-IN-THE-BLANKS

41. Glucocorticoids cause __retention__ (retention, excretion) of fluid.

42. To pass a nasogastric tube you should use a __water soluble__ lubricant.

43. Nasogastric suction is used for gastrointestinal __decompression__ in the presence of a bowel __obstruction__.

44. In a burn client fluid is lost by __third spacing__.

45. To pass a nasogastric tube, the client should be in the __high Fowlers__ position.

46. __Normal saline__ is the only acceptable irrigant for a nasogastric tube.

47. When selecting an IV site you should start with the most __distal__ (distal, proximal) vein that would support an intravenous catheter.

48. An __18__-gauge needle is used for a venipuncture if you have reason to believe the client may need blood.

49. To clean a site for venipuncture, start __at the site__ and clean in a circular motion __away from__ (toward, away from) the site.

50. When you make a venipuncture, you confirm that you are in the vein by observing __blood return__.

EXERCISING YOUR CLINICAL JUDGMENT

51. Six hours postsurgery your patient has signs of fluid volume deficit. The doctor orders a fluid challenge of 200 cc Lactated Ringers intravenously over 20 minutes STAT. You should assess for a positive response to this treatment by observing for:
    a. decrease in blood pressure.
    b. rales in lower lung bases.
    c. increase in specific gravity.
    d. increase in renal output.

52. Select the most appropriate nursing action for the patient with fluid volume excess.
    a. Assess breath sounds.
    b. Assess the diet for potassium content.
    c. Encourage increased fluid intake.
    d. Discourage use of salt substitutes.

53. Prior to administering a potassium supplement it is most important that the nurse assess:
    a. hepatic function.
    b. cerebral function.
    c. renal function.
    d. vascular function.

54. You determine that your client has been taking his diuretic when he thinks he needs it at home. A typical side effect of excess furosemide (Lasix) is signs and symptoms of:
    a. nephrosis.
    b. metabolic acidosis.
    c. hypokalemia.
    d. hypernatremia.

55. An 88-year-old man is admitted with an extracellular fluid volume excess. On admission, he is frightened and dyspneic. On assessment, the nurse would expect to identify:
    a. a weak thready pulse.
    b. sluggish skin turgor.
    c. neck vein distension.
    d. postural hypotension.

56. The nursing care plan for hypovolemia should include:
    a. increasing fluid intake to 2000cc/day.
    b. placing client in the supine position.
    c. increasing protein in the client's diet.
    d. auscultating for adventitious breath sounds.

TEST YOURSELF

57. Calcium and phosphate levels are primarily regulated by:
    a. kidneys.
    b. adrenal glands.
    c. parathyroid glands.
    d. pituitary glands.

58. The most accurate means of determining the amount of fluid retention in an individual is by:
    a. measuring edema with a mm tape.
    b. accurately measuring the client's intake.
    c. determining the amount of neck vein distention.
    d. classifying edema as 1+, 2+, 3+, or 4+.

59. The normal effects of Aldosterone include which of the following?
    a. sodium retention and water retention
    b. H_2O excretion and calcium retention
    c. chloride excretion and sodium retention
    d. magnesium retention and potassium excretion

60. The primary force at the arterial end of the capillary that moves fluid into the interstitial space is the:
    a. plasma colloid osmotic pressure.
    b. interstitial hydrostatic pressure.
    c. plasma hydrostatic pressure.
    d. interstitial colloid osmotic pressure.

61. Which one of the following vitamins plays the most important role in calcium absorption in the presence of hypocalcemia?
    a. vitamin A
    b. vitamin D
    c. vitamin B
    d. vitamin E

62. A 45-year-old client has just returned to your unit after major abdominal surgery. Based on the impact of antidiuretic hormone (ADH) released during the stress of surgery, select the most likely client response.
    a. increased urinary output for the first 24 hours
    b. decreased urinary output for the first 24 hours
    c. no change in output from the previous 24 hours
    d. intake equal to output for the first 24-hour period

63. Signs and symptoms of circulatory overload are:
    a. cold, clammy skin; decreased BP; SOB; hacking cough
    b. rales, moist cough, neck vein distention, increased BP
    c. decreased venous pressure, cyanosis, SOB, orthopnea
    d. decreased BP; pitting edema; cold, dry skin

64. While reviewing your patient's lab test you note a seriously low serum calcium. A nursing intervention to incorporate into your care would be:
    a. forcing fluid to 12 glasses per day.
    b. providing a quiet nonstimulating environment.
    c. monitoring intake and output.
    d. encouraging bananas and orange juice in diet.

65. Your client is to receive an intravenous infusion of 1000 D_5W over 10 hours. Your drip chamber delivers 1 cc per 15 gtts. How many drops per minute would you run the IV infusion?
    a. 33
    b. 25
    c. 20
    d. 16

32

Skin Integrity and Wound Healing

PURPOSE

This chapter discusses key concepts that relate to the nursing diagnoses Risk for impaired skin integrity, Impaired skin integrity, and Impaired tissue integrity. It describes the skin disruptions, wound health, and problems of wound healing.

LEARNING OBJECTIVES

After studying this chapter, you should be able to:

1. describe the skin disruptions, wound healing, and problems of wound healing.
2. discuss the staging of pressure ulcers.
3. explain the effects of lifestyle, age, and illness on skin integrity and wound healing.
4. assess the client who has Risk for impaired skin integrity or Impaired skin integrity.
5. evaluate the client's response to the diagnosed skin problem.
6. distinguish among the various nursing diagnoses for clients with alterations in skin integrity.
7. plan for goal-directed interventions to prevent Impaired skin integrity or promote wound healing.
8. evaluate the outcomes of interventions for Impaired skin integrity.

MATCHING

1. _f._ abrasion
2. _e._ blanchable erythema
3. _K._ debridement
4. _l._ dehiscence
5. _b._ eschar
6. _f._ epithelialization
7. _J._ evisceration
8. _C._ exudate
9. _h._ fistula
10. _d._ hematoma
11. _g._ hemorrhage
12. _m._ laceration
13. _a._ wound

a. a disruption of normal anatomical structure and function that results from bodily injury or a pathological process that may begin internally or externally to the involved organ or organs

b. thick, leathery, necrotic, devitalized tissue

c. refers to the fluid and cells that have escaped from blood vessels during the inflammatory response and are left in the surrounding tissues

d. an accumulation of bloody fluid beneath tissue

e. refers to a reddened area that turns white or pale temporarily when finger pressure is applied

(Continued on p. 130)

f.   a superficial injury caused by rubbing or scraping the skin against another surface

g.   bleeding from the wound bed or site

h.   an abnormal passage between two internal organs or between an organ and the external skin surface

i.   refers to a partial or total separation of the wound edges

j.   the protrusion of an internal organ (such as a bowel loop) through the incision

k.   the removal of dirt, foreign matter, and dead or devitalized tissue from a wound

l.   a process in which epithelial cells move to the wound bed

m.   open wound with jagged edges

TRUE OR FALSE

14. __ T __   Skin lesions are related to the client's medical condition. *May or may not be related*

15. __ F __   A black wound indicates that the wound is not yet ready to heal because it has fibrous slough or exudate that must be cleansed and removed. *yellow wound*

16. __ T __   Most acute wounds and surgical wounds close by primary intention.

17. __ T __   Internal hemorrhage can occur with no external evidence of bleeding.

18. __ F __   Wounds can heal when infection is present.

19. __ F __   Yellow drainage from a wound means the wound is infected. *does not always mean wound infected*

20. ____   Radiation is the least common mechanism of skin injury.

FILL-IN-THE-BLANKS

21. __ Protection __ is the primary function of the skin.

22. The __ red - yellow - black __ (RYB) classification system is based on wound bed color.

23. Typically, a __ pressure ulcer __ is located over a bony prominence or an area that sustains prolonged pressure.

24. The single most important factor in preventing wound infections and promoting wound healing is strict __ perioperative __ and __ postoperative __ asepsis.

25. Use the concept of the face of a __ clock __ to help define landmarks and areas of the wound or impaired skin area.

26. Surgical wounds and incisions are usually closed with __ sutures __ or stainless steel __ staples __ .

27. Interventions for a client with Impaired skin integrity are developed by the multidisciplinary team. A valuable resource to medical and nursing staff is the certified __ enterostomal __ therapist nurse.

EXERCISING YOUR CLINICAL JUDGMENT

28. Mrs. Jacan, the client from the chapter's case study, is bedridden after her hip surgery. She has developed a pressure ulcer that looks like a blister or shallow crater. Her pressure ulcer is most likely in which stage?
    a.   Stage I
    b.   Stage II
    c.   Stage III
    d.   Stage IV

29. Mrs. Jacan is given which one of the following diagnostic tests to help determine if she has inflammation, infectious, or necrotic processes?
    a.   complete blood count
    b.   erythrocyte sedimentation rate
    c.   prealbumin and albumin levels
    d.   blood panel

30. Mrs. Jacan had a reddened area on her sacrum and bilateral heels. Twenty-four hours after admission, you chart the following: Hydrocolloid dressing intact, no drainage (you had applied dressings to her sacrum and to her heels). Which of the following nursing diagnoses would be most appropriate for your evaluation of your client's care?
    a.   Impaired tissue integrity
    b.   Body image disturbance
    c.   Hopelessness
    d.   Impaired skin integrity

TEST YOURSELF

31. Your client was wounded by a knife. What type of wound is your client most likely suffering from?
    a. closed and clean wound
    b. abrasion and contusion
    c. open, contaminated, penetrating
    d. open, contaminated, abrasion

32. The area around your client's wound has edema, erythema, heat, and pain. His wound is one day old. This is an example of which phase of wound healing?
    a. inflammatory
    b. proliferative
    c. reconstruction
    d. maturation

33. If your client has an incision and dressing on the anterior part of the neck, you would check which of the following to determine if she was hemorrhaging externally?
    a. bloody drainage on dressing, distention of the affected area, a change in the amount or type of drainage from a drain
    b. distention of the affected area, a change in the amount or type of drainage from a drain, signs and symptoms of hypovolemic shock
    c. bloody drainage on dressing, signs and symptoms of hypovolemic shock
    d. bloody drainage on dressing and areas around the dressing and posterior to the wound site

34. Your client is a single 38-year-old female on her third postoperative day. She is very concerned about the large abdominal incision created during her hysterectomy and worries how this will affect her relationship with men she dates. Which of the following nursing diagnoses would be most appropriate?
    a. Impaired tissue integrity
    b. Body image disturbance
    c. Hopelessness
    d. Impaired skin integrity

35. For a wound to heal, the wound must be clean and free of bacteria. To cleanse a wound, you will need a wound cleaning solution. Which of the following is the preferred cleansing agent for most wounds?
    a. normal saline solution
    b. Dakin's solution
    c. Povidone iodine
    d. hydrogen peroxide

Body Temperature

PURPOSE

The purpose of this chapter is to introduce you to the concepts of thermoregulation and associated clinical problems.

LEARNING OBJECTIVES

After studying this chapter, you should be able to:

1. describe fever, hyperthermia, and hypothermia.
2. identify characteristics of clients with fever, hyperthermia, and hypothermia.
3. describe the assessment of the client with fever, hyperthermia, or hypothermia.
4. write a nursing diagnosis for the person with fever, hyperthermia, or hypothermia.
5. plan for nursing interventions for clients experiencing fever, hyperthermia, or hypothermia.
6. evaluate the effectiveness of interventions for clients with fever, hyperthermia, and hypothermia.

MATCHING

1. ____ fever
2. ____ heat exhaustion
3. ____ heat stroke
4. ____ hyperthermia
5. ____ hypothermia
6. ____ malaise
7. ____ pyrogen
8. ____ set-point

a. a nonregulated elevation in body temperature related to an imbalance between heat gain and heat loss

b. the temperature that thermoregulatory mechanisms attempt to maintain

c. an extreme elevation of body temperature, usually above 40.6°C (105°F), resulting in altered central nervous system function and shock

d. a feeling of indisposition; is thought to be an adaptive response which decreases most daily activities, thereby maintaining energy stores for fever generation

e. any agent that causes or stimulates a fever; the initial stimulus for fever is often exogenous

f. a regulated rise in body temperature that is mediated by a rise in temperature set-point

(Continued on p. 134)

133

g. a state in which body temperature is reduced below normal; severe reduction is temperature $\leq 32.2°C$ (90° F)

h. a rise in body temperature that is usually related to inadequate fluid and electrolyte replacement during physical activity

TRUE OR FALSE

9. ____ Fever is caused only by infection.

10. ____ During the initiation phase of a fever, pyrogens act on the hypothalamus to reset the temperature set-point higher than body temperature.

11. ____ Resolution of a fever by lysis is a gradual return to normal over several hours.

12. ____ A client with a fever is generally unable to sleep soundly.

13. ____ Hypothermia can be caused by infusion of a large volume of intravenous fluid in a short period of time.

14. ____ An immunosuppressed client is able to generate a fever.

15. ____ Fever may not develop as readily in the elderly as in the younger population.

16. ____ Treatment for arthritis may mask a fever.

17. ____ Blood cultures can be used to diagnose the causative organism for pneumonia.

18. ____ Blood cultures are best drawn through a central line IV site.

19. ____ An elderly client is more prone to heat stroke than a young adult.

20. ____ Febrile convulsions in infants are associated with temperatures over 105° F.

21. ____ Vasoconstriction decreases heat loss by radiation, convection, and conduction.

22. ____ Fever is a self-regulating phenomenon.

23. ____ A client with hypothermia will have decreased urinary output.

24. ____ The change in heart rate with hypothermia will depend on the degree of hypothermia.

25. ____ The height of a child's fever does not seem to trigger febrile convulsions as much as a sudden spike in body temperature.

FILL-IN-THE-BLANKS

26. The three phases of a fever are _____, _____, and _____.

27. During fever the metabolic rate increases by _____ for every degree of increase in temperature.

28. A client with a fever has a(n) _____ (increased, decreased) need for fluids.

29. The symptoms of heat stroke include _____ _____, _____, _____, _____, and _____.

30. Alcohol use contributes to hypothermia by providing a false sense of _____, inhibiting _____ and _____ of the skin.

31. _____ _____ or _____ _____ _____ _____ is defined as fever of 3 weeks duration with evaluation by a medical team for one week.

32. Side effects of aspirin include _____ and _____.

33. Acetaminophen should not be used in the presence of _____ disease.

34. Cooling blankets promote _____ heat loss.

35. Fans promote _____ heat loss.

36. Physical cooling is the standard for _____ (hyperthermia, fever).

37. _____ is the resolution of a fever.

38. The temperature control center is in the _____.

39. Three classes of medications that decrease the ability to sweat are _____-_____, _____, and _____.

40. To assess for tolerance before feeding a febrile client you would assess for _____ _____, _____ _____, and _____.

EXERCISING YOUR CLINICAL JUDGMENT

41. A mother calls the emergency room. Her six-year-old child has a fever of 101° F. Which information that she provides would prompt you to refer her to a physician?
    a. The child has not been exposed to a contagious disease.
    b. The child is having difficulty breathing.
    c. The child has clear drainage from the nose.
    d. The child is constipated.

42. You are making a home health visit to an elderly client in the middle of the summer. The outdoor temperature is 102° F. The client is complaining of weakness, headache, and diarrhea. You notice her skin is hot and dry, and she is not sweating despite a hot, closed house. She appears nervous and is somewhat confused. She has no fan. You would:
    a. call EMS.
    b. advise her to get a fan.
    c. call her daughter.
    d. help her take a cooling tub bath.

43. Mr. Stephen is 24 hours post a cardiac bypass surgical procedure. His temperature is 102° F. You find signs of postoperative atelectasis and encourage him to cough and deep breathe. How often should you recheck his temperature?
    a. q4h
    b. qid
    c. bid
    d. q8h

44. Your postsurgical client has a nasogastric tube. The physician has ordered acetaminophen per tube for temperature > 102° F. His temperature is 103° F. Select the best action.
    a. Administer the acetaminophen through the nasogastric tube and clamp the tube for 45 min.
    b. Administer the acetaminophen through the nasogastric tube and clamp the tube for 20 min.
    c. Call the physician to get the order changed to a rectal suppository.
    d. Administer the acetaminophen through the nasogastric tube and clamp the tube for 60 min.

45. A mother of a three-year-old asks for your advice about which antipyretic to use for her child's fever. Your best response would be:
    a. "Use acetaminophen. It is the best antipyretic."
    b. "Pediatricians often recommend avoiding aspirin in young children."
    c. "Never give your child antipyretics without the advice of a physician."
    d. "Acetaminophen can cause Reye's syndrome in young children."

TEST YOURSELF

46. A physician has written an order for acetaminophen for a temperature over 102° F. A rationale for not giving the antipyretic for a lower temperature is that:
    a. fever is a host defense response.
    b. normal temperature is variable.
    c. antipyretics only work on high temperatures.
    d. only a high fever produces a headache.

47. Cool saline gastric lavage may be more effective than a cooling blanket for hyperthermia because it:
    a. is a safer treatment.
    b. allows the skin to breathe.
    c. cools the body centrally rather than peripherally.
    d. does not directly stimulate vasoconstriction of the skin.

48. While it is a rare disorder, surgical nurses need to be aware of malignant hyperthermia. Malignant hyperthermia is:
    a. a result of carelessness with fluid administration in the operating room.
    b. an autosomal dominant genetic disorder that affects calcium levels.
    c. primarily associated with the administration of narcotics.
    d. a disorder that only occurs with bypass surgery.

49. A client with osteoarthritis has a painful swollen knee joint. Her temperature is 99.6° F. Select the best interpretation of her fever.
    a. Her knee has become infected.
    b. Her temperature is normally high.
    c. Her temperature is caused by inflammation.
    d. She is having a reaction to her medication.

50. Heat stroke results from:
    a. failure of the temperature regulating capacity of the body, caused by prolonged exposure to the sun.
    b. a rupture of a blood vessel in the brain from getting overheated.
    c. pyrogens building up in the blood stream because of kidney failure.
    d. a bacterial infection that attacks the temperature control center of the brain.

51. Your client has been admitted with bacterial pneumonia. She is having a chill. Select the best action to detect the highest point of fever.
    a. Check her temperature during the height of the chill.
    b. Check her temperature when the chill stops.
    c. Check her temperature one hour after the chill stops.
    d. Check her temperature six hours after the chill stops.

CHAPTER

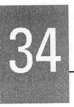

Bowel Elimination

PURPOSE

This chapter introduces you to alterations in bowel elimination such as constipation, diarrhea, and bowel incontinence. It describes a variety of factors that affect bowel function and uses the nursing process as a framework for caring for a client with an alteration in bowel elimination.

LEARNING OBJECTIVES

After studying this chapter, you should be able to:

1. describe the structure and function of the lower gastrointestinal tract.
2. discuss problems of bowel elimination, including constipation, diarrhea, and bowel incontinence.
3. explain how the client's diet and exercise, personal habits, cultural background, and age affect bowel elimination.
4. discuss the physiological and psychosocial factors affecting bowel elimination.
5. explain how to assess the client for manifestations of and responses to problems of bowel elimination.
6. distinguish among the variety of NANDA diagnoses for problems of bowel elimination.
7. plan for goal-directed interventions to prevent or correct problems of bowel elimination.
8. evaluate the outcomes that describe progress toward the goals of bowel elimination.

MATCHING

1. __f__ bowel incontinence
2. __h__ cathartic
3. __g__ colostomy
4. __i__ constipation
5. __r__ diarrhea
6. __o__ fecal impaction
7. __b__ feces
8. __e__ flatus
9. __c__ flatulence
10. __n__ guaiac test
11. __q__ ileostomy
12. __p__ laxative
13. __d__ occult blood
14. __l__ ostomy
15. __m__ paralytic ileus
16. __a__ peristalsis
17. __s__ steatorrhea
18. __k__ stoma

a. the rhythmic smooth muscle contractions of the intestinal wall that propel the intestinal contents forward

b. body waste discharged from the intestine

c. the presence of abnormal amounts of gas in the GI tract, causing abdominal distention and discomfort

d. an amount of blood that is too small to be seen without a microscope

e. an amount of gas that occurs normally in the GI tract

f. the inability to voluntarily control the passage of feces and gas

(Continued on p. 138)

g. a surgical procedure involving the creation of an opening between the colon and the abdominal wall.

h. medication used to induce emptying of the bowel; often used interchangeably with a laxative, although it has a stronger action

i. a condition in which feces are abnormally hard and dry and evacuation is abnormally infrequent

j. a gray stool mixed with observable fat and mucus, resulting from the malabsorption of fat

k. the opening between the abdominal wall and intestine through which fecal material passes

l. the surgical procedure used to create an opening through the abdominal wall and into the intestine

m. the absence of peristalsis for more than three days

n. a test to measure occult blood

o. a collection of putty-like or hardened feces in the rectum or sigmoid colon that prevents the passage of a normal stool and becomes more hardened as the colon continues to absorb water from it

p. medication used to induce emptying of the bowel; often used interchangeably with cathartic

q. a surgical procedure involving the creation of an opening between the ileum and the abdominal wall

r. the rapid movement of fecal matter through the intestine, resulting in poor absorption of water, nutrients, and electrolytes, and producing abnormally frequent evacuation of watery stools

TRUE OR FALSE

19. _T_ Constipation is a major complaint among the elderly.

20. _T_ Some risks of straining at stool include angina attacks, hemorrhoid development, and rupture of abdominal suture lines.

21. _F_ It is exceptionally difficult to train the bowel to evacuate at a certain time.

22. _T_ Spicy foods stimulate peristalsis by local reflex stimulation.

23. _F_ Exercise has no effect on bowel elimination.

24. _T_ Bowel elimination is usually not a problem for the adolescent unless there is a health problem.

25. _F_ Motor or sensory disturbances, such as with spinal cord injury or neurological disease, can lead to diarrhea. constipation

26. _T_ A medication that is given to prevent constipation can cause diarrhea in some clients.

27. _T_ The further down the bowel a colostomy is created, the greater the chance there is for being able to regulate the bowel.

28. _F_ Mental depression plays no role in the development of constipation.

FILL-IN-THE-BLANKS

29. A diet that is high in __fiber__ tends to prevent the occurrence of constipation.

30. Chocolate, coffee, and prune juice are foods that can __loosen__ the stool.

31. __Diverticulosis__ is an out-pouching of the intestinal wall that can occur after age 40.

32. Impaired dentition in the older adult impairs __mastication__, allowing food to enter the GI tract inadequately chewed.

33. A client is more at risk for cancer of the colon if the diet is high in __fat__ and low in __fiber__.

34. The consistency of ileostomy drainage is __liquid__.

35. As part of colon cancer screening, an annual digital rectal examination should be done every year after age __40__.

36. Beans, beer, and cucumbers are examples of foods that can cause __flatulence__.

37. How the GI tract reacts to a particular food depends on the __person__ or __individual__.

38. The overuse of laxatives can lead to physical and psychological __dependence__.

EXERCISING YOUR CLINICAL JUDGMENT

Dr. Daley, the 92-year-old retired neurosurgeon introduced in the chapter case study, has a nursing diagnosis of Constipation. He is living in a long-term care facility because he can no longer manage on his own with a diagnosis of bone cancer. He has begun limiting the use of his narcotic analgesic, morphine, because it could worsen the constipation. The nurse from the previous shift reports having just assessed Dr. Daley's abdomen and suspects impaction. You are now taking over the care of the clients on this unit.

39. Dr. Daley has chosen to use Milk of Magnesia as his laxative. You recall that this medication belongs to which of the following categories of laxatives?
    a. bulk-forming
    b. lubricant
    c. saline
    d. stimulant

40. The medication given to Dr. Daley has not worked and you obtain an order for an oil retention enema. When administering it to Dr. Daley, you ask him to try to retain it in the bowel for at least:
    a. 5 minutes.
    b. 15 minutes.
    c. 30 minutes.
    d. an hour.

41. The enema is successful and you are exploring with Dr. Daley strategies that can be used to prevent a recurrence. You both agree that he should try to walk to the toilet at which of the following times, when stimulation of the gastrocolic reflex is strongest?
    a. upon awakening
    b. after breakfast
    c. after lunch
    d. before bedtime

42. You begin an intake and output record to keep track of Dr. Daley's fluid intake. You encourage him to drink at least how much fluid per day to minimize the risk of constipation recurrence?
    a. 1.5 liters
    b. 3 liters
    c. 4 liters
    d. 5 liters

TEST YOURSELF

43. The nurse caring for a client with an ostomy would do which of the following to maintain the skin integrity around the stoma?
    a. use a skin barrier
    b. limit the use of skin paste
    c. wash peristomal skin but not dry it
    d. try to have the pouch last about 2 weeks

44. A client has abdominal pain related to flatulence. Which of the following items would the nurse suspect is contributing to the problem?
    a. walking
    b. eating slowly
    c. eating cauliflower
    d. drinking water

45. The nurse changing a client's ostomy bag should cut a new appliance how much larger than the size of the client's stoma to have a proper fit?
    a. 1/16 inch
    b. 1/8 inch
    c. 1/4 inch
    d. 1/2 inch

46. A client with diarrhea was treated with antibiotic therapy and now would benefit from recolonization of normal GI flora. The nurse should offer this client which of the following products?
    a. cheese
    b. yogurt
    c. skim milk
    d. raw apples

47. An older adult with multiple health problems has a severe case of diarrhea. The nurse would assess this client for which of the following common complications of diarrhea in this client population?
    a. thirst and ruddy skin color
    b. diverticulitis
    c. nausea and vomiting
    d. fluid and electrolyte imbalances

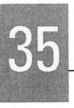

Urinary Elimination

PURPOSE

The purpose of this chapter is to review anatomy and physiology of the urinary system and to introduce you to basic nursing measures for clients with urinary problems. You will learn to recognize the signs and symptoms of urinary problems and intervene to improve urinary function. Additionally, you will be introduced to procedures for collecting an urine specimen from a Foley catheter, using a condom catheter, and inserting a Foley catheter.

LEARNING OBJECTIVES

After studying this chapter, you should be able to:

1. describe the normal structure and function of the urinary system.
2. identify common problems of urinary elimination.
3. discuss factors affecting urinary elimination.
4. assess urinary function and identify a client experiencing urinary elimination problems.
5. diagnose problems of urinary elimination that can be managed with nursing care.
6. plan goal-directed nursing interventions for managing problems in urinary elimination.
7. implement basic nursing care for a client experiencing problems with urinary elimination.
8. use expected outcomes as aids in evaluating care for a person experiencing problems with urinary elimination.

MATCHING

1. __I__ Kegel exercises
2. __K__ diuresis
3. __J__ dysuria
4. __f__ urinary retention
5. __h__ hematuria
6. __c__ urinary incontinence
7. __e__ frequency
8. __V__ micturition
9. __b__ nocturia
10. __Y__ oliguria
11. __d__ total incontinence
12. __v__ bacteriuria
13. __p__ urinalysis
14. __n__ ileal conduit
15. __o__ urgency
16. __e__ reflex incontinence
17. __J__ urination
18. __g__ stress incontinence
19. __l__ urge incontinence

a. recurrent involuntary urination that occurs during sleep

b. the term used for nighttime urination

c. involuntary passage of urine

d. the person is unaware of cues to a full bladder and may be unaware of the incontinence; the incontinence is either continual or unpredictable

e. incontinence associated with neurological damage to the spinal cord above the level of the third sacral vertebrae

f. the inability to pass all or part of the urine that has accumulated in the bladder

(Continued on p. 142)

20. __a__ enuresis

21. __m__ anuria

22. __s__ polyuria

g. incontinence reported or observed as dribbling with increased intra-abdominal pressure

h. the discharge of blood in the urine

i. incontinence reported or observed as a sudden desire to urinate and immediately seeking toileting facilities

j. the more commonly used term for the act of micturition; the term *void* is more common in clinical use

k. the increased secretion of urine

l. the symptom of difficulty with or painful urination; it may be accompanied by frequency, hesitancy, or urgency of urination

m. the absence of urine production

n. connects the distal ureters to a resected portion of the terminal ileum which is used in the formation of an ostomy or opening onto the surface of the abdomen

o. sudden, forceful urge to urinate; further assessment is needed to determine the cause

p. a physical, chemical, and microscopic examination of the urine

q. urination that occurs at shorter-than-usual intervals without an increase in daily urine output

r. a diminished, scanty amount of urine

s. a large amount of urine usually associated with diabetes mellitus or diabetes insipidus

t. exercises to strengthen the floor of the pelvis

u. bacteria in the urine

v. the process of emptying the bladder

TRUE OR FALSE

23. __F__ *Voluntary* The bladder is under the involuntary control of the sympathetic nervous system.

24. __T__ Enuresis occurs by the age of eight years in all but about 7% of children.

25. __T__ Urinary retention can be cause by obstruction or inability of the detrusor to contract.

26. __F__ Urinary incontinence is an expected or normal part of aging.

27. __F__ The client with a Kock pouch wears a bag for the collection of urine.

28. __T__ Six to eight glasses of water is equivalent to 1500 to 2000 cc.

29. __F__ The external urinary sphincter is smooth muscle under control of the parasympathetic nervous system. *Sympathetic*

30. __T__ A primary factor in incontinence for some elderly persons is urge incontinence in the presence of impaired mobility.

31. __T__ Constipation can be a factor in incontinence of urine.

32. __T__ Bilirubin is excreted in the urine when the biliary tract is obstructed.

33. __F__ There is no reason to test the urine for blood unless the urine is red or cloudy.

34. __F__ You need a minimum of 30 cc of urine to send for urinalysis. *1 cc*

35. __F__ All clients need an antibiotic after a cystoscopy.

FILL-IN-THE-BLANKS

36. The __vesicoureteral__ valve is the connection between the ureters and the bladder.

37. The __detrusor__ is the primary muscle of the bladder.

38. The kidneys control the excretion of these waste products: _____, _____, _____ _____, _____, and _____ ____ _____.

39. Among other electrolytes, the kidney controls the excretion of the two primary electrolytes, _sodium_ and _potassium_.

40. Urine moves through the ureters by gravity and _peristalsis_.

41. Dysuria is often related to _____, _____, or _____ of the lower urinary tract.

42. Voiding every hour would be described as _____.

43. The normal range for feeling the urge to urinate is _150_ to _500_ cc.

44. _voiding urogram_ measures the function of the bladder and urethra by measuring the flow rate of urine passing through the urethra.

45. _____ (creatinine, BUN) is the more specific test for renal function.

46. _Stress_ incontinence is associated with postmenopausal atrophy or the presence of a cystocele.

47. The Alzheimer's client who has progressed to the point of no neurological control over the bladder has _functional_ or _total_ incontinence.

48. As a means to control incontinence _prompted voiding_ is recommended for clients who can learn to recognize some degree of bladder fullness or the need to void.

49. As a means to control incontinence _habit training_ is recommended for clients for whom a natural pattern of voiding can be determined.

50. _Kegel exercises_ can help the client who has stress incontinence.

EXERCISING YOUR CLINICAL JUDGMENT

51. You are assessing a 57-year-old female client. She says she continues to have stress incontinence despite using the Kegel exercises regularly for six months. Her doctor has talked about surgery, but she is reluctant. She asks you if she should keep trying the exercises. Select the best response.
    a. "If you haven't had success in six months, you should see your doctor about surgery."
    b. "I can review the technique with you if you like; sometimes it is difficult to contract the right muscle."
    c. "Kegel exercises only work for a small number of women."
    d. "It is always best to follow your doctor's advice."

52. Select the technique to prevent the most serious complication of a condom catheter.
    a. To hold the catheter in place, use a soft flexible band that is snug but not tight.
    b. Inspect and clean the skin at least daily.
    c. Arrange the drainage tubing to ensure urine drains from the condom.
    d. Tape the catheter collecting tubing to the leg, allowing slack in the catheter.

53. You are assigned a client who has urinary incontinence. You see a nursing order on the care plan for prompted voiding. To correctly assist with this intervention you would:
    a. take the client to the bathroom every four hours or offer the bedpan.
    b. insist that the client go to the bathroom or use the bedpan every two hours.
    c. admonish the client for wetness and insist that the client use the call light.
    d. check the client for wetness every two hours and offer assistance to the bathroom or bedside commode.

54. Select the client for whom a Foley catheter may be used to prevent urinary retention.
    a. a client who has had bladder surgery where some bleeding is expected
    b. a client who has had surgery for a fractured hip
    c. a client who is in shock (blood pressure 88/50)
    d. a client with terminal cancer, who is expected to die within 24 hours

55. Select the method that is expected to reduce the incidence of urinary tract infections associated with the use of urinary catheters.
    a. changing the catheter every 48 hours
    b. taking a daily sitz bath
    c. placement of a suprapubic catheter
    d. emptying the drainage bag only when it is full

56. Your client is a 60-year-old male. He is 6′ 4″ tall and weighs 225 lbs. Select the catheter size that is most likely to be appropriate.
    a. 10 Fr
    b. 14 Fr
    c. 16 Fr
    d. 18 Fr

57. You are performing a Foley catheterization. You accidentally contaminate the connection tubing, but know the catheter is sterile. Select the action that would be most cost effective and still be correct.
    a. Ask someone to bring you a new sterile catheter.
    b. Obtain a new tray and start over.
    c. Ask someone to bring you a new sterile bag and tubing.
    d. Continue with the catheterization, avoiding the connection tubing until you have inserted the catheter.

TEST YOURSELF

58. The purpose of maintaining straight continuous gravity drainage from a Foley catheter is:
    a. to be more aesthetically pleasing to the client.
    b. to prevent the backflow of urine into the bladder.
    c. to keep the bladder empty of urine.
    d. to keep the catheter patent.

59. Your client has had a Foley catheter for three days after bladder surgery. The physician has written an order to discontinue the catheter. Which intervention would be the most important?
    a. Check to see if the client can void within 4 hours of removing the Foley.
    b. Push fluids to relieve irritation of the urethra.
    c. Have the client drink water rather than coffee or diet cola.
    d. Assist the client to take a sitz bath.

60. Your client has had bladder surgery. The surgeon has ordered a three-way Foley with continuous irrigation with normal saline. You enter the room and notice that the urine is dark red with only a small amount flowing through the drainage tubing. Select the best action.
    a. Call the surgeon immediately.
    b. Force fluids by mouth.
    c. Increase the flow of the irrigant until the urine clears.
    d. Turn the client in bed.

61. Your client has an urinary diversion that is well healed and has been functioning normally. She is currently admitted for pneumonia, is very weak, and needs assistance with caring for her elimination needs. You notice that urine is leaking under the stoma wafer applied to her skin. Select the best action.
    a. Use nonporous tape to secure the wafer.
    b. Remove the wafer and apply a new one.
    c. Pad the site to collect the leakage.
    d. Remove the wafer and insert a catheter to collect the urine.

62. Select the best method to acidify the urine.
    a. 500 mg vitamin C bid
    b. 4 glasses of diluted cranberry juice daily
    c. Sodium bicarbonate 1 tsp bid
    d. 4 glasses of orange juice daily

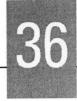

Hygiene

PURPOSE

This chapter discusses key concepts that relate to the nursing diagnoses Bathing/hygiene self-care deficit, Impaired skin integrity, Altered oral mucous membrane, Ineffective individual coping, and Powerlessness. It describes the structure and function of the skin, hair, nails, and oral cavity.

LEARNING OBJECTIVES

After studying this chapter, you should be able to:

1. describe the structure and function of the skin, hair, nails, and oral cavity.
2. discuss some problems of personal hygiene.
3. describe some cultural, developmental, socioeconomic, physical, and psychosocial factors affecting hygiene.
4. discuss assessment of a client who is at risk for or shows manifestations of self-care deficit for managing personal hygiene related to physical, psychological, or cognitive impairment.
5. differentiate among a variety of nursing diagnoses related to the client's bathing and hygiene.
6. plan client-centered outcomes to assist the client with meeting personal hygiene needs.
7. describe nursing interventions to promote hygiene of the skin, mouth, and hair.
8. evaluate outcomes of nursing care as being helpful in assisting the client to meet self-care needs for personal hygiene.

MATCHING

1. ____ alopecia
2. ____ caries
3. ____ cerumen
4. ____ dermis
5. ____ dentures
6. ____ epidermis
7. ____ gingivitis
8. ____ perineum
9. ____ plaque
10. ____ tartar

a. a waxy secretion of the glands of the external acoustic meatus; it is commonly called ear wax

b. a destructive process causing decalcification of the tooth enamel and leading to continued destruction of the enamel and dentin with resulting cavitation of the tooth

c. an inflammation of the gums usually manifested by the primary symptom of bleeding of the gums

d. a yellowish film of calcium phosphate, carbonate, food particles, and other organic matter deposited on the teeth by saliva

(Continued on p. 146)

e.   a complement of teeth, either natural or artificial, ordinarily used to designate an artificial replacement for the natural teeth

f.   loss of hair and baldness

g.   the pelvic floor and associated structures occupying pelvic outlet, bounded anteriorly by the symphysis pubis, laterally by the ischial tuberosities, and posteriorly by the coccyx

h.   a soft, thin film of food debris, mucin and dead epithelial cells that is deposited on the teeth and provides a medium for the growth of bacteria

i.   composed of stratified squamous epithelium and contains four kinds of cells

j.   composed of connective tissue containing collagenous and elastic fibers

TRUE OR FALSE

11. ____ The outer portion of the skin, the epidermis, is composed of stratified squamous epithelium that contains keratinocytes, which produce keratin, the substance that is responsible for the color of the skin.

12. ____ Hair grows faster at night than during the day and faster in warm weather than in cold.

13. ____ If your nails are thick and yellow, this may be indicative of bacterial infection.

14. ____ If you presuppose lack of ability when some ability may be present it can further reinforce a client's sense of independence and helplessness.

15. ____ Total hygiene care consists of bathing, skin care, oral care, hair care, perineal care, back massage, shaving, changing the bed linens and changing a client's gown or pajamas.

16. ____ Problems with nail and foot care usually occur because of neglect or abuse.

17. ____ The benefits of bathing in a tub or shower (instead of a sponge bath) for the client are so significant that if the option is available, you should use it even if it may be difficult and time consuming.

FILL-IN-THE-BLANKS

18. _____-_____ is the ability to meet hygiene needs without the assistance of another person.

19. The skin helps screen out ultraviolet (UV) rays from the sun, but it also lets in some necessary UV rays that convert a chemical in the skin call 7-dehydrocholesterol into _____.

20. If the origin of a client's halitosis is _____, oral hygiene will not remove the odor.

21. Dental _____ is a disease of the calcified structure of the tooth.

22. Body lice suck _____ from the skin and live in clothing, making them hard to detect.

23. Skin _____ are prominent in aging skin.

24. Complete _____ _____ is giving the complete bath without any assistance from the client.

EXERCISING YOUR CLINICAL JUDGMENT

25. Joy Wilson, the 78-year-old African-American client from the chapter's case study, suffers from a stroke (cerebrovascular accident). She is unable to bathe herself. Which nursing diagnosis would be most appropriate?
    a.   Ineffective individual coping
    b.   Bathing/hygiene self-care deficit
    c.   Activity intolerance
    d.   Impaired physical mobility

26. Ms. Wilson's daughter gives her a hot-water bath. The purpose of this type of bath is to:
    a.   decrease pain and inflammation.
    b.   relieve muscle spasm and muscle tension.
    c.   relax and soothe.
    d.   soothe skin irritation.

27. Ms. Wilson's cognitive status is impaired because of her short-term memory loss. She has difficulty caring for her basic needs. Which nursing diagnosis would be most appropriate?
    a.   Ineffective individual coping
    b.   Bathing/hygiene self-care deficit
    c.   Activity intolerance
    d.   Altered thought processes

TEST YOURSELF

28. You advise the client to do regular oral care and that dental intervention may be necessary. Which problem of the oral cavity is your client most likely suffering from?
    a. halitosis
    b. gingivitis
    c. periodontal disease
    d. stomatitis

29. Your client is having difficulty following through on doing self-care. A careful assessment of the client's cognitive status is essential because she may appear to be well-oriented and capable of doing self-care, but on a more careful assessment, you would most likely find she has:
    a. a short-term memory loss.
    b. a long-term memory loss.
    c. difficulty coping with stressors.
    d. lack of full range of motion.

30. Smegma is which of the following?
    a. loss of hair and baldness
    b. cheesy-like substance secreted by the sebaceous glands
    c. oily substance secreted by the sebaceous glands
    d. ascorbic acid

31. Your client is a 58-year-old poorly nourished woman who was diagnosed with Alzheimer's disease three years ago. She has shown rapid deterioration and now is unable to care for any of her basic hygiene. Which nursing diagnosis is most appropriate?
    a. Altered thought processes
    b. Sensory/perceptual alterations
    c. Activity intolerance
    d. Impaired physical mobility

32. Your client is a 43-year-old female who has had severe rheumatoid arthritis for 15 years. She has severe limitations of both her lower and upper extremities. She has difficulty grasping objects because of malformation of hand and fingers. Which nursing diagnosis is most appropriate?
    a. Altered thought processes
    b. Sensory/perceptual alterations
    c. Activity intolerance
    d. Impaired physical mobility

Physical Mobility

PURPOSE

This chapter discusses key concepts that relate to the nursing diagnoses Impaired physical mobility and Activity intolerance. It describes the concepts of the structure and function of the musculoskeletal system pertaining to mobility. It also discusses factors affecting mobility.

LEARNING OBJECTIVES

After studying this chapter, you should be able to:

1. describe the concepts of the structure and function of the musculoskeletal system pertaining to mobility.
2. discuss factors affecting mobility.
3. describe the assessment of a client with impaired mobility.
4. identify appropriate nursing diagnoses for clients with mobility problems.
5. identify expected outcomes for permanent and temporary mobility problems.
6. intervene to assist a client to restore or improve mobility.
7. evaluate nursing care for the nursing diagnoses Impaired physical mobility and Activity intolerance.

MATCHING

1. ____ flaccid
2. ____ hemiparesis
3. ____ hemiplegia
4. ____ isometric exercise
5. ____ isotonic exercise
6. ____ kyphosis
7. ____ paraparesis
8. ____ paraplegia
9. ____ PQRST model
10. ____ proprioception
11. ____ quadriparesis
12. ____ quadriplegia
13. ____ range-of-motion (ROM) exercises
14. ____ spastic
15. ____ synovium

a. the inner layer of the articular capsule surrounding a freely movable joint

b. sensation pertaining to stimuli originating from within the body regarding spatial position and muscular activity or to the sensory receptors that they activate

c. stands for: Provoking incidence, Quality, Region, Radiate, Relieve, Severity, and Timing of pain

d. an abnormal condition characterized by paralysis of the arms, legs, and trunk below the level of an associated injury to the spinal cord

e. a numbness or other abnormal or impaired sensation in all four limbs and the trunk

f. paralysis characterized by motor or sensory loss in the legs and trunk

(Continued on p. 150)

g. paralysis of one side of the body

h. a numbness or other abnormal or impaired sensation experienced on only one side of the body that limits mobility and activities of daily living (ADLs)

i. an abnormal condition of the vertebral column characterized by increased convexity in the thoracic spine when viewed from the side

j. the state of being weak, soft, and flabby, lacking normal muscle tone, or having no ability to contract

k. contraction of skeletal muscles below the injury by reflex activity rather than by central nervous system control

l. a form of active exercise that increases muscle tension by applying pressure against stable resistance

m. form of active exercise in which the muscle contracts and moves

n. any body action (active or passive) involving the muscles, joints, and natural directional movements, such as abduction, extension, flexion, pronation, and rotation

o. a numbness or other abnormal or impaired sensation in the legs and trunk

TRUE OR FALSE

16. ____ Widening your base of support by moving your feet apart helps you to maintain stability.

17. ____ Postmenopausal women's vertebral bone mass increases and the thoracic spine becomes more convex, or curved.

18. ____ The most common congenital spinal deformity is scoliosis.

19. ____ Some medications have side effects that cause muscle atrophy.

20. ____ If a client can perform ADLs, a slight limitation of ROM is still unacceptable, especially for older adults.

21. ____ The client with Impaired physical mobility is at risk for injury from falls and fractures as a result of osteoporosis.

22. ____ For the postoperative client with a total knee replacement, a realistic intermediate outcome is that the client is expected to walk in the hospital room using a walker.

FILL-IN-THE-BLANKS

23. At about the age of 35 years _____ activity becomes greater than osteoblastic activity which results in decreased bone which predisposes middle-aged and older adults to bone injury.

24. Muscle _____ causes weakness that can limit physical mobility.

25. An abnormal fixed position of the feet is _____ _____, or pigeon toe, a deformity that can worsen and delay physical development if not corrected.

26. The most common complaints associated with musculoskeletal health problems are pain, _____ _____, and inflammation.

27. _____ is a continuous grating sound caused by deterioration of a joint.

28. _____ and occupational therapists perform detailed assessments of muscle strength using various scales.

29. _____ nurses are specialists in helping clients return to or attain maximum function and a sense of well being and independence.

EXERCISING YOUR CLINICAL JUDGMENT

30. Kristina Lasauskas, the client from this chapter's case study, had an open reduction and internal fixation to repair her fractured left hip. What nursing diagnosis would be most appropriate?
    a. Impaired physical mobility
    b. Pain
    c. Activity intolerance
    d. Risk for injury

31. Ms. Lasauskas needs help to learn how to increase her mobility skills after her surgery for a fractured left hip. Which one of the following disciplines' primary role is improving clients' mobility skills?
    a. rehabilitation nurse
    b. physical therapist
    c. occupational therapist
    d. rehabilitation physician

32. Ms. Lasauskas will need range-of-motion exercises while she is bedridden. What type of exercises are these?
    a. isotonic
    b. isokinetic
    c. isometric
    d. muscle toning

TEST YOURSELF

33. Pulling is usually easier than pushing, so pull clients toward you rather then pushing them. This can help do which one of the following?
    a. reduce workload
    b. decrease opposition from gravity
    c. maintain stability
    d. prevent muscle strain

34. Your client is having problems with her ankle. To assess her ankle's range of motion, which ROM exercises will you have her do?
    a. flexion, extension, hyperextension
    b. flexion, extension, abduction, adduction
    c. extension, flexion, eversion, inversion
    d. external rotation, internal rotation

35. Your elderly client fell and fractured her hip and has degenerative arthritis in both knees. What nursing diagnoses would be most appropriate?
    a. Impaired physical mobility
    b. Pain
    c. Activity intolerance
    d. Risk for injury

36. Your teenaged client has rheumatoid arthritis. She uses a walker to ambulate short distances, but relies on a wheelchair most of the time. She becomes very fatigued when walking. What nursing diagnosis would be most appropriate?
    a. Impaired physical mobility
    b. Pain
    c. Activity intolerance
    d. Risk for injury

37. Which one of the following disciplines' primary role is improving clients' ADL abilities?
    a. rehabilitation nurse
    b. physical therapist
    c. occupational therapist
    d. rehabilitation physician

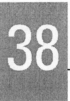
Disuse Syndrome

PURPOSE

This chapter discusses key concepts that relate to the nursing diagnosis Risk for disuse syndrome. It describes the physiological concepts underlying the diagnosis and the factors that may lead to immobility and disuse.

LEARNING OBJECTIVES

After studying this chapter, you should be able to:

1. describe the physiological concepts underlying the diagnosis of Risk for disuse syndrome.
2. discuss the factors that may lead to immobility and disuse.
3. assess a client who is at risk for complications from disuse.
4. diagnose the client at risk for disuse complications.
5. plan for goal-directed interventions to prevent complications of disuse.
6. describe interventions needed to prevent complications of disuse.
7. evaluate outcomes that describe progress toward managing immobility and preventing disuse.

MATCHING

1. ____ atrophy
2. ____ bedrest
3. ____ contracture
4. ____ deep vein thrombosis
5. ____ disuse
6. ____ excoriation
7. ____ footdrop
8. ____ friction injury
9. ____ hypostatic pneumonia
10. ____ immobility
11. ____ interface pressure
12. ____ maceration
13. ____ orthostatic hypotension
14. ____ osteoporosis
15. ____ pressure ulcer
16. ____ pulmonary embolus
17. ____ renal calculi
18. ____ shear
19. ____ wrist drop

a. the inability to move the whole body or a body part

b. a prescribed or self-imposed restriction to bed for therapeutic reasons

c. a decrease in the size of a normally developed tissue or organ as a result of inactivity or diminished function

d. the abnormal shortening of muscle fibers or their associated connective tissue, resulting in resistance of stretching and eventually to flexion and, thereby resulting in permanent fixation

e. a contracture deformity in which the muscles of the anterior foot lengthen

f. a condition in which there is a decreased mass per unit volume of normally mineralized bone, primarily from a loss of calcium, that makes bones brittle and porous

(Continued on p. 154)

g. a local defect or excavation of the surface of an organ or tissue that is produced by sloughing of necrotic inflammatory tissue created by impaired local circulation

h. pressure created in tissues that are compressed between the bones and a support surface by the weight of the body

i. a mechanical action in which an applied force exerted against the skin causes the tissue layers to slide in opposite but parallel directions, resulting in torn blood vessels

j. the epidermal layer of skin is rubbed off, possibly by a restraint, a dressing, or a tube

k. an injury to the epidermis caused by abrasion; scratching; a burn or chemicals, such as sweat; wound drainage; or feces or urine coming in contact with skin

l. a softening of the epidermis caused by prolonged contact with moisture, such as from a wet sheet or diaper

m. a drop in systolic blood pressure of 20mm Hg or more and a drop in diastolic blood pressure of 10 mm Hg or more for 1 or 2 minutes after a client stands up

n. results when a piece of a deep vein thrombus breaks free, floats in the bloodstream to the pulmonary circulation, and lodges in a pulmonary blood vessel

o. the condition caused when a blood clot (thrombus) develops in the lumen of a deep leg vein, such as the tibial, popliteal, femoral, or iliac vein

p. an inflammation of the lungs, caused by stasis of secretions, that becomes a medium for bacterial growth

q. stones formed in the kidney when the excretion rate of calcium or other minerals is high, as when osteoclastic activity releases calcium from the bones during immobility

r. means to cease or decrease use of organs or body parts, to restrict activities, or to be immobile

s. a contracture of the wrist in the flexed position

TRUE OR FALSE

20. _____ Inactivity and immobility have a cyclic relationship with the development of complications.

21. _____ When muscles atrophy, they lose size and strength.

22. _____ Length of immobilization of a client is not directly related to a higher risk of complications for the client of disuse.

23. _____ A pressure ulcer is a local defect or excavation of the surface of an organ or tissue that is produced by sloughing of necrotic inflammatory tissue creating impaired systemic circulation.

24. _____ Orthostatic hypotension is a rise in systolic blood pressure of 20 mm Hg or more and a drop in diastolic blood pressure of 10 mm Hg or more for 1 or 2 minutes after a client stands up.

25. _____ Clients who are at minimal Risk for disuse syndrome should be assessed every 4–6 hours.

26. _____ Constant contact with a bed made wet by perspiration causes maceration of the skin.

FILL-IN-THE-BLANKS

27. _____ can affect a single body part or multiple interrelated body systems.

28. The _____ the person is immobile, the higher the risk of complication of disuse.

29. When a client is immobile, her body breaks down muscle mass to obtain _____.

30. Pressure _____ account for a large proportion of skin injuries that result from bed rest.

31. Low blood pressure and _____ _____ increase the client's risk of falling.

32. Stasis of the urine and infection increase the risk for _____ to form in the kidneys, renal pelvis, or urinary bladder.

33. You should assess and intervene every _____-_____ _____ with clients who have high Risk for disuse syndrome.

EXERCISING YOUR CLINICAL JUDGMENT

34. Mr. Jackson, the 48-year-old African American with a compound fracture of the left tibia and a fractured left clavicle from this chapter's case study, develops a friction injury. This type of injury occurs when:
    a. the epidermal layer of skin is rubbed off.
    b. the client is neither very young or very old.
    c. there is a decrease in range of motion.
    d. there is maximal inactivity of long duration.

35. Mr. Jackson has moderate inactivity of moderate duration, is middle-aged, has normal-to-slight increased body weight, no chronic illnesses, minimal discomfort, and low environmental risk. Your client is at moderate risk for disuse syndrome. How often should you assess and intervene with this client?
    a. every 4–6 hours
    b. every 2–4 hours
    c. every 1–2 hours
    d. every shift

36. You encourage Mr. Jackson to exercise his right arm and leg against resistance three times daily. Which nursing diagnosis does Mr. Jackson have?
    a. Altered role performance
    b. Sensory/perceptual alterations
    c. Risk for disuse syndrome
    d. Self-care deficit

TEST YOURSELF

37. Your client has been immobile for several weeks. Once he begins ambulating he is more susceptible to ambulation problems and injury caused by what?
    a. footdrop
    b. contracture
    c. osteoporosis
    d. falling

38. Your client has a deformity that involves flexion of the wrist and fingers and opposition of the thumb. What is this called?
    a. hand drop
    b. wrist drop
    c. osteoporosis
    d. ankylosis

39. Your client has softening of the epidermis caused by prolonged contact with a wet sheet. What type of injury is this?
    a. maceration
    b. shear
    c. friction injury
    d. excoriation

40. There are two purposes in assessing the immobile client. One is to detect the risk of complication of immobility. What is the second?
    a. to determine the client's needs
    b. to determine how much assistance the client will need to manage the activities of daily living and prevent complications
    c. to determine the client's emotional well-being
    d. to determine the client's level of understanding of his situation

41. To relieve pressure, how often do you turn the client to a new position?
    a. every 1–2 hours
    b. every hour
    c. twice a shift
    d. every 3 hours

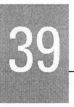
Respiratory Function

PURPOSE

The purpose of this chapter is to review anatomy and physiology of the respiratory system and to introduce you to basic respiratory nursing measures. You will learn to recognize the signs and symptoms of respiratory distress and intervene to improve respiratory function. Additionally you will be introduced to some advance procedures such as managing a chest tube, suctioning the airways, and caring for a tracheostomy.

LEARNING OBJECTIVES

After studying this chapter, you should be able to:

1. describe the physiological concepts underlying the respiratory nursing diagnoses.
2. discuss the most common lifestyle, environmental, developmental, and physiological factors affecting respiration, as well as contributing pathologies.
3. assess the client who has risk for experiencing a respiratory problem and the client's responses to the respiratory problem.
4. diagnose the client's respiratory needs that are amenable to nursing care.
5. plan for goal-directed interventions to prevent or correct respiratory diagnoses.
6. describe and practice key interventions for respiratory care, including positioning, suctioning, providing supplemental oxygen, and maintaining a patent airway.
7. evaluate the outcomes that describe progress toward the goals of respiratory nursing care.

MATCHING

1. _i_ chest physiotherapy
2. _h_ diaphragmatic (abdominal) breathing
3. _d_ cough
4. _c_ chest percussion
5. _k_ hyperventilation
6. _j_ dyspnea
7. _a_ cyanosis
8. _e_ diffusion
9. _b_ bronchospasm
10. _w_ hemoptysis
11. _g_ hypercapnia
12. _l_ pulse oximetry
13. _f_ hypoventilation
14. _m_ postural drainage
15. _n_ pursed-lip breathing
16. _q_ incentive spirometer
17. _v_ hypoxia

a. a blue color to the skin that results from the concentration of deoxygenated hemoglobin close to the surface of the skin

b. spasm of the smooth muscles of the bronchi and/or the bronchioles that result in decreased airway diameter

c. using cupped hands to rhythmically clap on the chest wall over various segments of the lungs to mobilize secretions

d. a sudden audible, forceful expulsion of air from the lungs, usually an involuntary, reflexive action in response to an irritant

(Continued on p. 158)

18. __o__ hypoxemia

19. __t__ vibration

20. __p__ sputum

21. ____ respiration

22. __s__ ventilation

23. __f__ endotracheal tube

e. the process in which molecules move from an area of higher concentration to an area of lower concentration without the expenditure of energy, resulting in even distribution of the particles in a fluid

f. a catheter passed through the nose or mouth into the trachea for the purpose of establishing an airway

g. high carbon dioxide level in the blood, usually resulting from failure of the lungs to remove carbon dioxide

h. breathing in which the majority of ventilatory work is accomplished by the diaphragm and abdominal muscles; deliberate use of the diaphragm and abdominal muscles to control breathing

i. an approach to mobilizing and draining secretions from gravity-dependent areas of the lung that uses a combination of postural drainage, chest percussion, and vibration

j. the subjective sensation of difficulty in breathing

k. increase in the rate and depth of breathing, clinically defined as $PaCO_2$ less than 35 mm Hg

l. a method of measuring the oxygen saturation of functional hemoglobin in the blood

m. a technique in which the client assumes one or more positions that will facilitate the drainage of secretions from the bronchial airways

n. a technique of mouth breathing that creates slight resistance to exhalation by contracting the lips to reduce the size of the opening, thus maintaining an even reduction of intrathoracic pressure during exhalation

o. deficient oxygenation of the blood

p. mucus secreted from the lungs, bronchi, and trachea; may include epithelial cells, bacteria, and debris

q. a device that provides a visual goal for and measurement of inspiration, thus encouraging the client to execute and sustain maximal inspiration

r. decrease in the rate and depth of breathing, clinically defined as $PaCO_2$ greater than 45 mm Hg

s. the process of exchanging air between the ambient air and the lungs; *pulmonary ventilation* refers to the total exchange of air, whereas *alveolar ventilation* refers to the effective ventilation of the alveoli

t. a technique of chest physiotherapy whereby the chest wall is set in motion by oscillating movements of the hands or a vibrator for the purpose of mobilizing secretions

u. the exchange of oxygen and carbon dioxide between the atmosphere and the cells of the body; a series of metabolic activities by which living cells break down carbohydrates, amino acids, and fats to produce energy in the form of ATP (adenosine triphosphate)

v. deficient oxygenation of body tissues

w. coughing and spitting up blood as a result of bleeding from any part of the lower respiratory tract

TRUE OR FALSE

24. _T_ The accessory muscles of respiration become more active during forceful expiration.

25. _T_ The work of breathing is directly related to the amount of airway resistance.

26. _F_ Tidal volume is the amount of air inhaled with a deep inspiration.

27. _T_ Oxygen and carbon dioxide are exchanged through the alveolar membrane by the passive process of diffusion.

28. _F_ Fowler's position is the position of optimum ventilation/perfusion ratio. *sitting standing*

29. _T_ In the older adult, decreased compliance and elasticity increases the risk for respiratory complications during illness or surgery.

30. _F_ Nicotine patches have a 50% success rate in helping people quit smoking.

31. _F_ Fractured ribs are a type of obstructive respiratory disease.

32. _T_ Asthma is more common where there is a history of asthma in the family.

33. _T_ Ambulation is an efficient, noninvasive, inexpensive method of stimulating respiration.

34. _F_ Endotracheal suctioning is a sterile procedure without regard to the client's condition or setting.

35. _F_ Oxygen therapy is given in the lowest possible dose to maintain arterial oxygen saturation above 90%.

FILL-IN-THE-BLANKS

36. The primary muscle of respiration is the _diaphragm_.

37. _Elastic recoil_ is the tendency of the lungs to return to a nonstretched state.

38. _Surfactant_ is a lipoprotein secreted by the alveolar epithelium and acts like a detergent to reduce the surface tension and hold the alveoli open.

39. _Sighing_ stimulates the production of surfactant.

40. _Dead space_ is any surface of the airways that contains air but does not participate in gas exchange.

41. The _glottis_ is the opening at the top of the larynx between the resting vocal cords.

42. A _Complete blood count_ is the diagnostic test that provides information about the oxygen carrying capacity of the blood.

43. The _forced vital capacity_ is the volume of air forcefully (with maximum effort) exhaled after a maximum inhalation.

44. The pulse oximetry measurement is used to ensure that oxygen saturation is maintained above _95_ %.

45. _Obtundation_ describes the client rendered insensitive to painful stimuli by reducing the level of consciousness with a narcotic or anesthetic. This client has rapid shallow breathing.

46. _Thick_, _tenacious_ sputum is difficult to cough out and may be associated with dehydration.

47. The client with pain from a high abdominal surgical incision is at risk for the nursing diagnosis of _Altered breathing pattern_.

48. Cyanosis represents the presence of increased amounts of _deoxygenated hemoglobin_ in the blood.

49. _Narcan (naloxone)_ is a medication used to reverse the action of narcotics, thus stimulating respiration.

50. Three actions that are necessary to produce an effective cough are _take a deep breath_ _hold it_, _force exhalation_ and _____ _____.

EXERCISING YOUR CLINICAL JUDGMENT

51. Your client had a thoracentesis 30 minutes ago. He is complaining of shortness of breath. You listen to his lungs. Which finding indicates the possibility of the complication of atelectasis?
    a. bilateral crackles (rales) in the bases
    b. diminished breath sounds on the side where the thoracentesis was performed
    c. harsh sonorous sounds over the bifurcation of the bronchi
    d. wet, bubbling sounds over the mid-sternum

52. Select the client description that fits the definition of hypoventilation.
    a. respiratory rate of 36, with visible chest wall movement in the upper third of the chest
    b. a measured tidal volume of 500 with a rate of 12
    c. arterial carbon dioxide level of 43, oxygen saturation of 94%
    d. Respiratory rate of 10, no dyspnea, color good, skin warm and dry

53. Your client is having an asthma attack. You hear wheezes throughout the lung fields. You can attribute the sounds to:
    a. mucus in the bronchioles.
    b. atelectasis.
    c. bronchospasms.
    d. inflammation of the pleura.

54. A client who has a dry, hacking cough and wheezes throughout the lung fields would be given the nursing diagnosis of
    a. Ineffective airway clearance.
    b. Ineffective breathing pattern.
    c. Impaired gas exchange.
    d. Obstructive airway disease.

55. Your postoperative client has an order for an incentive spirometer treatment q2h for the 72 hours following surgery. He asks you why he needs this treatment when his surgery was on his abdomen. Select the best answer that represents the primary purpose of an incentive spirometer.
    a. "It will help you use all of your lungs when you breathe and prevent a respiratory infection."
    b. "It helps you maintain a maximal inspiration, thus preventing atelectasis."
    c. "It will increase the perfusion to your lungs for better arterial oxygen saturation."
    d. "It will increase the blood flow to your lungs so you can get more oxygen from the air that you breathe."

56. Your client with chronic obstructive pulmonary disease has chronic inflammation in her lungs. She is taking a corticosteroid by metered dose inhaler. She asks why she can't just take a pill. Your most accurate response would be:
    a. "Your doctor prefers a metered dose inhaler."
    b. "You can use the metered dose inhaler anytime you need it."
    c. "The medication in a pill form won't reach your lungs."
    d. "You are less likely to have the complication of failure of your adrenal glands to produce corticosteroids."

57. You observe all of the following in your client with a chest tube. Select the finding that represents the most serious complication of a chest tube.
    a. 100 cc of serosanguineous drainage in an eight-hour period
    b. itching under the pressure dressing around the chest tube
    c. air from the pleural space bubbling in the water-sealed drainage system
    d. sucking air into the pleural space through the chest tube.

TEST YOURSELF

58. The primary purpose of pursed-lip breathing is to:
    a. increase the resistance to expiration to maintain functional residual volume.
    b. help the client focus on the respiration during times of stress.
    c. increase the inspiratory capacity thus improving exercise tolerance.
    d. produce the relaxation response during times of dyspnea.

59. To correctly use a metered dose inhaler, the client should:
    a. activate the inhaler and then take a deep breath.
    b. take a deep breath and then activate the inhaler.
    c. simultaneously activate the inhaler and take a deep breath.
    d. activate the inhaler, close the mouth, and take a deep breath.

60. The primary purpose of learning diaphragmatic breathing is to:
    a. increase the strength and use of the diaphragm for exhalation.
    b. increase the strength and use of the diaphragm for inhalation.
    c. produce the relaxation response and reduce stress.
    d. increase the strength and use of the accessory muscles of respiration.

61. You are suctioning the client's airway through a tracheostomy. Select the action that is correct.
    a. Apply suction continuously as you enter the airway.
    b. Apply suction intermittently as you enter the airway.
    c. Apply suction continuously as you exit the airway.
    d. Apply suction intermittently as you exit the airway.

62. The Yankauer tip suction device is used for safety in oral suctioning because:
    a. the tip has multiple openings thus preventing damage to the oral mucosa.
    b. it can only be attached to low-suction devices.
    c. the hard plastic catheter cannot be swallowed by the client.
    d. the openings are not large enough to cause mucosal damage.

63. The primary principle of assisting the client to clear the airway is:
    a. to use the most aggressive procedure first to reduce the time needed for treatment.
    b. to use the least invasive procedure necessary to produce the desired results.
    c. to avoid invasive suctioning until the secretions are life threatening.
    d. to suction when the level of need is preventive.

64. The most serious complication of suction is represented by which of the following data?
    a. streaks of blood in the sputum
    b. oxygen saturation of 88%
    c. large amount of watery sputum
    d. moderate amounts of yellow sputum

65. Select the statement that is true of a low-flow oxygen delivery system, such as a nasal cannula.
    a. The wall mounted oxygen flow meter delivers 35–45% oxygen to the nasal cannula.
    b. 100% oxygen from the wall is mixed precisely with room air to deliver the ordered percentage of oxygen.
    c. A low-flow system can only deliver 28% oxygen.
    d. The client supplements the flow of oxygen with room air to maintain the minute ventilation.

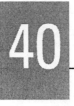
Cardiovascular Function

PURPOSE

This chapter discusses concepts of and factors affecting cardiovascular function. It uses the nursing process as a framework to discuss management of decreased tissue perfusion due to common cardiovascular problems.

LEARNING OBJECTIVES

After studying this chapter, you should be able to:

1. describe the anatomical and physiological concepts underlying the three tissue perfusion diagnoses.
2. discuss some common problems of cardiovascular function.
3. identify the lifestyle, developmental, physiological, and psychological factors affecting tissue perfusion and cardiac function.
4. explain how to assess the client at risk for problems of tissue perfusion or cardiac function, how to detect the manifestations of an actual problem, and how to recognize the client's responses to problems.
5. differentiate among nursing diagnoses used for clients with cardiovascular problems amenable to nursing care.
6. plan for goal-directed interventions to prevent or correct problems of tissue perfusion and cardiac function.
7. evaluate the outcomes of cardiac nursing care and interventions to ensure tissue perfusion.

MATCHING

1. __f.__ afterload
2. __g__ antidiuretic hormone
3. __f__ atherosclerosis
4. __a__ baroreceptors
5. __i__ cardiac output
6. __b__ claudication
7. __J.__ diastole
8. __l.__ dysrhythmias
9. __m__ edema
10. __o__ inotropic agent
11. __d__ ischemia
12. __n.__ necrosis
13. __h.__ preload
14. __q__ stroke volume
15. __e.__ systole
16. __c__ tachycardia
17. __K.__ viscosity

a. specialized cells located in the aorta and carotid bodies that detect pressure changes in the vascular system

b. cramp-like pains in the calves caused by poor circulation of blood to the leg muscles

c. a heart rate above 100 beats per minute

d. a decreased supply of oxygenated blood to tissues

e. contraction of the ventricles

f. the pressure against which the left ventricle pumps

g. a hormonal compensatory mechanism that is also called vasopressin

h. the amount of blood in the left ventricle immediately before contraction

(Continued on p. 164)

163

i. the amount of blood pumped by the ventricles in one minute

j. refers to the relaxation of the ventricles

k. the relative ability of a fluid to flow that results from the thickness of the fluid

l. abnormalities of heart rate or rhythm

m. an abnormal accumulation of fluid in the interstitial spaces of tissues, commonly known as swelling

n. localized death of tissues caused by disease, oxygen deficit, or injury.

o. medication that increases the contractility of the heart muscle, thereby increasing cardiac output

p. a pathological condition in which fat and plaque form deposits on the intimal (inner) surface of the arteries

q. the amount of blood ejected from the heart with each contraction

26. __T__ Excessive intake of high-fat foods can lead to elevated serum cholesterol levels.

27. __T__ Lack of circulation destroys nerves and impairs motor function in the involved extremity.

FILL-IN-THE-BLANKS

28. The average cardiac output is __5__ - __6__ liters per minute.

29. __Cocaine__ and __amphetamines__ are stimulants that increase heart rate and oxygen demand.

30. The primary effect of aging as a developmental factor on the circulation is the development of __atherosclerosis__.

31. Hypertension is a condition in which the blood pressure is persistently higher than __140__ / __90__ mm Hg.

32. A __cerebrovascular accident__ is the blockage of a blood vessel in the brain through thrombus, embolus, or hemorrhage, which results in ischemia or death of brain tissue distal to the insult.

33. Fluid in the lungs is a prominent symptom in __left__-sided heart failure.

34. __Iron__ is needed to manufacture oxygen-carrying hemoglobin molecules.

35. Clients who take __aspirin__ and warfarin have a dangerous risk of bleeding.

36. Antihistamines and appetite suppressants are contraindicated for clients with hypertension because they cause __vasoconstriction__

37. Lifestyle choices such as __diet__, __exercise__, and __smoking__ have direct effects on circulation.

TRUE OR FALSE

18. __T__ Highly viscous blood encounters more resistance while moving through blood vessels.

19. __F__ Starling's Law indicates that stronger recoil of cardiac muscle tissue produces weaker stroke volume. _greater_

20. __T__ Elevated blood glucose is a modifiable risk factor for cardiovascular disease.

21. __F__ Nicotine produces vasodilatation, which increases blood flow to tissues, and increases the oxygen-carrying capacity of hemoglobin.

22. __T__ Women have an increased incidence of Raynaud's disease, while men are more likely to have Buerger's disease.

23. __T__ Atherosclerotic plaque deposits create a rough spot on the normally smooth inner surface of the blood vessel.

24. __F__ Bacterial and viral infections of the heart are minor problems that leave no permanent heart damage as a result.

25. __T__ Stress increases the heart rate and blood pressure, which, in turn, raise the body's oxygen demands.

EXERCISING YOUR CLINICAL JUDGMENT

Mr. Yoder, the man introduced in the chapter case study, is a 74-year-old Amish client who has a medical diagnosis of angina pectoris and a nursing diagnosis of Altered cardiopulmonary tissue perfusion. He was admitted two days ago with chest pain and underwent cardiac catheterization yesterday. You are assigned to take care of Mr. Yoder today and must develop and implement a teaching plan before his discharge, which is planned for later this afternoon.

38. To help Mr. Yoder conserve energy in order to decrease oxygen demand, you should encourage him to:
    a. take rest breaks between daily activities such as eating, bathing, and walking.
    b. do all of his chores early in the morning provided he has had a good night's sleep.
    c. save chores for late in the day so endurance will be greater.
    d. stop all exertional activities and turn over responsibility for them to his son.

39. You would encourage Mr. Yoder to limit which of the following food items that typically has a high salt content?
    a. vegetables
    b. fresh water fish
    c. sauces
    d. fruits

40. Knowing that Mr. Yoder is being discharged with a prescription for an antihypertensive medication, which of the following general teaching points would you include in a discussion with him?
    a. take the medication when eating a heavy meal
    b. wear slippers or shoes at all times
    c. the medication should be taken whenever chest pain occurs
    d. rise out of bed or out of a chair slowly

41. In teaching Mr. Yoder to avoid the Valsalva maneuver, you would tell him it is important to avoid:
    a. drinking lots of fluids.
    b. bearing down hard when having a bowel movement.
    c. walking up and down stairs.
    d. lying flat in bed.

TEST YOURSELF

42. To determine the presence of jugular vein distention, the nurse would:
    a. raise the head of the bed to 45 degrees.
    b. turn the client onto the right side.
    c. lie the client supine in bed.
    d. turn the client onto the left side.

43. A client has had a cardiac catheterization using the right femoral artery as the access site. The nurse would report which of the following peripheral vascular findings in the client's right leg following the procedure?
    a. strong palpable pedal pulse
    b. pink skin
    c. warmth
    d. numbness and tingling

44. The nurse would assess for which of the following peripheral vascular manifestations in a client with venous disease of the lower extremities?
    a. pale, cool skin
    b. decreased pulses
    c. edema
    d. tingling and burning sensations

45. A nurse has signed out a unit of blood from the blood bank at 2 p.m. The unit must be hung by which of the following times in order to prevent bacterial contamination of the unit?
    a. 6:00 p.m.
    b. 4:00 p.m.
    c. 3:30 p.m.
    d. 2:20 p.m.

46. A nurse who has administered care to a client in shock interprets that the shock state is resolving. The nurse bases this conclusion on which of the following pieces of client data?
    a. urine output 45 mL/hour
    b. pulse rate 128 beats per minute
    c. blood pressure 92/48 mm Hg
    d. neurological confusion

Sleep and Rest

PURPOSE

This chapter introduces you to concepts central to normal sleep and rest, and the variations from normal that can occur. It describes how to use the nursing process to assist the client in meeting personal needs for sleep and rest.

LEARNING OBJECTIVES

After studying this chapter, you should be able to:

1. describe the physiological concepts underlying normal rest and sleep.
2. distinguish between dyssomnias and parasomnias and give examples of each.
3. discuss the lifestyle, environmental, developmental, and physiological factors that affect rest and sleep.
4. describe the general assessment of rest and sleep, including the sleep diary.
5. assess clients for a risk of sleep problems, manifestations of actual sleep problems, and responses to sleep problems.
6. distinguish between related diagnoses for problems of rest and sleep that are amenable to nursing care.
7. plan for goal-directed interventions that address sleep pattern disturbances and meet rest needs.
8. Evaluate outcomes of nursing care for clients with sleep pattern disturbances.

MATCHING

1. __k__ bruxism
2. __a__ circadian rhythm
3. __m__ dyssomnia
4. __v__ hypersomnia
5. __s__ hypnotic
6. __c__ insomnia
7. __h__ multiple sleep latency test
8. __g__ narcolepsy
9. __t__ nightmare
10. __p__ nonrapid eye movement sleep
11. __e__ obstructive sleep apnea
12. __r__ parasomnia
13. __f__ polysomnography
14. __x__ rapid eye movement sleep
15. __i__ rest
16. __w__ restless legs syndrome
17. __u__ sedative

a. a biorhythmic pattern that is regularly scheduled at 24-hour intervals

b. the state that results from a person not getting enough sleep

c. difficulty initiating or maintaining sleep

d. occur during slow-wave sleep and are characterized by arousal, agitation, and signs of sympathetic nervous system activity, such as dilated pupils, sweating, tachypnea, and tachycardia

e. a sleep disorder manifested by periodic cessation of airflow at the nose and mouth during inspiration, which arouses the person from sleep

(Continued on p. 168)

18. ___g___ sleep
19. ___b___ sleep deprivation
20. ___n___ sleep enuresis
21. ___a___ sleep terrors
22. ___j___ slow-wave sleep
23. ___l___ somnambulism
24. ___o___ sundowning

f. the continuous measurement and recording of physiological activity during sleep by using electroencephalogram, electro-oculogram, electrocardiogram, and electromyogram.

g. a reversible behavioral state in which perceptions of and responses to environmental stimuli are decreased, and the body is relatively quiet

h. a direct, objective measure of sleepiness used to evaluate excessive somnolence and daytime sleepiness.

i. a state of being physically and mentally relaxed while being awake and alert

j. characterized by high-voltage EEG activity and a high arousal threshold

k. a parasomnia characterized by violent, repetitive grinding of the teeth that occurs during the lighter stages of sleep or during partial arousals

l. a slow-wave sleep parasomnia associated with stereotypical "sleep-walking" behaviors

m. any sleep disturbance that involves the amount, quality, or timing of sleep

n. a parasomnia characterized by bed-wetting during sleep

o. a sleep disruption involving the nocturnal exacerbation of disruptive behaviors and agitation associated with clients who have dementia

p. a state in which a quiet brain functions in an active body

q. a striking hypersomnia characterized by abnormal sleep tendencies as well as by pathological REM sleep, manifested as excessive daytime sleepiness, disturbed nighttime sleep, cataplexy, sleep paralysis, and hypnagogic hallucinations

r. sleep disorders that are not difficulties with sleep themselves, but rather abnormal movements and behaviors that occur during sleep

s. a drug that acts on the CNS to shorten sleep onset, reduce nighttime wakefulness, or decrease anxiety when insomnia is associated with increased anxiety

t. a vivid or frightening dream that occurs during REM sleep, awakens the sleeper, and can be vividly recalled

u. a type of hypnotic drug that exerts a soothing, tranquilizing effect on the CNS, resulting in shortened sleep onset and alleviation of anxiety

v. a sleep disorder characterized by excessive sleepiness

w. an intrinsic sleep disorder characterized by intense, abnormal, lower extremity sensations and irresistible leg movements that delay sleep onset

x. a state in which a highly active brain functions in an immobilized body

TRUE OR FALSE

25. __T__ Wrist actigraphs are a newer means of measuring sleep in the client's home by application of a bracelet that records wrist movements that signal restlessness during sleep.

26. __F__ A client who is physically rested is therefore also mentally rested.

27. __T__ An electroencephalogram (EEG) can be used to distinguish among coma, sleep, and wakefulness when other assessment results are inconclusive.

28. __T__ Current thought is that a complex network of neurons passing through the medulla, pons, midbrain, thalamus, hypothalamus, and basal forebrain maintains homeostatic balance between sleep and wakefulness.

29. __F__ Restless legs syndrome is an extrinsic sleep disorder. _intrinsic_

30. __F__ A person experiencing a night terror should be awakened by others nearby.

31. __T__ The half-life of nicotine is 1–2 hours.

32. __T__ Chronic fatigue syndrome is a long-standing fatigue that lasts for six months or more.

FILL-IN-THE-BLANKS

33. A ___Zeitgeber___ is an environmental trigger or synchronizer that adjusts the body's internal clock to a 24-hour day.

34. ___Melatonin___ is the "hormone of darkness" that regulates the circadian phase of sleep.

35. A person should avoid excess coffee, tea, or chocolate near bedtime because they contain the stimulant ___Caffeine___.

36. ICU psychosis is an iatrogenic complication that is strongly correlated with ___REM___ sleep deprivation in ICUs.

37. The sleep-wake cycle is fully developed by the age of ___2___.

38. ___Narcolepsy___ is one of the few sleep disorders with a demonstrated genetic link.

39. A person with sleep apnea should avoid sleeping on the ___back___.

40. The only spice or herb that has been shown in some studies to improve the subjective quality of sleep is ___Valerian___.

EXERCISING YOUR CLINICAL JUDGMENT

Ms. Weiss, the woman introduced in the chapter case study, is experiencing transient situational insomnia that she attributes to a new job and enrollment in graduate school courses. Personal habits include drinking a glass of wine to help with sleep, and smoking cigarettes and drinking coffee throughout the day. The nurse practitioner has asked you to counsel Ms. Weiss about nonprescription treatments for her sleep disorder.

41. Knowing that caffeine has stimulant properties, you would encourage Ms. Weiss to refrain from drinking coffee after which of the following times?
    a. Noon
    b. 2 p.m.
    c. 4 p.m.
    d. 8 p.m.

42. To reduce the interference of nicotine with Ms. Weiss's sleep, you would advise her to continue to try to have the last cigarette no later than:
    a. mid-morning.
    b. at lunchtime.
    c. at suppertime.
    d. an hour before bed.

43. When discussing the Bootzin technique with Ms. Weiss, you would include which of the following points?
    a. Adjust the alarm clock nightly to a time that allows for eight hours of continuous sleep.
    b. If you cannot get to sleep after 30 minutes of trying, get up and go into another room until sleepy.
    c. Take a nap at mid-day to make up for sleep lost the previous night.
    d. Go to bed at the same time each night, regardless of whether you feel sleepy.

44.   You are instructing Ms. Weiss about progressive relaxation techniques as a method to promote sleep onset. Which of the following points would you include?
   a.   The exercises should be practiced for 45–60 minutes before going to bed.
   b.   They should be used only at bedtime but not during the night if wakefulness occurs.
   c.   They are not to be used in conjunction with deep breathing exercises.
   d.   Relaxation begins with voluntary muscles in the feet and progresses upward to the face.

TEST YOURSELF

45.   A client reports an inability to fall asleep, which is followed by awakening at night and a sense of not feeling well rested in the morning. The nurse interprets that these symptoms are defining characteristics of which of the following nursing diagnoses?
   a.   Fatigue
   b.   Sleep pattern disturbance
   c.   Anxiety
   d.   Altered thought processes

46.   The nurse who is planning behavioral outcomes for a client who has a problem with interrupted sleep would include which of the following suggestions?
   a.   does not eat heavy or fat-filled foods just before going to sleep
   b.   refrains from drinking milk before bedtime
   c.   drinks a glass of wine or beer just prior to bedtime
   d.   keeps a bedside lamp on during the night

47.   When teaching a client cognitive strategies to reduce insomnia, the nurse would encourage the client to spend 20 minutes reflecting on daytime activities and achievements:
   a.   just after getting home from work, such as around 4 p.m.
   b.   just prior to going to bed.
   c.   just after getting into bed for the night.
   d.   in the early evening after dinner.

48.   The nurse would encourage the client who has an order for a prn sleep medication to take it:
   a.   just after supper.
   b.   two hours before going to bed.
   c.   shortly before going to bed.
   d.   an hour after going to bed if not successful falling asleep.

49.   The nurse would evaluate that interventions to treat a Sleep pattern disturbance were most effective if the client states:
   a.   compliance with the interventions prescribed.
   b.   feeling well rested after sleep.
   c.   obtaining four hours of uninterrupted sleep per night.
   d.   using at least half of the methods suggested by the nurse.

Pain

PURPOSE

This chapter discusses key concepts that relate to the nursing diagnoses Chronic pain and Pain. It describes the physiological concepts supporting pain-related nursing diagnoses. It also describes the physiological concepts supporting pain-related nursing diagnoses and pathophysiological, cognitive, affective, sensory, cultural, environmental, and other variables that affect the pain experience.

LEARNING OBJECTIVES

After studying this chapter, you should be able to:

1. describe the physiological concepts supporting pain-related nursing diagnoses.
2. discuss the pathophysiological, cognitive, affective, sensory, cultural, environmental, and other variables that affect the pain experience.
3. assess the client at risk for or experiencing a pain problem and the client's responses to the experience.
4. diagnose the client's pain management needs that will respond to nursing care.
5. plan for goal-directed interventions to prevent or correct the pain diagnoses.
6. describe and practice key nonpharmacologic and pharmacologic interventions for pain management.
7. evaluate outcomes that indicate progress in providing effective pain management.

MATCHING

1. _S_ acute pain
2. _dd_ adjuvant analgesic
3. _l-_ agonist analgesic
4. _hh_ analgesia
5. _M_ antagonist
6. _V_ atypical analgesic
7. _Y_ breakthrough pain
8. _t_ chronic pain
9. _ff_ endorphin
10. _w_ epidural analgesia
11. _aa_ equianalgesia
12. _bb_ first pass effect
13. _ll_ gate control theory
14. _v_ intrathecal analgesia
15. _h_ mixed agonist-antagonist analgesic
16. _h_ modulation
17. _d_ neuropathic pain

a. an unpleasant sensory and emotional experience associated with actual and potential tissue damage

b. the process of transmitting a pain signal from a site of tissue damage to areas of the brain where perception occurs

c. pain transmitted from a site of injury to the higher brain centers along an intact nervous system

d. the transmission of a pain signal from the site of injury to the higher brain centers via a nervous system that has been temporarily or permanently damaged in some way

(Continued on p. 172)

18. ___b___ nociception
19. ___c___ nociceptive pain
20. ___ee___ nociceptor
21. ___k___ nonopioid analgesic
22. ___j___ opioid analgesic
23. ___cc___ opioid naive
24. ___i___ opioid receptor
25. ___a___ pain
26. ___r___ pain behavior
27. ___x___ patient-controlled analgesia
28. ___p___ physical dependence
29. ___q___ psychological dependence
30. ___g___ referred pain
31. ___z___ rescue dose
32. ___e___ somatic pain
33. ___q___ suffering
34. ___o___ tolerance
35. ___f___ visceral pain

e. well-located pain, usually bone or spinal metastases or from injury to cutaneous or deep tissues

f. poorly localized pain

g. pain experienced at a site distant from the injured tissue

h. an internal or external restraining of the nociceptive process that inhibits transmission of the pain signal at any place along the transmission pathway

i. a portion of a nerve cell to which an opioid or opiate-like substance can bind

j. morphine-like drug that attaches to an opioid receptor and produces analgesia by blocking substance P

k. a drug that provides analgesia at the peripheral level by a mechanism other than the opioid receptor sites

l. an opioid that stimulates activity at an opioid receptor to produce analgesia

m. blocks activity at *mu* and *kappa* opioid receptors by displacing opioid analgesics that are currently attached

n. formulation that attaches to both the *kappa* and *mu* receptor sites

o. an involuntary physiological phenomenon that occurs after repeated exposure to an opioid analgesic; it involves a decreased-level pain relief despite a stable or escalating opioid dosage

p. an involuntary physiological phenomenon that occurs after repeated exposure to an opioid analgesic

q. a chronic disorder demonstrated by overwhelming involvement with obtaining and using a drug for its mind-altering effects

r. anything a person says or does that infers the presence of pain

s. short-term, self-limiting pain with a probable duration of less than six months

t. long-term, constant or recurring pain without an anticipated or predictable end and a duration of more than six months

u. drugs not primarily indicated for pain but used to treat specific types of pain

v. a catheter is placed in the subarachnoid space between the dura mater and the spinal cord to allow immediate drug diffusion into the cerebrospinal fluid

w. a catheter is placed between the spinal vertebrae and the dura mater to allow the diffusion of an analgesic drug across the dura mater into the cerebrospinal fluid

x. a drug-delivery approach that uses an external infusion pump to deliver an opioid dose on a "client-demand" basis

y. intermittent episodes of pain that occur despite continued use of an analgesic

z. as-needed dose of an immediate-release analgesic in response to breakthrough pain and in addition to the scheduled analgesic dosage

aa. the dosage that provides the same amount of pain relief independent of the drug or the route bb. the partial metabolism of opioid analgesics by the liver before they reach the systemic circulation, thereby resulting in a decrease in opioid availability (dosage)

cc. those who have had minimal or no exposure to opioid analgesics

dd. any medication that may increase analgesic efficacy, thus allowing for a smaller opioid dosage

ee. the primary afferent fibers that initiate the pain experience when stimulated by tissue damage

ff. a group of internally secreted opiate-like substances released by a signal from the cerebral cortex

gg. unpleasant emotional response to pain

hh. a reduction in the perception or experience of pain

ii. hypothesizes an alteration in the transmission of the ascending pain signal by a spinal gating mechanism located in the dorsal horn; the pain signal may be inhibited or facilitated by multiple variables

TRUE OR FALSE

36. __T__ Pain is primarily a protective mechanism, but it is also a complex biopsychosocial phenomenon.

37. __F__ Visceral pain is well-localized pain, usually from bone or spinal metastases or from injury to cutaneous or deep tissues. _somatic_

38. __T__ A single disorder may have components of both nociceptive and neuropathic pain.

39. __T__ Educating a client about what to expect during a painful procedure decreases the pain's intensity and controls pain behaviors.

40. __T__ Pain is the actual physical sensation of discomfort, while suffering is the unpleasant emotional response.

41. __F__ Pain is a normal part of aging.

42. __T__ The administration schedule of analgesia should be based on the known half-life of the drug.

FILL-IN-THE-BLANKS

43. Pain functions as a __diagnostic__ tool, an assessment variable, and a measure of __response__ interventions.

44. __Referred__ pain is experienced at a site distant from the injured tissue.

45. Behavioral expressions of pain are __learned__ from others.

46. __Chronic__ pain can quickly deplete a person's physical and emotional resources, immobilize the person, and lead to physical disability and subsequent loss of employment.

47. Once you choose a __pain rating scale__ for a client, continue to use the same scale throughout your ongoing assessment to keep the responses as comparable as possible over time.

48. Clients with __neuropathic__ pain commonly have trouble finding adequate words to describe the sensation.

49. Nonmalignant etiologies are more likely to produce __neuropathic__ pain, which tends to be difficult to treat and, at times, more disabling than cancer pain.

EXERCISING YOUR CLINICAL JUDGMENT

50. Mr. Joseph Valdez, the client from the chapter's case study, was born in Mexico City. He has recurrent gastric carcinoma and he hurts most of the time. His brothers told him to be tough and that he could "beat this thing." They were encouraging him to remain stoic even in the presence of severe pain. This is an example of which of the following?
    a. religious beliefs
    b. psychosocial modifiers
    c. cultural norms
    d. aggravating and relieving variables

51. Mr. Valdez is being admitted to an oncology unit for epidural catheter placement. He is experiencing unrelieved and severe pain. Which of the following nursing diagnoses would be appropriate?
    a. Ineffective individual coping
    b. Hopelessness
    c. Pain
    d. Chronic pain

52. Mr. Valdez experiences breakthrough pain, which is an intermittent episode of pain that occurs despite continued use of an analgesic. You treat him with rescue dosing, which means that you:
    a. call his physician and request he receive a more effective analgesic.
    b. give him a one-time extra dose of his analgesic.
    c. change the schedule of his analgesic to be more effective.
    d. give him as-needed doses of an immediate-release analgesic in response to the breakthrough pain in addition to the scheduled analgesic dosage.

TEST YOURSELF

53. Which type of pain is described as squeezing, pressure, cramping, distention, or deep stretching?
    a. somatic
    b. visceral
    c. referred
    d. neuropathic

54. Your client develops withdrawal symptoms if the opioid is abruptly withdrawn or an opioid antagonist is administered. This is considered which of the following?
    a. tolerance
    b. physical dependence
    c. psychological dependence
    d. pseudo-addiction

55. You use a pain rating scale that is a 10-centimeter horizontal line. At its left endpoint is written *No pain at all*. At its right endpoint is written *Worst pain imaginable*. What type of pain rating scale is this?
    a. self-report rating scale
    b. verbal descriptor scale
    c. numerical rating scale
    d. a visual analog scale

56. In the frail elderly the most sensitive indicator of pain may be which of the following?
    a. crying out in pain
    b. moaning
    c. an observed decrease in the client's usual level of functioning
    d. facial grimacing

57. If your client is receiving an opioid analgesic for acute or chronic pain and her respiratory rate is significantly affected (fewer than 8 breaths per minute), the appropriate intervention is which of the following?
    a. stop the opioid analgesic until respiratory rate returns to normal
    b. slowly push intravenously 0.4 of Narcan which has been diluted in normal saline to equal 10 cc until an adequate respiratory rate returns but pain relief remains intact
    c. quickly push intravenously 0.4 of Narcan which has been diluted in normal saline to equal 10 cc until an adequate respiratory rate returns but pain relief remains intact
    d. give an intramuscular (IM) injection of 0.4 of Narcan which has been diluted in normal saline to equal 10 cc

Sensory / Perceptual Function

PURPOSE

This chapter discusses key concepts that relate to the nursing diagnoses Sensory/perceptual alteration (visual, auditory, kinesthetic, gustatory, tactile, olfactory). It describes the normal physiology of sensation and perception, and a variety of factors affecting sensory/perceptual function.

LEARNING OBJECTIVES

After studying this chapter, you should be able to:

1. describe the normal physiology of sensation and perception.
2. differentiate among sensory deficit, sensory deprivation, and sensory overload.
3. discuss a variety of factors affecting sensory/perceptual function.
4. describe techniques for assessing a client at risk for sensory/perceptual alterations, the manifestations of a sensory/perceptual alterations, and the client's responses to sensory/perceptual alterations.
5. differentiate among the related diagnoses for the problems of sensory/perceptual alterations that are amenable to nursing care.
6. plan goal-directed nursing interventions to manage sensory/perceptual alterations.
7. evaluate outcomes for sensory/perceptual alterations to determine effectiveness of nursing care.

MATCHING

1. _i_ auditory
2. _e_ chemoreceptors
3. _c_ exteroceptors
4. _j_ gustatory
5. _o_ interoceptors
6. _m_ kinesthetic
7. _l_ olfactory
8. _s_ ototoxic
9. _b_ perception
10. _d_ proprioceptors
11. _g_ presbycusis
12. _f_ presbyopia
13. _p_ reticular activating system
14. _a_ sensation
15. _q_ sensory deprivation
16. _r_ sensory overload
17. _n_ somesthetic
18. _k_ tactile
19. _h_ visual

a. the reception of stimulation through receptors of the nervous system

b. the conscious mental recognition or registration of a sensory stimulus; for example, when a person smells a sweet fragrance and gets a mental image of a cherry

c. sensory receptors located in the skin and mucous membranes and are stimulated by touch, light, pressure, pain, temperature, odor, sound, and light

d. sensory receptors located chiefly in muscle, tendons, and inner ear

e. specialized cells adapted for excitation or simulation by various chemicals

(Continued on p. 176)

f. a loss of near vision in older people; develops because the crystalline lens loses elasticity and the ciliary muscles, which focus the lens by changing its shape, begin to weaken

g. a sensorineural hearing loss of high frequency tones that occurs in the elderly and may lead to a loss of all hearing frequencies

h. for the sensation of sight

i. for the sensation of hearing

j. for the sensation of taste

k. for the sensation of touch

l. for the sensation of smell

m. for the sensation of position

n. pertains to sensations and sensory structures of the body

o. sensory receptors located in the viscera and blood vessels

p. located in the midbrain and thalamus, keeps the brain aroused

q. inadequate reception or perception of environmental stimuli

r. results from excessive environmental stimuli or a level of stimuli beyond the person's ability to absorb or comprehend it

s. having a damaging effect on cranial nerve VIII or the organs of hearing and balance

TRUE OR FALSE

20. _F_ Nurses observe sensory deficits more commonly in infants because of age-related changes in their sense organs. *elderly*

21. _T_ The cerebral cortex must be alerted or aroused to perceive and produce a conscious act in response to stimuli.

22. _T_ Taste sensations decline normally with age.

23. _T_ Adolescents are at risk for hearing loss if they are exposed to chronic loud noise.

24. _F_ The Weber and Rhinne tests are auditory screening tests used to evaluate the client for high-frequency hearing loss. *Conduction or sensory neural hearing loss*

25. _T_ Ageusia is the complete loss of taste.

26. _F_ A hearing aid will not be damaged by x-ray examinations.

FILL-IN-THE-BLANKS

27. The human body has six types of _Somesthetic_ receptors, which pertain to sensations and sensory structures of the body.

28. _Extero receptors_ are sensory receptors located in the skin and mucous membranes and are stimulated by touch, light pressure, pain, temperature, odor, sound, and light.

29. _Strabismus_ is commonly called crossed eyes and occurs in about 5% of children under the age of four years.

30. A _Conductive_ loss results from a problem in the outer and middle ear that reduces sensitivity to tones received by air conduction.

31. The sensation of smell declines with _age_, nerve damage, or the presence of other odors in the nasal passages.

32. The _Snellen_ alphabet chart is used most commonly and appropriately for adults and older children to test their visual acuity.

33. Corneal _staining_ is indicated for diagnosis of corneal trauma, foreign bodies, corneal abrasions, or corneal ulcers.

34. The client hospitalized in an intensive care unit following major trauma or surgery is at risk for sensory _overload_.

EXERCISING YOUR CLINICAL JUDGMENT

35. Mrs. Pfannenstiel, the client from the chapter's case study, was most likely having difficulty doing which of the following things if she was scheduled for cataract surgery?
    a. driving at night
    b. selecting clothes that matched
    c. reading a book since letters appeared small
    d. reading a book because she had double vision

36. Mrs. Pfannenstiel was scheduled for cataract surgery. Which nursing diagnosis would be most appropriate?
    a. Social isolation
    b. High risk for injury
    c. Sensory/perceptual alterations: visual
    d. Self-care deficit

37. You instructed Mrs. Pfannenstiel to wear glasses, tape the metal shield over her operated eye at night, and not do heavy work, such as moving her furniture. Which nursing diagnosis would be most appropriate?
    a. Social isolation
    b. Risk for injury
    c. Sensory/perceptual alterations: visual
    d. Self-care deficit

TEST YOURSELF

38. Your client has double vision, which is also called:
    a. presbyopia.
    b. emmetropia.
    c. diplopia.
    d. ametropia.

39. Your elderly client has a hearing loss of high-frequency tones that may lead to a loss of all hearing frequencies. What type of hearing loss is this?
    a. presbycusis
    b. partial deafness
    c. conductive loss
    d. sensorineural

40. During your general assessment of your client's sensory/perceptual status, you asked your client if she was experiencing any numbness or tingling. Which of the following areas were you assessing?
    a. hearing
    b. sensation
    c. vision
    d. taste

41. You assessed bone condition by placing the base of a vibrating tuning fork on the client's mastoid process and noting how many seconds passed before he could no longer hear it. Which of the following tests were you performing?
    a. Weber
    b. Rinne
    c. whisper
    d. finger-rubbing

42. Your 80-year-old client has had a progressive hearing loss over the past 8 months, has refused to participate in activities at the skilled nursing facility, and has often been found alone in his room. Which nursing diagnosis would be most appropriate?
    a. Social isolation
    b. Altered thought processes
    c. Sensory/perceptual alterations: auditory
    d. Self-care deficit

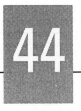
Impaired Verbal Communication

PURPOSE

This chapter introduces you to the physiological and behavioral concepts underlying impaired verbal communication. The chapter explores factors that affect communication and uses the nursing process as a framework for working with a client who has impaired verbal communication.

LEARNING OBJECTIVES

After studying this chapter, you should be able to:

1. describe the physiological and behavioral concepts underlying impaired verbal communication.

2. discuss the most common lifestyle, developmental, physiological, and psychological factors affecting communication.

3. assess the client who is at risk for impaired communication, who has actual impaired communication, or who has a related nursing diagnosis.

4. diagnose the problems of impaired communication that are amenable to nursing interventions.

5. plan nursing interventions to prevent or correct impaired verbal communication based on client goals.

6. implement key interventions for a client with impaired verbal communication.

7. evaluate outcomes for impaired verbal communication to determine the effectiveness of nursing care.

MATCHING

1. ____ aphasia
2. ____ articulation
3. ____ Broca's area
4. ____ communication
5. ____ dysarthria
6. ____ dysphagia
7. ____ dysphonia
8. ____ neologism
9. ____ paraphasia
10. ____ phonation
11. ____ resonance
12. ____ Wernicke's area

a. difficulty swallowing

b. a word substitution problem of the aphasic client who speaks fluently

c. helps control the content of speech and affects auditory and visual comprehension

d. the process of molding sounds into enunciated words and phrases

e. the production of sound by the vibration of the vocal cords

f. the forced vibration of a structure that is related to a source of sound and results in changes in the quality of the sound

g. a complex process in which information is exchanged between two or more people

(Continued on p. 180)

h. difficulty produc-
    ing vocal sounds

i. a language disorder
    that results from
    brain damage or
    disease that in-
    volves speech
    centers in the brain

j. the creation of
    words that are
    meaningless to the
    listener; a com-
    mon language
    problem of the
    aphasic client

k. the center of
    motor speech
    control

l. impaired articula-
    tion

TRUE OR FALSE

13. ____ Most voice disorders result from vocal
    abuse, which can cause such problems as
    vocal nodules, polyps, and traumatic
    laryngitis.

14. ____ Although verbal communication varies
    from culture to culture, nonverbal commu-
    nication remains the same.

15. ____ A stimulating environment for a very
    young child aids in language acquisition.

16. ____ Since it is difficult to hide emotions from
    other people, including clients, the nurse's
    emotions can and should be discussed with
    clients.

17. ____ Self-concept plays a major role in communi-
    cation patterns with other people.

18. ____ The use of a team approach is often neces-
    sary when working with a client who has
    impaired verbal communication.

19. ____ Active listening, when used with the client
    with impaired verbal communication,
    focuses on the feelings of the client as well
    as nonverbal cues.

20. ____ Psychiatric illnesses do not affect communi-
    cation with others.

21. ____ During verbal communication, a nurse
    should speak slowly and naturally to a
    client.

22. ____ The risk for misunderstanding is greatest
    when the client and nurse speak each
    other's languages somewhat, but not
    fluently.

FILL-IN-THE-BLANKS

23. Adult loss of language usually stems from
    _____ diseases.

24. _____ speech is telegram-like
    speech that lacks grammatical elements, such as
    articles, prepositions, and conjunctions.

25. When the client cannot comprehend spoken
    language and cannot articulate or write words,
    it is called _____ aphasia.

26. A disorder of voice volume, quality, or pitch,
    known as _____, can result from
    damage or disease of the larynx or vagus nerve.

27. A _____ is a temporary or permanent
    upper airway diversion that results in altered
    speech production.

28. The nurse should allow ample time for the
    client with _____ aphasia to respond
    verbally to the nurse.

29. An alternative communication method for the
    client who has had a laryngectomy is the use of
    _____ speech, which involves eructa-
    tion of swallowed air.

30. Limiting environmental stimuli and reducing
    distractions may increase comprehension in the
    client with _____ aphasia.

31. A client who is unable to communicate due to
    language barrier, and who has no one who can
    interpret, is likely to have a nursing diagnosis
    of _____.

32. An endotracheal tube, tracheostomy or tumor is
    considered to be a _____ barrier to
    communication.

EXERCISING YOUR CLINICAL JUDGMENT

Señor Martinez, the man identified in the chapter case
study, is a Mexican-American client who has tuberculosis, a communicable disease. You have been asked
by the nurse who admitted this client to provide information needed to manage this health problem.

33. If you become concerned that Señor Martinez is responding "yes" to your questions without fully understanding them, you should:
    a. look for incongruity between the responses and the client's facial expressions.
    b. assume that he will answer the important questions correctly.
    c. ask the same question of his wife after the client answers.
    d. refrain from asking any further questions.

34. After obtaining an interpreter to assist with communication, you would direct your attention to which of the following individuals when obtaining information from Señor Martinez?
    a. the interpreter
    b. Señora Martinez
    c. Señor Martinez
    d. attend equally to all three

35. If Señor Martinez speaks English to some extent, it would be most appropriate for you to communicate about which of the following before an interpreter becomes available?
    a. reason for coming to the hospital
    b. informed consent
    c. reason for procedures
    d. medication information

36. You would formulate which of the following expected outcomes for the nursing diagnosis of Impaired verbal communication for this client?
    a. answers all questions correctly
    b. expresses satisfaction with the communication process
    c. provides nurse with sufficient information
    d. adheres to instructions given while in the hospital

TEST YOURSELF

37. A nurse would assess the client with a tentative diagnosis of laryngitis for speech that is:
    a. hoarse or soft.
    b. spoken in a monotone.
    c. garbled.
    d. hesitant or deliberate.

38. A client is scheduled to have a tracheostomy performed. The nurse should make alternate plans for communication with this client:
    a. before the surgery is done.
    b. just after the client returns from surgery.
    c. on the day following surgery.
    d. as part of the discharge planning process.

39. The home health nurse notes that a client with Impaired verbal communication is frustrated about ineffective communication skills and does not interact with family and friends as frequently as before. The nurse would tentatively make which of the following nursing diagnoses for this client?
    a. Anxiety
    b. Powerlessness
    c. Impaired social interaction
    d. Altered role performance

40. The nurse is communicating with a client who has Broca's aphasia. It would be most appropriate to do which of the following to enhance the client's ability to speak?
    a. Give directions in concise, quick, and sharp tones.
    b. Ask the client several questions at once so the client can formulate answers to all.
    c. Give lengthy, detailed explanations.
    d. Allow ample time for the client to respond to the nurse's communications.

41. The nurse is providing health teaching to adolescents about the risk of brain and spinal cord injuries, which often result in impaired verbal communication. The nurse would encourage these individuals to avoid using which of the following?
    a. drugs and alcohol
    b. seatbelts
    c. helmets
    d. protective sports equipment

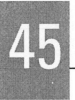

Confusion

PURPOSE

This chapter explores factors that affect normal cognition and concepts that underlie acute and chronic confusion. It describes how to use the nursing process to work with the client experiencing either acute or chronic confusion.

LEARNING OBJECTIVES

After studying this chapter, you should be able to:

1. describe the physiological concepts underlying acute or chronic confusion.
2. identify the lifestyle, environmental, developmental, psychological, and physiological factors affecting normal cognition.
3. assess a client at risk for confusion, the manifestations of confusion, and client responses to confusion.
4. diagnose the problems of a confused client that are amenable to nursing care.
5. plan for goal-directed interventions to prevent, correct and support a client with confusion.
6. describe interventions designed to prevent or reduce confusion.
7. evaluate the outcomes of nursing care for the confused client and the client's caretakers.

MATCHING

1. _e_ affect
2. _g_ agnosia
3. _n_ apraxia
4. _f_ attention
5. _c_ awareness

6. _j_ cognition
7. _i_ confusion
8. _a_ consciousness
9. _o_ delirium
10. _c_ delusions
11. _k_ dementia
12. _m_ hallucinations
13. _p_ judgment
14. _b_ memory
15. _d_ orientation
16. _h_ pseudo-dementia

a. the state of being awake and alert enough to react to stimuli; also called awareness

b. the retention or storage of information learned about the world

c. false personal beliefs

d. an awareness of person, place, and time

e. the observable expression of feelings or emotions

f. the ability to focus on an object or activity

g. the failure to recognize or identify objects despite an intact sensory ability

h. depression that is misinterpreted as dementia

i. the state in which the individual experiences or is at risk of experiencing a disturbance in cognition, attention, memory, and orientation of an undetermined origin or onset

(Continued on p. 184)

j. the process of knowing and interacting with the world; also called thought

k. involves multiple cognitive deficits including impairment of memory and judgment, and resulting in a progressive decline in intellectual functioning

l. the state of being awake and alert enough to react to stimuli; also called consciousness

m. sensory reactions in the absence of real stimuli

n. the inability to carry out motor activities despite the functional ability to perform them

o. a disturbance in consciousness or a change in cognition that develops over a short period of time

p. the ability to make rational decisions

TRUE OR FALSE

17. _F_ Confusion is a condition that occurs only in the older adult.

18. _T_ Acute confusion in the older adult usually develops over hours or days.

19. _T_ Perceptual difficulties, such as illusions and hallucinations, may occur in acute confusion.

20. _F_ Because cognitive changes occur more slowly with chronic confusion, the client does not lose the ability to judge his or her own safety.

21. _T_ The loss of ability to perform activities of daily living occurs in the third stage of chronic confusion.

22. _T_ Lack of an appropriate and complete mental status examination can be a barrier to identifying confusion.

23. _T_ A child who develops a high fever is at risk for experiencing acute confusion.

24. _F_ The nurse should not include attention span when conducting a mental status exam.

25. _T_ Anxiety is a common client reaction in both acute and chronic confusion.

26. _F_ The nurse should use pale muted colors on symbols used to identify the room of a client with chronic confusion.

FILL-IN-THE-BLANKS

27. Pick's disease is characterized by the formation of Pick's cells in the _frontal_ and _temporal_ lobes of the brain.

28. Cerebral hypoxia due to a medical condition can cause _acute_ confusion.

29. Acute confusion in the older adult typically occurs at _night_.

30. A disrupted _circadian_ rhythm is a classic symptom of acute confusion.

31. Dementia of the _Alzheimers_ type is the most common in older adults.

32. A person who cannot interpret proverbs during an assessment has a loss of _abstract_ thinking.

33. A client who does not brush the hair due to lack of recall about the purpose of the hairbrush is said to have an _apraxia_.

34. Often an older adult will exhibit a change in mental status with a serious infection instead of a _fever_.

35. A client who can recall people and events from 30 years ago is said to have an intact _remote_ memory.

36. A client who is unaware of environmental hazards due to confusion may have the nursing diagnosis Risk for _injury_.

EXERCISING YOUR CLINICAL JUDGMENT

Mr. Tellis, the man identified in the chapter case study, has a nursing diagnosis of *Acute confusion related to disturbances in cerebral metabolism secondary to urinary tract infection as evidenced by agitation, inattention, and fluctuating consciousness.* You have been assigned to work with Mr. Tellis on the day after hospital admission.

37. One of the expected outcomes formulated for Mr. Tellis in relation to this nursing diagnosis is "client will experience no injury." Which of the following actions would be most helpful in achieving this outcome?
    a. Restrict visitors as much as possible.
    b. Assist with ambulation and toileting as needed.
    c. Leave bed side rails lowered at all times.
    d. Encourage him to stay in bed by obstructing the path to the bathroom with chairs.

38. Which of the following approaches to communicating with Mr. Tellis will be helpful in minimizing confusion and maintaining the client's dignity?
    a. Divide his care among several staff members.
    b. Give directions quickly and with a firm tone of voice.
    c. Focus on his real message and concerns during conversation.
    d. Quiz him about orientation level with each encounter.

39. Mr. Tellis lost most of his last night's sleep with the events surrounding admission. Which of the following strategies should be used to help re-establish his sleep-wake pattern?
    a. Schedule medications and care to allow for at least one uninterrupted four-hour block of sleep each night.
    b. Make sure all visitors go home for the night by at least 8 p.m.
    c. Keep the door to his room open with the hall lights on.
    d. Encourage frequent naps during the day in case there are unexpected interruptions to sleep at night.

40. Mr. Tellis requires intermittent re-orientation to his environment. Which of the following environmental cues would be most helpful?
    a. bright lighting 24 hours a day
    b. no lighting during nighttime hours
    c. name of caregivers written on a small pad on the night table
    d. clock and calendar on wall at foot of bed

TEST YOURSELF

41. A nurse is conducting a mental status examination for a client newly immigrated to the United States. Which of the following questions, if asked by the nurse, would be least helpful in determining whether confusion is present?
    a. "What is your name?"
    b. "What did you eat for breakfast?"
    c. "Did any family members visit you today?"
    d. "Who was the first president of the United States?"

42. The nurse who is working with a client with chronic confusion would not assess which of the following factors?
    a. impaired socialization
    b. a change in level of consciousness
    c. long-standing cognitive impairment
    d. altered response to stimuli

43. A client has been placed in a protective environment due to chronic confusion and irreversible dementia. The client has been disoriented to person, place, and time for at least six months. The nurse would choose which of the following most precise nursing diagnoses for this client?
    a. Acute confusion
    b. Chronic confusion
    c. Impaired environmental interpretation syndrome
    d. Altered thought processes

44. A nurse is caring for a client who seems confused, and also lost a spouse three months ago. The nurse would determine that the client is experiencing feelings of depression more than confusion if the client:
    a. is worse in the morning than any other time of day.
    b. has visual hallucinations.
    c. is not preoccupied by certain people or events.
    d. does not exaggerate and is unaware of inabilities.

45. A confused client is hallucinating that someone is trying to steal the client's clothing in the closet. The nurse who is looking for a deeper meaning to this episode would pursue which of the following themes in conversation with this client?
    a. money
    b. safety
    c. food
    d. loneliness

Self-Concept

PURPOSE

This chapter introduces you to self-concept, self-esteem, personal identity, role performance, and body image as they relate to clients. It provides direction in using the nursing process in caring for a client with an alteration in one or more of the components of self-concept.

LEARNING OBJECTIVES

After studying this chapter, you should be able to:

1. differentiate among self-concept, self-esteem, personal identity, role performance, and body image.
2. discuss factors affecting self-concept.
3. assess responses of clients who may be at risk for changes in self-esteem or body image.
4. write a nursing diagnosis and develop a care plan for a client experiencing a problem with alterations in the components of self-concept.
5. plan for goal-directed interventions that address the identified nursing diagnoses.
6. describe and practice key interventions for clients who are experiencing alterations in self-esteem and body image.
7. evaluate the client's progress versus expected outcomes for alterations in self-esteem and body image.

MATCHING

1. ____ body image
2. ____ personal identity
3. ____ role performance
4. ____ self-concept
5. ____ self-esteem

a. a relatively enduring set of attitudes and beliefs about both the physical self and the psychological self

b. includes the roles a person assumes or is given

c. the organizing principle of the personality that accounts for the unity, continuity, consistency, and uniqueness of a person.

d. the degree to which a person has a positive evaluation of self based on perceptions of how one is viewed by others as well as view of the self.

e. a person's perception of his or her body

TRUE OR FALSE

6. ____ Self-concept is not a static state but one that develops and changes over time.

7. ____ Low self-esteem can result in lack of confidence and inability to act in one's own best interest.

8. ____ According to Maslow, self-esteem develops before the need for belonging and being loved by others is met.

9. ____ Erikson describes the development of self-esteem in eight stages that correspond to a period in the life span.

10. ____ Research has demonstrated a negative correlation between positive self-esteem and positive health practices.

11. ____ An inability to perform role responsibilities can negatively affect other aspects of self-concept, especially self-esteem.

12. ____ Socioeconomic status has no relationship to self-concept.

13. ____ Loss of a spouse, good job, or previous good health can easily lower self-esteem.

14. ____ Fatigue, illness, and surgery are examples of physiological factors that can affect self-esteem.

15. ____ Nurses should conduct an in-depth assessment of self-concept with all clients.

FILL-IN-THE-BLANKS

16. The four components of self-concept are self-esteem, personal identity, role performance, and _____ _____.

17. At the top of Maslow's hierarchy of needs is _____-_____.

18. According to Erikson's stages of development, adolescence involves development of _____.

19. The ability to influence and control others, according to Coopersmith, is termed _____/_____.

20. The components of personal identity are _____, _____, and _____ images.

21. Self-esteem in infants and preschoolers can be related to the type of _____ a child receives.

22. Behaviors such as smoking, overeating, substance abuse, school difficulties, and early sexual experimentation can be associated with low _____-_____.

23. The client's affective experience of the self, manifested as any negative self-feelings, is the defining characteristic for the nursing diagnosis of _____-_____ _____.

24. A sense of powerlessness can result in the nursing diagnosis of _____ low self-esteem.

25. If the client has a major change in body structure or function, the nurse should assess that client for the presence of the nursing diagnosis _____ _____ _____.

EXERCISING YOUR CLINICAL JUDGMENT

Nancy Ward, the 43-year-old Navajo woman introduced in the chapter case study, has a nursing diagnosis of Self-esteem disturbance due to a breast mass that requires biopsy. Recall that Nancy's husband, who died six months ago from complications of alcohol abuse, diabetes, and heart disease, abused her physically and emotionally during their marriage. You see Nancy in the clinic when she comes to receive the biopsy results.

26. If you were focusing on the influence of her husband's behavior on Nancy's self-concept, you might have selected which of the following alternate nursing diagnoses?
    a. Situational low self-esteem
    b. Chronic low self-esteem
    c. Altered role performance
    d. Body image disturbance

27. If you were to focus on how to promote Nancy's feelings of acceptance/worthiness as part of her self-esteem, you would include which of the following people in her care?
    a. physician and nurse manager of the clinic
    b. tribal medicine man (Shaman) and friend that came to clinic with her
    c. clinic social worker and billing clerk
    d. radiologist and continuing care nurse from the affiliated hospital

28. Nancy is told by the physician that the breast mass is cancerous and that surgery will be needed. You would interact with Nancy expecting that her first reaction will be one of:
    a. shock and disbelief.
    b. anger.
    c. depression.
    d. acceptance.

29. In trying to assist Nancy to adjust to the idea of the loss of a breast, you could inquire whether she is interested in talking to:
    a. the surgeon who took the breast biopsy.
    b. the pathologist who did the examination of the breast tissue.
    c. someone from Reach to Recovery who has loss a breast herself.
    d. the staff who will be doing her pre-admission testing before surgery.

30. To foster a sense of power and control in Nancy about her upcoming surgery, you would use which of the following approaches?
    a. Remind Nancy that emotional healing is a matter of determination and courage.
    b. Tell her of the scheduled date for surgery as soon as it is known.
    c. Give her a list of instructions that must be followed before the surgery.
    d. Allow her to make as many decisions about the upcoming procedure as possible.

TEST YOURSELF

31. The nurse who is teaching a client with a new colostomy about colostomy care and management is indirectly increasing the client's sense of:
    a. competence/mastery.
    b. power/control.
    c. moral worth/virtue.
    d. acceptance/worthiness.

32. To reduce the impact of a recent loss on the client's self-concept, the nurse would assist the client to focus on:
    a. past religious habits.
    b. personal successful coping skills.
    c. the importance of forgetting negative events.
    d. the negative attributes of the object of the loss.

33. The nurse would look for other evidence of low self-esteem in a client who:
    a. accepts compliments with grace and ease.
    b. takes negative feedback from others in stride.
    c. continually seeks acceptance from others.
    d. is proud of personal accomplishments, but not boastful.

34. The nurse would determine that the client most at risk for developing issues with self-concept is one who:
    a. must take medication for allergies.
    b. gets short of breath after walking up two flights of stairs.
    c. has a gallbladder that must be removed.
    d. has suffered facial burns.

35. A postoperative client who is also the mother of four is overexerting herself with housework and childcare responsibilities. In working with this client, the nurse incorporates the understanding that this client is experiencing a values conflict in which of the following areas of self-esteem?
    a. competence/mastery
    b. power/control
    c. moral worth/virtue
    d. acceptance/worthiness

36. The nurse is evaluating effects of an intervention on a client's self-concept. If the nurse were interested in using a subjective approach to evaluation, that nurse would select which of the following methods as most appropriate?
    a. the client's self-report of progress
    b. a standardized questionnaire
    c. a rating scale
    d. observation of the client's behavior

Anxiety

PURPOSE

This chapter introduces you to concepts of anxiety as they are manifested in the health care setting. It uses the nursing process as a framework for interacting with clients experiencing anxiety.

LEARNING OBJECTIVES

After studying this chapter, you should be able to:

1. describe the concepts of anxiety as manifested in the health care setting.
2. assess the anxious client to determine level of anxiety.
3. differentiate between normal and pathological anxiety.
4. plan for goal-directed interventions to prevent, reduce, or manage anxiety.
5. evaluate achievement of the expected outcomes for the client who is experiencing anxiety.

MATCHING

1. _d_ anxiety
2. _a_ anxiety disorder
3. _b_ anxiolytics
4. _c_ pathological anxiety

a. a disorder that is accompanied by a relentless, ineffective mechanism designed to compel the person to lessen the supposed danger that is triggering the anxiety response

b. anti-anxiety medications used primarily to treat anxiety disorders

c. a disproportionate anxiety response to a given stimulus by virtue of its intensity or duration

d. a diffuse, highly uncomfortable, sometimes vague sense of apprehension or dread accompanied by one or more physical sensations

TRUE OR FALSE

5. _T_ Anxiety is caused by interplay of factors that can be internal, external or both.

6. _T_ A person can actually create or worsen his or her own anxiety.

7. _T_ When a client is in a state of panic, he or she may faint or freeze.

8. _F_ Anxiety disorders are fairly uncommon in today's society due to the number of medications available.

9. _T_ A phobia is a specific type of fear that is often exaggerated and incapacitating.

10. __T__ A healthy lifestyle does not make us immune to stress, but may help us to weather it better.

11. __F__ Learning theory suggests that anxiety is not a learned behavior.

12. __T__ Cognitive characteristics of anxiety can include blocking of thoughts, forgetfulness, and impaired concentration or problem-solving ability.

13. __T__ The nursing diagnosis of Fear is appropriate when the client has an intense feeling of dread related to an identifiable source that the client can verify.

14. __F__ A panic attack is a repetitive, stereotyped behavior that one feels compelled to carry out despite some conviction that the behavior is unrealistic.

FILL-IN-THE-BLANKS

15. Anxiety can be considered as falling into one of two primary categories, either a threat to __Biological__ integrity or a threat to __ego__ integrity.

16. A core dynamic theme found at all levels of anxiety is a sense of __vulnerability__.

17. In the level of anxiety that is __Severe__, the person's perceptual field is completely distorted.

18. If anxiety impedes daily living and productivity, it is labeled as __pathological__.

19. A client who has a persistent thought, image, or impulse that causes anxiety, and that the client cannot set aside, is said to have an __obsession__.

20. __Psychoanalytic__ theory proposes that anxiety comes from unconscious conflicts that arose from real or symbolic events and situations that were threatening in infancy or childhood.

21. __Powerlessness__ is the nursing diagnosis that applies when the client believes that he or she has no control over situations or events.

22. Being admitted to a hospital can be considered to be an __environmental__ factor that produces anxiety.

23. An __obsessive-compulsive__ disorder is marked by uncontrollable thoughts, images, or impulses and behavioral rituals that the client cannot dismiss.

24. Lack of access to health care services due to inadequate insurance is considered to be an __economic__ factor contributing to anxiety.

EXERCISING YOUR CLINICAL JUDGMENT

Ms. Adkins, the 42-year-old divorced woman introduced in the chapter case study, has a history of cardiac disease and panic attacks. Her 16-year-old son told her before the onset of symptoms that he wishes to move in with his father. While she is being evaluated for a cardiac cause of chest pain, she is also given the nursing diagnosis Anxiety by the admitting nurse. You come on duty to relieve the admitting nurse and take over the care of Ms. Adkins.

25. Ms. Adkins tells you that she cannot convince her son to remain living in her home. She goes on to say that she feels that she has no control over her situation or life events. Based on these statements, you might also consider which of the following viable alternate nursing diagnoses for Ms. Adkins?
    a. Sensory-perceptual alterations
    b. Powerlessness
    c. Fear
    d. Altered thought processes

26. You identify a short-term goal with Ms. Adkins, which is to identify her own anxiety symptoms and participate in care planning. You determine that she has met the first expected outcome when she is able to:
    a. verbally identify signs and symptoms of escalating anxiety.
    b. sleep at least in six-hour blocks.
    c. demonstrate relaxation techniques.
    d. use problem-solving skills.

27. While you are talking with Ms. Adkins, you try to "tune in" to the feelings behind her words. In this instance, you are using which of the following interventions to reduce anxiety?
    a. communicating a sense of caring
    b. giving permission
    c. listening actively
    d. modifying the environment

28. Ms. Adkins has a new order to begin medication therapy with an anxiolytic drug, buspirone. You would teach her that the full effects of this new medication may not be felt for:
    a. 1–2 weeks.
    b. 2–3 weeks.
    c. 4–6 weeks.
    d. 8–10 weeks.

TEST YOURSELF

29. The nurse who is assessing for physiological evidence of anxiety in a client would look for:
    a. bradycardia.
    b. excessive salivation.
    c. constricted pupils.
    d. urinary frequency.

30. If a client with anxiety also has an illness-related loss of control over physical integrity, the most appropriate nursing diagnosis in this situation would most likely be:
    a. Ineffective individual coping.
    b. Altered thought processes.
    c. Sensory-perceptual alterations.
    d. Ineffective denial.

31. The nurse would formulate which of the following expected outcomes to measure whether a client has experienced a reduction in anxiety?
    a. use of problem-solving skills
    b. identification of stressors associated with anxiety
    c. reduced tension, irritability, tremors, and sweating
    d. participation in decision making

32. The nurse would offer which of the following forms of complementary therapy as a means of offering hope and decreasing feelings of aloneness in a client?
    a. relaxation
    b. music therapy
    c. spiritual support
    d. touch therapy

33. The nurse who assesses energy fields and uses appropriate interventions to modulate and balance the energy field is using which of the following forms of complementary therapy?
    a. relaxation
    b. music therapy
    c. spiritual support
    d. touch therapy

Vulnerability

PURPOSE

This chapter describes the domains of the Vulnerable Populations Conceptual Model. It identifies factors affecting vulnerability and describes the key components of assessing a vulnerable population. It also describes key interventions for the diagnoses of Hopelessness and Powerlessness in vulnerable populations.

LEARNING OBJECTIVES

After studying this chapter, you should be able to:

1. describe the domains of the Vulnerable Populations Conceptual Model.
2. describe how poverty, social inequality, and poor educational and vocational resources affect health problems.
3. identify factors affecting vulnerability.
4. describe key components of assessing a vulnerable population.
5. describe planning for the nursing diagnoses Hopelessness and Powerlessness in vulnerable populations.
6. describe key interventions for Hopelessness and Powerlessness.
7. discuss the elements of evaluation for Hopelessness and Powerlessness.

MATCHING

1. ____ community approach
2. ____ health status
3. ____ hope
4. ____ human capital
5. ____ personal control
6. ____ social integration
7. ____ relative risk
8. ____ resource availability
9. ____ social status
10. ____ vulnerable populations

a. the belief that through one's own actions, behaviors, or personal characteristics the person can affect outcomes

b. the images that person forms for him- or herself concerning the future

c. considered to be the ratio of the risk of poor health among populations who do not receive resources and are exposed to risk factors compared with those populations who do receive resources and are not exposed to risk factors

d. having a harmonious relationship with society in which the person participates as a full member of the society

e. refers to the availability of socioeconomic and environmental resources

f. includes age- and gender-specific morbidity and mortality

(Continued on p. 196)

195

g. position of an individual in relation to others in the society

h. includes income, jobs, education, and housing

i. social groups who have limited resources and consequently are at high risk for myriad health-related problems

j. a nursing approach for vulnerable populations that emphasizes the provision of resources for disease prevention, treatment, and rehabilitation, with a consequent decrease in exposure to risk factors for health-related problems; necessary for vulnerable populations

TRUE OR FALSE

11. ____ Resource availability includes human capital, social integration, social status, and access to health care.

12. ____ For adolescent girls, the combination of high socioeconomic status, poor academic achievement, lack of available jobs, and the resultant feelings of low self-esteem may lead to pregnancy as the only reasonable alternative.

13. ____ For a person to have hope there must be a desire and some expectation that the desire will be fulfilled.

14. ____ A client who has a perception of power seeks knowledge and takes action to affect the outcome of the illness or to manage health.

15. ____ Hope cannot be present when the client feels no ability to control a situation.

16. ____ Both hope and power have to do with clients' ability to achieve goals.

17. ____ Only clients can empower themselves.

FILL-IN-THE-BLANKS

18. The Vulnerable Populations Conceptual Model provides a framework for understanding the relationships among the limited resource availability, the health-related _____ factors, and the _____ status of vulnerable populations.

19. Human capital includes income, jobs, education, and _____.

20. _____ _____ is reflected in power to control the political process and the distribution of resources.

21. _____ isolation is one of the well-known risks of elderly persons who live alone in the community.

22. Hope on the unconscious level is a life force that provides the _____ to drive the individual forward.

23. The primary distinction between Hopelessness and Powerlessness rests in the concept of _____.

24. To empower another individual you need to respect the individual's capacity for _____-_____.

EXERCISING YOUR CLINICAL JUDGMENT

Brenda Carter, referred to in this chapter's case study, is a single mother living alone with her two-year-old child. She tells you, "I am just stuck here with this baby with no chance to do anything." She is socially isolated and has been in abusive relationships.

25. During your nursing assessment, you asked Brenda about her safety in her neighborhood. This would be an example of which type of needs assessment?
a. physical
b. psychological
c. general
d. social

26. Brenda has broken off relations with her parents. She tells you she misses them. A potential nursing intervention would be to:
a. acknowledge her parent's disappointment with her.
b. help her contact her parents.
c. encourage her to make a new life for herself and baby.
d. have her attend group counseling for pregnant teenagers.

27. You have been working with Brenda to help her deal with her feelings of hopelessness due to her parents refusing to allow her to return home. She says that they told her, "you wanted to be an adult, now act like one." Brenda was diagnosed as suffering from Hopelessness. A few weeks later, she tells you that she has accepted living at the local home for unwed mothers and no longer feels hopeless about her situation. Your evaluation of Hopelessness may mean that she:
    a. needs to continue trying to win her parents back.
    b. has achieved acceptance of her situation, which cannot be changed.
    c. be referred to mental health for counseling about her parents' rejection of her.
    d. is unrealistic about her situation.

TEST YOURSELF

28. Vulnerable social groups include which of the following?
    a. persons subjected to intolerance, the poor, and those associated with a stigma
    b. teenagers and people living in rural areas
    c. infants and clients over 60 years of age
    d. those with resources, and children and the elderly

29. Your client has been diagnosed with breast cancer. She believes that through her own actions, behaviors, or personal characteristics she can affect her outcome. She feels in control of her situation. This is an example of which concept?
    a. "power over"
    b. human capital
    c. hope
    d. personal control

30. At the health department's teen clinic, adolescent girls and teen mothers are routinely screened for symptoms of conflict with their parents and with their partners. This is an example of which type of assessment of vulnerability?
    a. hopelessness
    b. physical needs
    c. social needs
    d. psychological needs

31. As a nurse, you can offer a client hope by:
    a. offering empathy or understanding of the client's feelings associated with being in a desolate situation.
    b. calling the mental health center and getting the client an appointment.
    c. referring the client to the public health department for follow-up care.
    d. telling the client to improve his or her self-esteem.

32. Your client has been diagnosed with diabetes. You can empower the client by:
    a. helping the client to develop, obtain, and use resources.
    b. calling the diabetes association to obtain information for the client.
    c. referring the client to the outpatient diabetic program.
    d. waiting until the client requests help.

Roles and Relationships

PURPOSE

The purpose of this chapter is to describe the concepts underlying roles and relationships, and the factors affecting the health of clients' relationships. It discusses the four relationship nursing diagnoses presented and appropriate nursing care to prevent, alleviate, or correct problems of relationships.

LEARNING OBJECTIVES

After studying this chapter, you should be able to:

1. describe the concepts underlying the four relationship nursing diagnoses presented.
2. identify a variety of factors affecting the health of clients' relationships.
3. discuss the assessment of clients who are at risk for, or who have, one of the four relationship problems discussed in this chapter.
4. differentiate among the various diagnoses for clients with relationship problems that are amenable to nursing care.
5. plan for goal-directed interventions to prevent, alleviate, or correct problems of relationships.
6. evaluate the outcomes that describe the degree of progress toward meeting the goals of relationship-oriented nursing care.

MATCHING

1. ____ learned help-lessness
2. ____ relocation stress syn-drome
3. ____ role
4. ____ role conflict
5. ____ role distance
6. ____ role failure
7. ____ role perfor-mance
8. ____ role strain
9. ____ role transition
10. ____ social isolation

a. homogeneous sets of behaviors, attitudes, beliefs, principles, and values that are normatively defined and expected of a person in a given social position or status in a group

b. a condition in which a person carries out role behaviors that differ from those expected in the person's current cultural or societal situation

c. the absence of role behaviors or ineffective role behaviors resulting in a lack of success in a role

d. a state in which a person has started to take on behaviors of a role but has not fully developed the expected behaviors

(Continued on p. 200)

e. the perception that further efforts would be useless based on the failure of previous attempts

f. the condition in which a person feels unable to accomplish the tasks required of a role or of multiple roles; this results in feelings of frustration, tension, and overload

g. refers to a person's perceptions of her roles and her current responsibilities in her life situations

h. the experience of aloneness, usually with the perception of it being imposed by others and viewed as a negative or threatened state

i. occurs when a person has incompatible expectations for behavior within a role or between two or more roles, or when a role is incongruent with the person's beliefs and values

j. a set of physiological or psychosocial disturbances (or both) caused by transferring a person from one environment to another

TRUE OR FALSE

11. ____ The roles of nurse and teacher are prescribed, not acquired.

12. ____ Learned helplessness is perceived by a person with a sense of powerlessness and feelings of insecurity.

13. ____ Parental expectations affect the roles of children.

14. ____ Older adults are no more at risk for developing Relocation stress syndrome than are younger adults.

15. ____ You will need to assess clients with health problems for social isolation and clients who are socially isolated for health problems.

16. ____ Defining characteristics for the diagnosis Social isolation are objective, not subjective.

17. ____ To qualify for a Relocation stress syndrome diagnosis the client must have been recently relocated.

18. ____ A goal for a client with Impaired social interaction is to practice redefined roles.

FILL-IN-THE-BLANKS

19. Some roles are _____ by age, gender, or position in the family.

20. _____ role performance refers to a change in the way a person perceives or enacts the role.

21. _____ social interaction is a state in which a person engages in social exchange of insufficient or excessive quantity or insufficient quality.

22. Everything we have experienced from the moment of conception to the present, along with our _____ of those experiences, affects our relationships with other.

23. In families in which one parent is emotionally or physically unavailable because of alcohol, drug abuse, or physical or mental illness, the child may have to take on the role of _____ to one or both parents and to any siblings.

24. _____ helps define the various roles a person assumes and the rules for interpersonal relationships.

25. A client with Altered role performance is experiencing conflict in the _____ and _____ of a role.

EXERCISING YOUR CLINICAL JUDGMENT

Maria, the 22-year-old single mother described in the chapter's case study, was born and raised in Honduras.

26. If Maria raised her son according to Honduran customs rather than U.S. customs, she would likely experience which of the following?
    a. role transition
    b. learned helplessness
    c. acquired role
    d. role distance

27. Maria feels unable to accomplish the tasks required of her as a mother of two. She is consequently feeling frustrated, tense, and overloaded. This is an example of which type of Altered role performance?
    a. role transition
    b. learned helplessness
    c. role strain
    d. role distance

28. Maria is suffering from Social isolation related to the loss her husband, separation from family and country, lack of training, and inability to communicate in English. She says, "I feel so alone and different from everyone here. I wish I had family and friends." Appropriate nursing intervention would be which of the following?
    a. help Maria write some goals for dealing with her social isolation
    b. have her clarify her roles
    c. recommend that she return to Honduras
    d. call her parents and ask them to help her

TEST YOURSELF

29. Your clinical instructor's roles of teacher and nurse are considered which type of roles?
    a. prescribed
    b. acquired
    c. transition
    d. role performance

30. When a person has several roles and one of the roles requires behavior that is incompatible or incongruent with another role, the person will most likely be experiencing which of the following types of Altered role performance?
    a. role conflict
    b. role failure
    c. role stress
    d. role distance

31. Your hospitalized client was transferred to a nursing home. She experienced psychological problems as a result of the move. She is most likely experiencing which of the following?
    a. relocation stress syndrome
    b. burnout
    c. role failure
    d. role strain

32. Social factors related to the diagnosis Altered role performance include which of the following?
    a. inadequate role preparation, development level, poverty, domestic violence, lack of a role model
    b. inadequate linkage with the health care system, job demands, development level, poverty, domestic violence
    c. cognitive deficits, substance abuse, low self-esteem, pain
    d. inadequate linkage with the health care system, job demands, low self-esteem, pain

33. Your client was recently moved from her home to a nursing home. Her adjustment will depend largely on which of the following?
    a. her expectations about the move
    b. feelings about her family
    c. her perception of problems living at home
    d. adequacy of her support system and her preparation for the move

50

Loss

PURPOSE

This chapter discusses key concepts that relate to the nursing diagnoses of Anticipatory grieving and Dysfunctional grieving. It describes a focused assessment of a dying client. It also discusses interventions to help the client and family feel understood and facilitate grief work.

LEARNING OBJECTIVES

After studying this chapter, you should be able to:

1. define the concepts of loss, grief, mourning and bereavement, death, and thanatology.
2. compare and contrast the types of loss and grieving.
3. identify a variety of factors affecting the grief response.
4. describe the assessment of a client or family member who is experiencing grief.
5. describe the focused assessment of a dying client.
6. differentiate among nursing diagnoses that describe problems associated with loss.
7. plan for interventions to help the client and family feel understood and facilitate grief work.
8. evaluate the outcomes of caring for a person experiencing grief.

MATCHING

1. _n_ anticipatory grief
2. _a_ bereave
3. _f_ code status
4. _k_ disenfranchised grief
5. _j_ dysfunctional grieving
6. _i_ grief
7. _e_ grief attack
8. _h_ grief work
9. ____ hospice
10. ____ intrusive memory
11. ____ loss
12. ____ mourning
13. ____ searching
14. ____ selective attention
15. ____ sense of presence
16. ____ thanatology

a. to rob or make desolate; traditionally defined as being deprived through death, such as a widow who is deprived by the death of her husband

b. discipline of study and research that deals with death and death-related topics

c. the act of choosing when and how a person will attend to a loss and allow thoughts and feelings to enter the conscious mind

d. a vivid, realistic memory of events surrounding the death that return to the bereaved unexpectedly or unintentionally, overriding existing conscious thinking

(Continued on p. 204)

e. an unexpected, involuntary resurgence of acute grief-related emotions and behaviors triggered by routine events and sometimes accompanied by uncontrollable crying or emotional display

f. a term used to identify the specific orders for a client regarding whether to begin resuscitative actions and the extent of those actions at the time of a cardiac or respiratory arrest

g. a nonthreatening, comforting perception by the bereaved of the deceased's presence through one or more of the senses or in dreams, fortuitous events, or conversations

h. the effort by a grieving person to acknowledge the physical and psychological pain associated with bereavement and to integrate the loss into the future

i. includes emotional, physical, cognitive, and behavioral responses to bereavement, separation, or loss

j. an extended, unsuccessful use of intellectual and emotional responses with which individuals, families, and communities attempt to work though the process of modifying self-concept based on the perception of potential loss

k. grief that lacks social acknowledgment, validation, and support for the bereaved

l. used to describe social and cultural acts used by a bereaved person to express thoughts and feelings of sorrow

m. a philosophical concept of providing palliative or supportive care to dying persons in which the goal of care in the last stages of life is to accentuate living and enhance the quality of life

n. involves the intellectual and emotional responses and behaviors by which individuals, families, and communities attempt to work through the process of modifying self-concept based on the perception of potential loss

o. the removal, change, or reduction in value of something valued or held dear and the feelings that result

p. refers to conscious and unconscious efforts by bereaved to negate the reality of the loss through finding the deceased alive and well

TRUE OR FALSE

17. ____ Mourning honors the dead and helps manage emptiness after death.

18. ____ Normal grieving can lead to life-long problems and breakdowns in psychological and physical health.

19. ____ The ultimate loss a person faces is his own death.

20. ____ Normal anticipatory grief includes making plans for living after an ill person dies.

21. ____ Until the reality of the loss has been acknowledged, further grief work is constrained.

22. ____ Seldom do people have feelings of relief or emancipation from burdens after a person's death.

23. ____ If you are comfortable facing the reality of your own future death, you will find it difficult to provide support to others facing these same circumstances and issues.

FILL-IN-THE-BLANKS

24. Acts of mourning include _____ rituals, expressions of _____, and _____ practices.

25. The loss of _____ is recognized as the ultimate loss.

26. Cultural and societal mores commonly govern the behavioral responses associated with the _____ phase of grieving.

27. During the _____ phase the mind comes to clearly understand that the loss is irreversible and life has changed irrevocably.

28. When planning care for a terminally ill client, you are really caring for two clients, the dying person and the immediate _____ unit.

29. The most important intervention during the Recognition: Shock and Denial phase of grief may be simply your _____.

30. _____ by other nurses or health care team members about attachments and feelings for clients in your care is detrimental both to you and to team dynamics.

EXERCISING YOUR CLINICAL JUDGMENT

31. Mr. Hashimoto, the 54 year-old first generation Japanese-American client who was referred to in this chapter's case study, died with his family with him. After his death his wife became nauseated, had abdominal cramping, and vomited. She felt heart palpitations and had trouble swallowing. She was in which phase of the grieving process?
    a. Dysfunctional grieving
    b. Recognition: Shock and Denial
    c. Reflection: Physical, Emotional, and Spiritual Suffering
    d. Redirection: Reorganizing and Moving Forward

32. Mr. Hashimoto did not talk to staff about his loss because he felt that they were not receptive to his concerns. This is an example of which type of cognitive denial?
    a. selective attention
    b. deception
    c. true denial
    d. anger

33. A year after Mr. Hashimoto's death, Mrs. Hashimoto continues to experience periods of acute grief-related emotions and behaviors triggered by routine events and sometimes accompanied by uncontrollable crying or emotional display. Which type of psychological response is she experiencing?
    a. sense of presence
    b. intrusive memories
    c. grief attacks
    d. dysfunctional grief

TEST YOURSELF

34. Nurses wore a black band on their nurses' caps at the time of Florence Nightingale's death. This is an example of what?
    a. bereavement
    b. mourning
    c. loss
    d. grief

35. Which researcher presented a model of grief that compared the mental trauma of grief to the physical trauma sustained with injuries?
    a. George Engel
    b. Sigmund Freud
    c. Elisabeth Kubler-Ross
    d. Erich Lindemann

36. This phase of the grief reaction has been called the "listen now, hear later" phase because it grants the grieving person time to buffer the truth while mobilizing coping resources to face the truth of a loss.
    a. Reflection: Physical, Emotional, and Spiritual Suffering
    b. Anticipatory Grieving
    c. Recognition: Shock and Denial
    d. Redirection: Reorganization and Moving Ahead

37. Sometimes a person develops physical symptoms experienced earlier by the deceased person, especially pains or specific somatic symptoms associated with the death. This is an example of which type of dysfunctional grief?
    a. chronic
    b. delayed
    c. exaggerated
    d. masked

38. Meeting the client's physical needs promptly, scheduling pain medications so they are being delivered to the client at the exact administration times, and touching and talking to the dying person are interventions to promote healthy grieving during which phase?
    a. Reflection: Physical, Emotional, and Spiritual Suffering
    b. Anticipatory Grieving
    c. Recognition: Shock and Denial
    d. Redirection: Reorganization and Moving Ahead

Sexuality and Reproductive Function

PURPOSE

This chapter discusses key concepts that relate to the nursing diagnoses Altered sexuality patterns and Sexual dysfunction. It discusses the concepts and biological, psychological, social, and cultural influences related to development of sexuality. It also describes issues in the health care of gay men and lesbians.

LEARNING OBJECTIVES

After studying this chapter, you should be able to:

1. describe the biological, psychological, social, and cultural influences in the development of sexuality.
2. discuss concepts related to sexual development.
3. assess the client who is at risk for or is experiencing alterations in sexuality patterns or sexual dysfunction.
4. diagnose sexual problems that are amenable to nursing care.
5. use a standard model of care to provide goal-directed interventions to prevent or correct sexuality diagnoses.
6. evaluate the outcomes that describe progress toward the goals of sexuality nursing care.
7. discuss sexual health promotion across the life span.
8. describe issues in the health care of gay men and lesbians.

MATCHING

1. _s_ androgyny
2. _m_ arousal
3. _j_ bisexual
4. _b_ gender
5. _c_ gender identity
6. _e_ gender role
7. _h_ heterosexual
8. _g_ homophobia
9. _i_ homosexual
10. _o_ libido
11. _n_ orgasm
12. _l_ sexual desire
13. _p_ sexual dysfunction
14. _d_ sexual identity
15. _a_ sexuality
16. _g_ sexual orientation
17. _k_ sexual patterns

a. the state or quality of being sexual, including the collective characteristics that distinguish male and female

b. refers to a person's sex, either male or female

c. may be referred to as sexual identity, which is the internal belief or sense that one is male or female

d. may be referred to as gender identity, which is the internal belief or sense that one is male or female

e. refers to the outward appearance, behaviors, attitudes, and feelings deemed appropriate for males and females

(Continued on p. 208)

f.   an anthropological term; means that a person may display both male and female characteristics and may relate to both a male and female gender identity and role

g.   refers to a person's sexual attraction and feelings of erotic potential toward a partner or toward members of either sex

h.   type of sexual orientation in which one is attracted to members of the opposite gender

i.   type of sexual orientation in which one is attracted to members of the same gender

j.   type of sexual orientation in which one may be attracted to members of either gender

k.   person's chosen expressions of sexuality

l.   a wish to participate in sexual intimacy that is activated by thoughts, fantasies, emotions, and psychological wants and needs

m.   physical and emotional stimuli heighten desire and begin the physiological changes that mark the sexual response cycle

n.   a highly pleasurable involuntary response in which the clitoris, vagina, and uterus of the female or the penis of the male undergo repeated muscular contractions

o.   the conscious or unconscious sex drive or desire to pleasure or satisfy

p.   implies a change or disruption in sexual health or function that the affected person views as unrewarding or inadequate

q.   a fear of becoming homosexual through contact with lesbians and gay men or of having close or intimate feelings toward someone of the same sex

TRUE OR FALSE

18. __T__ Puberty is a physiologically stressful time.

19. __F__ Gender identity is an external belief that one is either male or female. internal

20. __F__ Sexual patterns generally fit with the prevailing expectations of a particular culture or society. may not precisly fit

21. __T__ A characteristic of being sexually healthy includes a person's willingness to make adjustments in sexual functioning when limitations of illness, injury, unavailability of a partner, or other situations occur.

22. __F__ Nurses routinely discuss their client's sexual health and concerns.

23. __T__ Numerous health problems can have a biochemical effect on sexual energy and the ability to engage in sex.

24. __T__ It is a myth that it is best for a man to be on the bottom during sex after a heart attack.

FILL-IN-THE-BLANKS

25. A person's sexuality is a vital component of health and is influenced by __biological__, psychological, social, and __cultural__ forces.

26. Awareness of sexual feelings usually does not occur until __adolescence__, at the onset of mature sexuality.

27. __Orgasm__ is a highly pleasurable involuntary response in which the clitoris, vagina, and uterus of the female or the penis of the male undergo repeated muscular contractions.

28. The World Health Organization describes sexual health as the integration of somatic, __emotional__, intellectual, and social aspects of sexual being in ways that are enriching and that enhance personality, communication, and __love__.

29. Your anxiety and __embarassment__ in discussing sexual concerns will be communicated to your client.

30. A vital part of your assessment of a client with altered sexuality patterns is to understand the client's __sexual__ knowledge and attitudes.

31. You should encourage children to tell a parent, teacher, or other trusted adult when a __touch__ is uncomfortable for them.

EXERCISING YOUR CLINICAL JUDGMENT

32. Lisa Simelli, the 46-year-old client from this chapter's case study who was diagnosed with breast cancer, expresses concern regarding her sexuality. Which of the following nursing diagnoses would be most appropriate?
    a. Altered sexuality patterns
    b. Sexual dysfunction
    c. Ineffective individual coping
    d. Hopelessness

33. Ms. Simelli states that she is feeling unattractive and expresses concern about the results of her biopsy. She reports she has had no intercourse with her husband for the past three months. Which of the following nursing diagnoses would be most appropriate?
    a. Altered sexuality patterns
    b. Sexual dysfunction
    c. Ineffective individual coping
    d. Hopelessness

34. Ms. Simelli is fearful of disclosing her personal anxieties and beliefs about sex. You assure her that sometimes sharing personal information is necessary to provide the best possible health care. This is an example of which step of the PLISSIT model?
    a. permission
    b. limited information
    c. specific suggestions
    d. intensive therapy

TEST YOURSELF

35. Gender roles (e.g., whether a wife is encouraged to cut the wood for the fireplace), refer to which of the following?
    a. outward appearance, behaviors, attitudes, and feelings deemed appropriate for males and females
    b. internal belief that one is male or female
    c. awareness and feelings of being male or female
    d. a person's chosen expressions of sexuality

36. During which phase of the sexual response cycle does a male experience the following: the head of the penis enlarges slightly, the scrotum thickens further and tenses, and two to three drops of pre-orgasmic fluid emerge from the head of the penis?
    a. excitement
    b. plateau
    c. orgasm
    d. resolution

37. Your client was raised to think that sexual intercourse is disgusting and dirty. This is an example of what kind of factor that affects sexuality?
    a. developmental
    b. psychological
    c. physiological
    d. psychiatric disorder

38. After your client had heart surgery, which advice would you give him about maintaining his sexual patterns?
    a. "It is best for you to be on the bottom during sex."
    b. "Impotence and lack of sex drive always occur after a heart attack."
    c. "If angina occurs during sex, you should permanently stop having sex."
    d. "You can safely resume sex within a few weeks or as soon as you feel ready."

39. Your client, a 12-year-old boy, masturbates. His minister says that masturbation is sinful. He is concerned that he is not normal. Which of the following nursing diagnoses would be most appropriate?
    a. Altered sexuality patterns
    b. Sexual dysfunction
    c. Ineffective individual coping
    d. Hopelessness

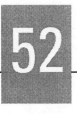

Coping–Stress Tolerance

PURPOSE

This chapter introduces you to the concepts of physiological and psychological stress, and the factors affecting one's ability to cope with stress. It provides guidelines on using the nursing process to work effectively with clients who are experiencing stress in their lives.

LEARNING OBJECTIVES

After studying this chapter, you should be able to:

1. describe physiological and psychological concepts of stress.
2. identify two challenges to coping skills and a variety of commonly used methods of coping.
3. describe at least three factors affecting coping skills, including physiological, developmental, and psychological factors.
4. discuss the assessment of a client's stress tolerance and coping skills.
5. write a stress-related nursing diagnosis for a client and distinguish among related diagnoses.
6. plan for goal-directed interventions to reduce stress.
7. evaluate a client's progress toward stress tolerance and coping.

MATCHING

1. _M_ adaptation
2. _g_ coping
3. _i_ crisis
4. _C_ defense mechanisms
5. _J_ developmental crisis
6. _K_ eustress
7. _L_ hardiness
8. _b_ homeostasis
9. _a_ psychoneuroimmunology
10. _d_ resilience
11. _F_ situational crisis
12. _e_ stress
13. _h_ stressor

a. the study of the interface between the brain and immunology

b. the tendency of biological systems to maintain relatively constant conditions in the internal environment while continuously interacting with and adjusting to changes originating within or outside the system

c. mental processes used to protect or defend one's psychological self from stress and maintain psychological homeostasis

d. the process of identifying or developing resources and strengths to flexibly manage stressors to gain a positive outcome; a sense of confidence, mastery, and self-esteem

(Continued on p. 212)

e. a physiological response produced by the normal wear and tear of bodily processes and external and internal demands

f. a physically or psychologically hazardous situation that is not easily anticipated and for which a person is inadequately prepared

g. any effort directed toward management of dangerous, threatening, or challenging situations

h. a description of a stress-causing agent

i. an upset in a balanced or stable state for which the usual methods of adaptation and coping are not sufficient

j. occurs when a person is unable to complete the tasks needed for a particular developmental level

k. stress that results in positive outcomes

l. the ability to survive stress

m. a process through which individuals accommodate changes in the internal or external environment to preserve functioning and pursue goals

TRUE OR FALSE

14. _T_ Stress results from attempts to balance internal and external environmental demands.

15. _F_ *exhaustion stage* In the resistance stage of the physiological stress response, the body cannot function defensively against the stressor.

16. _T_ Negative moods, such as anxiety and depression, are associated with reduced immune function and are considered to be distress.

17. _T_ A birthday, job promotion, or holiday can precipitate a situational crisis.

18. _F_ Sublimation involves using an excuse to justify behavior while disguising an unconscious motive. *Rationalization*

19. _T_ When assessing for stress tolerance and coping, it is helpful to ask whether the client has had any changes in lifestyle, health, or finances within the last month. *(year)*

20. _T_ Stress can cause some diseases and exacerbate others.

21. _F_ What is stressful for one person in almost all cases is also stressful for another.

22. _T_ Lack of unconditional love can precipitate a developmental crisis in infancy.

23. _T_ While all people react uniquely to stress, some have more reserve or capacity to resist challenges to self-integrity.

FILL-IN-THE-BLANKS

24. The first stage of the physiological stress response is the _alarm_ _reaction_ stage.

25. Mild stress, such as occurs with regular exercise, is known as _eustress_.

26. A person in _crisis_ is faced with overwhelming adaptive tasks.

27. Because of its emergency qualities, a crisis usually lasts no more than _24_– _48_ hours.

28. A person who attributes unacceptable thoughts or feelings to others is using the defense mechanism of _projection_.

29. The body's natural tranquilizers, called _beta_-_endorphins_, correlate closely with self-esteem, hardiness, and affective stability.

30. The fight-or-flight response, a physiological response to stress, is mediated by the _sympathetic_ nervous system.

31. Both anxiety- and crisis-provoking situations challenge a person's _coping_ skills.

32. An inability to have children is generally considered to be a developmental crisis of _adulthood_.

33. At certain stages of coping, _denial_ is a useful and healthy defense mechanism that permits the client to retain hope.

EXERCISING YOUR CLINICAL JUDGMENT

Billy Osceola, the Native American of the Seminole tribe identified in the chapter case study, is diabetic, drinks alcohol, and has developed signs of stump infection following a recent left below-knee amputation. He was using a special herbal concoction made by the tribe's medicine man to treat the painful stump area. After resisting attempts by a home health nurse to work with him in his home, he is ultimately re-admitted to the hospital for treatment of the infection. You are now assigned to Mr. Osceola's care.

34. Based on your knowledge of Mr. Osceola thus far, you would select which of the following nursing diagnoses as most appropriate for him at this time?
    a. Altered thought processes
    b. Ineffective denial
    c. Ineffective family coping
    d. Anxiety

35. As a first step to assisting Mr. Osceola work through the stress of the amputation and its consequences, you would try to:
    a. confront his denial of the infection before admission.
    b. get a consult with a psychiatrist.
    c. establish a therapeutic relationship.
    d. make him identify past coping strategies.

36. If you wish to help Mr. Osceola cope by helping him gain control through knowledge, you would focus on teaching him:
    a. relaxation and deep breathing techniques.
    b. the relationship of his diabetes and drinking to the surgery he just had.
    c. that the medicine man, or shaman, is not very helpful in matters such as these.
    d. how to prevent further infection, control diabetes, and increase mobility.

37. Mr. Osceola shares with you that he finds comfort in listening to tribal music, especially the beat of the drums. Using knowledge of various coping methods, you would teach and encourage him to use which of the following while listening to this music?
    a. relaxation
    b. adaptive thinking
    c. self-suggestion
    d. coping thoughts

TEST YOURSELF

38. A coping method that is not conducive to alleviating stress in a healthy way would be:
    a. listening to music.
    b. overeating.
    c. talking to others about the stressor.
    d. crying or singing as an emotional release.

39. When working with a client experiencing a major stressor, the nurse would protect the client's "vulnerable self" by doing which of the following?
    a. immediately break down any denial
    b. enlist the help of the client's social supports
    c. help the client identify inner strengths that can be used in this situation
    d. tell the client about the negative physiological effects of stress

40. The nurse who is teaching relaxation techniques to a client would most likely incorporate which of the following methods in discussions with the client?
    a. deep breathing and guided imagery
    b. self-suggestion and coping thoughts
    c. coping thoughts and inner dialogue
    d. adaptive thinking and self-suggestion

41. A nurse who is teaching a client about the stress-reducing benefits of meditation would include which of the following?
    a. increased oxygen consumption
    b. increased heart rate
    c. increased blood pressure
    d. improved immune system function

42. A client under extreme stress has come to the emergency room expressing thoughts of suicide. The nurse should take which of the following most appropriate actions?
    a. Locate and obtain resources to help with the crisis.
    b. Document the findings and then discharge the client to home.
    c. Encourage the client to resume antidepressant medications.
    d. Leave the client alone in a room to provide opportunity for reflective thought.

Family Coping

PURPOSE

This chapter describes the concepts of family, family function, family relationships, and factors affecting family coping. Family assessment criteria are identified, as are goal-directed interventions to prevent or correct family problems.

LEARNING OBJECTIVES

After studying this chapter, you should be able to:

1. describe the concepts of family, family function, and family relationships.
2. discuss the factors affecting family coping.
3. assess the family, especially noting major stressors that may interfere with healthy coping, place the client at risk, or both.
4. diagnose family problems that respond to nursing care.
5. plan for goal-directed interventions to prevent or correct family problems identified by nursing diagnoses.
6. evaluate outcomes that describe progress toward or resolution of family problems.

MATCHING

1. ____ binuclear family
2. ____ closed system
3. ____ communal family
4. ____ extended family
5. ____ family
6. ____ family-centered nursing
7. ____ family household
8. ____ family systems theory
9. ____ heterosexual cohabiting family
10. ____ intergenerational family
11. ____ lesbian or gay family
12. ____ nuclear family
13. ____ open system
14. ____ role conflict
15. ____ role stress
16. ____ single-parent family
17. ____ system

a. two or more people united by a common goal to create a physical, cultural, spiritual, and nurturing bond that will promote the physical, mental, spiritual, and social development of each of its members, while maintaining cohesiveness as a unit

b. unit includes the nuclear family as well as other relatives such as aunts, uncles, cousins, and grandparents who are committed to maintaining family ties

c. contains the householder and at least one other person related to the householder by birth, marriage, or adoption

(Continued on p. 216)

d. exchanges matter, energy, and information with other systems and with the environment

e. includes more than one generation of a family living together in one residence or within a small geographical area

f. includes either a female or male couple living together with or without children

g. is a set of integrated, interacting parts that function as a whole and do not interact with other systems or the environment

h. health care that focuses on the health of the family as a unit, as well as the maintenance and improvement of the health and growth of each person in that unit

i. composed of husband, wife, and offspring living in a common household with one or both partners gainfully employed

j. the study of a system (family) with subsystems (individual members) interacting with each other

k. a household of more than one monogamous couple with children, each of which shares and socializes the children as a group activity

l. opposition between two simultaneous feelings or demands that prevents successful fulfillment of the tasks associated with a role

m. households in which the children live with one parent, usually because of divorce, out-of-wedlock births, or death of a spouse

n. an emotion that occurs when a person has difficulty meeting the demands of a role

o. exists when children are part of two nuclear families with co-parenting and joint custody

p. is a set of integrated, interacting parts that function as a whole, with structure and patterns of function that accomplish the work of the whole

q. an unmarried couple living together with or without children

TRUE OR FALSE

18. _____ The family is the basic social unit of society and has needs as a unit.

19. _____ The healthy family is an open system with complex interactions both within the family and in the external world.

20. _____ Stress is the ability of the family to achieve a balance or equilibrium with the stressors that affect it.

21. _____ An unhealthy family will show genuine interest in learning to help the client.

22. _____ The family may or may not recognize that their coping is compromised.

23. _____ An appropriate nursing intervention to establish a nurse-family relationship is active listening.

24. _____ Interventions provided when a family is stressed or not focused are more easily remembered and accepted.

FILL-IN-THE-BLANKS

25. You will have to assess clients as _____, as members of _____, as members of geographical communities, as members of _____ groups, and as spiritual beings.

26. The primary functions of a family include the _____, _____ and social placement, reproductive, economic, and _____ care function.

27. During the senescence family stage, children are planning or assuming care of _____.

28. Family _____ is the family unit's method of managing the stressors of family life.

29. Your first visit to the family is definitive in establishing a _____ relationship.

30. You will need to group all the _____ collected about a family into clusters to arrive at appropriate nursing diagnoses.

31. Resistance can be _____ by having the family assume control through the process of mutual _____ setting.

EXERCISING YOUR CLINICAL JUDGMENT

32. You carefully listen to the concerns the family is expressing about their family member who suffers from alcoholism. What type of intervention are you using?
    a. interventions to help solve family problems
    b. interventions to deal with destructive behaviors
    c. interventions to change family behaviors
    d. interventions to establish a nurse-family relationship

33. One of the clients mentioned in the chapter's case study is suffering from alcoholism. You educate his family members about alcoholism. This is an example of which type of nursing intervention?
    a. interventions to help families with problem solving
    b. interventions to establish a nurse-family relationship
    c. interventions to change family behaviors
    d. interventions to deal with destructive behaviors

34. You ask the family to recall all past concrete events that caused them worry, concern, or grief that were related to the alcoholic member of the family. You have a "family session" to discuss the personal growth and goals of each family member that has been affected by the alcoholic family member. You allow time for them to vent their feelings and respect the perspective of each family member. This is an example of which type of nursing intervention?
    a. interventions to help solve family problems
    b. interventions to establish a nurse-family relationship
    c. interventions to change family behaviors
    d. interventions to deal with destructive behaviors

TEST YOURSELF

35. Your client's family is very supportive of her. This is an example of which family function?
    a. health care
    b. socialization
    c. affective
    d. cognitive

36. The husband and wife could not agree on whose responsibility it was to clean their house. The husband believed it was his wife's responsibility to do the house cleaning, and his wife believed that the household duties should be shared. They are experiencing which one of the following stressors?
    a. developmental stress
    b. economic stress
    c. role stress
    d. role conflict

37. Your client is interested in learning about a low-salt diet. Both he and his wife have hypertension and want to change their eating habits. The most appropriate nursing diagnosis would be which of the following?
    a. Altered parenting
    b. Family coping: potential for growth
    c. Ineffective family coping: compromised
    d. Ineffective family coping: disabling

38. A client, 80, has been living with her middle-aged son and his wife, who have been providing financial and emotional support. The relationship has been mutually satisfying and beneficial. Unfortunately, the client fell and fractured her hip. The family does not know how to manage the client's care. Which nursing diagnosis would be most appropriate?
    a. Altered parenting
    b. Family coping: potential for growth
    c. Ineffective family coping: compromised
    d. Ineffective family coping: disabling

39. The family has agreed to confront an alcoholic family member about his drinking. You help the family identify his destructive behaviors and arrange a convenient date and private space for the confrontation to occur. What type of nursing intervention is this?
    a. interventions to help solve family problems
    b. interventions to establish a nurse-family relationship
    c. interventions to change family behaviors
    d. interventions to deal with destructive behaviors

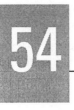

The Caregiver Role

PURPOSE

This chapter discusses key concepts of caregiving and Caregiver role strain. It discusses a variety of factors affecting an individual's ability to provide care. It also provides potential nursing diagnoses that may be appropriate for caregiving clients and goal-directed nursing interventions directed at preventing Caregiver role strain.

LEARNING OBJECTIVES

After studying this chapter, you should be able to:

1. describe the concepts of caregiving and Caregiver role strain.
2. discuss a variety of factors affecting an individual's ability to provide care.
3. describe the assessment of caregivers, including clients experiencing or at risk for role strain.
4. differentiate among the variety of diagnoses that may be appropriate for caregiving clients.
5. plan for goal-directed nursing interventions directed at preventing or reducing Caregiver role strain.
6. evaluate the outcomes of nursing care provided to clients experiencing Caregiver role strain.

MATCHING

1. _____ caregiver
2. _____ caregiver burden
3. _____ caregiver burnout
4. _____ caregiver stress
5. _____ caring
6. _____ coping patterns
7. _____ family dynamics
8. _____ objective caregiver burden
9. _____ stress
10. _____ subjective caregiver burden

a. refers to the caregiver's reaction to physical, emotional, sociocultural, financial, and environmental stressors brought on by the caregiving experience

b. forces at work within the family that result in particular coping behaviors

c. one who provides care to a dependent or partially dependent family member or friend

d. refers to the caregiver's personal appraisal of a caregiving situation and the extent to which the person perceives it to be a burden

e. the specific protective behaviors used by an individual or a family to respond to stressful situations

(Continued on p. 220)

f. refers to the unrelenting physical, psychological, social, or financial problems that occur when a caregiver provides for the health needs of an impaired family member or friend

g. a depletion of physical and mental energy caused by providing care for a chronically ill person over a long period of time

h. a universal behavior observed in human beings and influenced by society, culture, values, and gender

i. refers to the observable, tangible costs to the caregiver in behaviors required or disruptions experienced

j. a stimulus that a person perceives as challenging or harmful

20. Caregiver _____ refers to the caregiver's reaction to physical, emotional, sociocultural, financial, and environmental stressors brought on by the caregiving experience.

21. The _____ serious and demanding the care is, the greater the likelihood the caregiver will experience psychological problems.

22. To determine the needs of a caregiver, you will need to _____ his _____ of the caregiving processes.

23. Many caregivers do not have _____ into the role responsibilities involved in the day-to-day care of a dependent care receiver.

24. Encourage caregivers to use a social _____ system to help them manage their emotional needs.

TRUE OR FALSE

11. ____ Caregivers may experience a greater burden when they also hold a job.

12. ____ Caregiver role strain may be increased when the recipient and the caregiver predetermine how and by whom the care will be provided.

13. ____ Caregivers are more likely to experience Caregiver role strain when they have adequate support systems.

14. ____ An example of a cue that a family is at risk for Caregiver role strain is resurfacing of childhood issues with siblings.

15. ____ Financial costs associated with caregiving can cause many families to experience financial difficulties.

16. ____ In most health care settings, caregivers are considered clients, so their specific needs are met.

17. ____ Many caregivers are unaware of the resources available to them in the community or how to request help from others.

FILL-IN-THE-BLANKS

18. In many cases, caregivers enter their roles with _____ feelings.

19. Caregiver role strain can occur when a caregiver _____ her own health and lets existing conditions worsen.

EXERCISING YOUR CLINICAL JUDGMENT

25. Mrs. Roddy's daughter, the client referred to in this chapter's case study, quits work to care for her ill mother. As a result, she experiences a financial hardship. Her stress originates from which one of the following sources?
    a. interfamily
    b. extrafamily
    c. intrafamily
    d. community

26. Mrs. Roddy is deteriorating physically and mentally. She is currently hospitalized, but her daughter insists that she be discharged to her home as opposed to a skilled nursing facility. The daughter is going to have to learn how to care for her mother's tracheotomy, gastrostomy tube feedings, Foley catheter, heparin lock, and multiple medications. Her daughter is currently:
    a. at Risk for caregiver role strain.
    b. experiencing Caregiver role strain.
    c. at Risk for Injury.
    d. experiencing Ineffective management of therapeutic regimen.

27. As a home health nurse, you develop a plan of care with Mrs. Roddy's daughter that includes having a home health aide bathe Mrs. Roddy three times a week. This is an example of which nursing intervention?
    a. engaging the assistance of family and friends
    b. encouraging social support
    c. setting realistic goals
    d. providing direct assistance

TEST YOURSELF

28. Typical family caregivers are:
    a. married, young adult, female, and living with the person receiving care.
    b. married, middle-aged, female, living with the person receiving care, and managing multiple responsibilities.
    c. widowed, elderly, female, and living with the person receiving care.
    d. married, elderly, male, and living with the person receiving care.

29. Your client is experiencing caregiver burnout. What is the recommended nursing intervention?
    a. Have her and the ill family member placed in a skilled nursing facility.
    b. Help her recognize her unrealistic expectation of herself and get respite care.
    c. Have her and the ill family member placed in assisted living facility for respite care.
    d. Help her recognize that she is experiencing burnout, then proceed with nursing intervention.

30. Picot studied the physiological aspect of caregiving on African-American female caregivers. What did her research discover that may help other caregivers and professionals working with them?
    a. There were no differences between the African-American female caregivers and Caucasians.
    b. Caregivers with a higher level of education reported more rewards than those with less education.
    c. African-American males were the primary caregivers in the family.
    d. African-American female caregivers perceived greater levels of reward, mediated by the comfort of religion and prayer, than Caucasians.

31. You praise your client's family caregiver for doing a good job in taking care of the client. This is an example of what type of nursing intervention to reduce Caregiver role strain?
    a. promoting a realistic appraisal
    b. allowing the client to ventilate
    c. providing direct care
    d. providing empathy

32. Your client's family caregiver has given you some indications that she may be becoming stressed in caring for her husband. To prevent this from occurring you encourage her to contact the Internet site "Caregiver Survival Resources." This is an example of what type of nursing intervention?
    a. providing direct assistance
    b. providing empathy
    c. allowing the client to ventilate
    d. providing assistance from friends

Spirituality

PURPOSE

This chapter discusses key concepts that relate to the nursing diagnoses Spiritual distress, Risk for spiritual distress, and Potential for enhanced spiritual well-being. It discusses the concepts of spirituality, religion, and faith with the idea of providing spiritual care in nursing.

LEARNING OBJECTIVES

After studying this chapter, you should be able to:

1. relate the concepts of spirituality, religion, and faith with the concept of providing spiritual care in nursing.
2. discuss the factors affecting a client's spiritual needs.
3. assess a client for spiritual well-being.
4. make a nursing diagnosis for a client in Spiritual distress.
5. plan care for a client experiencing Spiritual distress.
6. discuss nursing interventions for enhancing spiritual well-being.
7. evaluate interventions for relieving Spiritual distress.

MATCHING

1. ____ agnostic
2. ____ atheist
3. ____ faith
4. ____ hope
5. ____ monotheism
6. ____ polytheism
7. ____ religion
8. ____ spiritual distress
9. ____ spirituality
10. ____ spiritual well-being

a. a process and sacred journey, the essence or life principle of a person, a belief that relates a person to the world, and a way of giving meaning to existence

b. a belief system, including dogma, rituals, and traditions

c. the belief in the existence of one God who created and rules the universe

d. the belief in more than one god

e. a person who believes there is no God or higher power

f. a person who is undecided about the existence of God or a higher power

(Continued on p. 224)

g. belief in or commitment to something or someone that helps a person realize purpose

h. a process of being and becoming that surrounds the totality of a person's inner resources, the wholeness of spirit and unifying dimension, a process of transcendence, and the perception of life having meaning

i. an interpersonal process created through trust and nurtured by a trusting relationship with others, including God

j. a disruption that pervades the entire being and that integrates and transcends biological and social nature resulting in distress of human spirit

TRUE OR FALSE

11. ____ Religion can mean a social institution in which people participate together, rather than an individual searching alone for meaning in life.

12. ____ Spiritual and religious expressions are synonymous.

13. ____ By definition, faith is belief with proof. Each person chooses what to believe.

14. ____ Several research studies confirm that nurses commonly address spirituality.

15. ____ The fundamental teachings of Judaism are grouped around the concept of monotheism.

16. ____ Children do not have spiritual crises in the same sense as adults.

17. ____ Clients who despair or feel hopeless are more likely to die, or die sooner, even when there is little physiological disease to justify the death.

FILL-IN-THE-BLANKS

18. Religion can be viewed as a service to _____, organized within a specified set of beliefs and practices.

19. _____ is belief, expectancy, or trust that things will be better.

20. _____ believe in three gods, including the originator Lao Tzu.

21. Protestant churches have many _____ with a variety of differing beliefs.

22. All religious _____ and practices are bound to the culture and guide the group's lifestyle.

23. Clients who are experiencing a crisis are susceptible to _____ distress.

24. Many clients use _____ as an effective coping strategy for dealing with health crises.

EXERCISING YOUR CLINICAL JUDGMENT

25. Mr. Groves, the 56-year-old Mexican-American client from this chapter's case study, states that he is going to ask his priest why God causes diseases like cancer. You ask him if his wife is going to be present when he discusses his feelings with the priest. You tell him that you think he might be able to express himself more openly if his wife was not present during his conversation with the priest. What were you taking into consideration during your discussion with Mr. Groves?
    a. his religion
    b. his culture
    c. his family
    d. his psychological well-being

26. You ask Mr. Groves what has bothered him most about being sick. This is an example of which element of a spiritual assessment?
    a. to determine client's beliefs, values, and concept of God or divine being
    b. to determine client's sources of hope and strength
    c. to determine client's religious practices
    d. to determine client's perceived relationship between spiritual beliefs and health

27. If the expected outcome for Mr. Groves is to establish a meaningful relationship with himself, God, and others, the most likely nursing diagnosis is which of the following?
    a. Ineffective individual coping
    b. Potential for enhanced spiritual well-being
    c. Risk for spiritual distress
    d. Spiritual distress

TEST YOURSELF

28. Activities such as prayer and going to church are examples of which characteristic of spirituality?
    a. general
    b. being
    c. knowing
    d. doing

29. Your client acknowledges and respects the beliefs, symbols, rituals, and traditions of other faith groups. What development of faith stage is she in?
    a. polar-dialectical
    b. universalizing
    c. individuating-reflective
    d. synthetic-conventional

30. Which nursing theorist stated that one assumption about the healing process is the premise that human nature is rooted in relatedness to the absolute truth of the creator?
    a. Watson
    b. Roy
    c. Travelbee
    d. Newman

31. If you help your client examine his life experiences to discover new meanings or reconnect to forgotten moments that represent significant meaning, which nursing intervention are you using?
    a. life review
    b. reminiscence
    c. counseling
    d. visualization

32. Your client who recently lost her infant expresses disbelief in God. Which nursing diagnosis would be most appropriate?
    a. Ineffective individual coping
    b. Potential for enhanced spiritual well-being
    c. Risk for spiritual distress
    d. Spiritual distress

The Client with Functional Limitations

PURPOSE

This chapter discusses key concepts that relate to the concepts related to rehabilitation, common conditions that require rehabilitative services, and the roles of members of the interdisciplinary team. It cites assessment tools that can be used for a person with a functional disability and major nursing diagnoses for a person with a spinal cord injury.

LEARNING OBJECTIVES

After studying this chapter, you should be able to:

1. discuss several concepts related to rehabilitation.
2. distinguish among the following terms: functional limitation, disability, impairment, and handicap.
3. state three major goals of rehabilitation.
4. identify some common conditions that require rehabilitative services.
5. contrast the roles of the members of the interdisciplinary team.
6. compare a variety of care settings in which rehabilitation may be practiced.
7. discuss the current costs and funding sources for those with disabilities.
8. describe factors affecting ability and disability, including the client's environment, lifestyle, and culture.
9. cite two assessment tools that could be used for a person with a functional limitation.
10. list three major nursing diagnoses for a person with a spinal cord injury.
11. implement nursing interventions to provide quality care for people with physical limitations.
12. state several ways to evaluate whether rehabilitation outcomes have been met.

MATCHING

1. _____ activities of daily living
2. _____ chronic illness
3. _____ chronicity
4. _____ community reintegration
5. _____ functional limitations
6. _____ handicap
7. _____ impairment
8. _____ instrumental activities of daily living
9. _____ rehabilitation
10. _____ rehabilitation nurse

a. the process of adaptation or recovery, through which an individual suffering from a disabling condition, whether temporary or irreversible, participates to regain or attempts to regain maximum function, independence, and restoration

b. difficulties people may experience in performing activities of daily living (ADLs) or instrumental activities of daily living (IADLs)

c. the basic activities usually performed in the course of a normal day in a person's life such as eating, toileting, dressing, bathing, or brushing the teeth

(Continued on p. 228)

d. food preparation, housekeeping, laundry, transportation, using the telephone, shopping, and handling finances

e. limitations resulting from any one of a variety of conditions, whether related to disease, trauma, or birth defect.

f. a disadvantage experienced by a person as a result of impairment that limits the person's "normal" function

g. all impairments or deviations from normal that have one or more of the following characteristics: are permanent, leave residual disability; are caused by a nonreversible pathological condition; require special training of the client for rehabilitation; or are expected to require a long period of supervision, observation, or care

h. a broad term that encompasses chronic illnesses, as well as disease or congenital defects, that permanently alter a person's previous health status

i. nurses who specialize in caring for people with disabilities or functional limitations

j. the return and acceptance of a disabled person as a participating member of the community

14. ____ Assisted living facilities provide interdisciplinary care to people who do not require hospitalization but whose needs for care exceed availability from informal community resources.

15. ____ Environmental factors that can affect ability and disability of clients with functional limitations include the person's living situation, workplace, or time spent in leisure activities.

16. ____ For a client who has functional limitations, you have primary responsibility for documentation of his overall health status and functional assessment.

17. ____ The client with sensory neglect may have minor neglect or be experiencing a more severe form, in which a body part, most often a paralyzed arm, is not recognized.

FILL-IN-THE-BLANKS

18. Disabilities can be a result of _____, chronic illness, congenital defect, or _____ _____.

19. Nurses who care for those with functional limitations become experts in _____ and psychosocial assessment, _____ and bladder management, _____ care, nutrition, behavior, teaching, and family participation.

20. Clients with long-term health alterations often use prayer as a _____ mechanism and look to God or another spiritual being as a source of comfort.

21. _____ living facilities combine shelter with other support services, such as meals, housekeeping, and personal care.

22. The _____ with _____ Act is a significant piece of legislation that advocates for those with disabilities.

23. The _____ _____ _____ (FIM) scale is one of the most reliable and valid tools for measuring functional status.

24. Goals in rehabilitation are aimed at _____ function and preventing _____.

TRUE OR FALSE

11. ____ It is estimated that about 13% of the world's population is disabled.

12. ____ The Association of Rehabilitation Nurses (ARN) is the specialty organization for rehabilitation nurses.

13. ____ A prosthetist helps fit braces, orthoses, and adaptive equipment to assist with normal movement and prevent secondary complications of corrective braces.

EXERCISING YOUR CLINICAL JUDGMENT

25. Which type of health care professional would most likely assess the range of motion, mobility, strength, balance, and gait of Robert, the 18-year-old student referred to in this chapter's case study, who has a complete C5-6 spinal cord injury?
    a. recreational therapist
    b. physical therapist
    c. rehabilitation nurse
    d. occupational therapist

26. Robert receives respite care. What type of service does this represent?
    a. help with home maintenance
    b. comprehensive services requiring medical care that can be managed at home
    c. assistance with personal care
    d. temporary service enabling informal caregivers to take a break from their caregiving responsibilities

27. Robert is unable to perform most of the basic self-care activities such as feeding, bathing, and toileting. What nursing diagnosis would be appropriate?
    a. Self-care deficit
    b. Impaired physical mobility
    c. Activity intolerance
    d. Risk for injury

TEST YOURSELF

28. Which term is appropriate to describe the difficulties that your clients who have functional disabilities face with their physical challenges in performing activities of daily living?
    a. impairment
    b. functional limitations
    c. chronicity
    d. handicap

29. Your client receives assistance from homemaker services. What type of help does she receive?
    a. help with home maintenance
    b. comprehensive services requiring medical care that can be managed at home
    c. assistance with personal care
    d. temporary service enabling informal caregivers to take a break from their caregiving responsibilities

30. When your client's family is evaluating a nursing home for their frail, elderly family member, they ask the staff what infection control measures are enforced. This question helps to evaluate which area of a nursing home assessment?
    a. social, educational, recreational, and religious activities
    b. location
    c. safety
    d. living environment

31. Your client with hemiplegia as a result of a stroke has tactile impairments. Which nursing diagnosis would be most appropriate for the problems associated with tactile impairments?
    a. Self-care deficit
    b. Impaired physical mobility
    c. Sensory/perceptual alterations
    d. Risk for injury

32. Falls are a common problem among older adults with reduced functional capacity and a major factor contributing to dependence. Which nursing diagnosis would be appropriate?
    a. Self-care deficit
    b. Impaired physical mobility
    c. Sensory/perceptual alterations
    d. Risk for injury

The Surgical Client

PURPOSE

This chapter describes the perioperative phases and factors that affect the surgical experience for a client. It discusses how you can use the nursing process to care for a client before, during, and after surgery.

LEARNING OBJECTIVES

After studying this chapter, you should be able to:

1. describe the surgical experience using the perioperative phases as a framework.
2. identify factors that may affect the surgical outcome of a perioperative client.
3. conduct a preoperative nursing history and physical assessment to identify client strengths and factors that increase risks for perioperative complications.
4. describe the nursing role in the psychological and educational preparation of the surgical client.
5. differentiate among general, regional, and local anesthesia.
6. discuss the role of the perioperative nurse when managing the intraoperative care of the surgical client.
7. identify priority intraoperative nursing diagnoses.
8. design an intraoperative nursing care plan.
9. list factors that may affect a postoperative client in the immediate recovery period.
10. explain the nursing management of potential complications the client faces postoperatively.

MATCHING

1. ____ ambulatory surgery
2. ____ anesthesia
3. ____ anesthesiologist
4. ____ certified registered nurse anesthetist
5. ____ circulating nurse
6. ____ general anesthesia
7. ____ intraoperative phase
8. ____ local anesthesia
9. ____ malignant hyperthermia
10. ____ perioperative
11. ____ perioperative nursing
12. ____ postanesthesia care unit
13. ____ postoperative phase
14. ____ preoperative phase

a. can be divided into two segments of care: the immediate and the ongoing periods

b. any agent that induces a temporary loss of feeling due to the inhibition of nerve endings in a specific part of the body

c. an area where clients remain until they regain consciousness from the effects of anesthesia; formerly called recovery room

d. a specialized area of practice that describes the provision of care for the surgical client throughout the continuum of care

(Continued on p. 232)

15. ____ regional anesthesia

16. ____ registered nurse first assistant

17. ____ scrub nurse

e. a registered nurse with special qualifications that include knowledge of aseptic technique, instruments and equipment, anatomy and physiology, surgical procedures, and promotion of client safety

f. a type of anesthesia in which medication is instilled into or around the nerves to block the transmission of nerve impulses in a particular area or region

g. a medical physician who specializes in anesthesiology

h. same-day or outpatient surgery that can be performed with general or local anesthesia, usually takes less than two hours, and requires less than a three-hour stay in a recovery area

i. a rare, autosomal dominant inherited syndrome that is life-threatening, triggered by general anesthesia agents, and characterized by a rapid rise in temperature

j. begins when the decision for surgical intervention is made and ends when the client is safely transported into the operating room (OR) for the surgical procedure

k. an expanded nursing role requiring additional education, in which the perioperative nurse works as a first assistant during the surgical procedure

l. an advanced practice registered nurse who has been specifically educated in the administration of anesthetic agents

m. begins with the client's entrance into the OR and ends when the client is transferred to the recovery room or other areas where immediate postsurgical attention is given

n. the partial or complete loss of sensation with or without a loss of consciousness that results from administration of an anesthetic agent

o. produced by inhalation or injection (or a combination of both) of anesthetic drugs into the bloodstream; causes the client to lose all sensation and consciousness

p. a registered nurse who assists the client to meet individual needs during all three phases of the surgical experience

q. the term used to describe the preoperative, intraoperative, and postoperative phases of the surgical experience

TRUE OR FALSE

18. ____ Palliative surgery is done to reduce intensity of disease or illness symptoms but does not effect a cure.

19. ____ The scrub nurse coordinates client care, is the client advocate, and manages all activities outside the sterile field.

20. ____ In a life-threatening situation when family cannot be contacted to give consent, it is assumed that consent is given; this is labeled implied consent.

21. ____ Normal tissue repair and resistance to infection after surgery depend on good nutrition.

22. ____ With effective preoperative teaching the client will express new knowledge and decreased anxiety about the surgical procedure.

23. ____ Pain is an unexpected and abnormal response to the surgical procedure.

24. ____ Turning in bed postoperatively improves venous return and respiratory function.

25. ____ In addition to the skin incision, there are many other risk factors that can influence a surgical client's risk for infection.

26. ____ Acetaminophen (Tylenol) is the drug of choice to treat malignant hyperthermia.

27. ____ Urinary retention and urinary tract infections are two common postoperative complications of the urinary system.

FILL-IN-THE-BLANKS

28. A surgery that is performed according to the client's preference with no ill effects occurring due to postponement would be classified as _____ surgery.

29. The _____ phase of anesthesia is begun as soon as the client is brought into the operating room.

30. One advantage of _____ anesthesia is that it can be used for clients of any age and for any surgical procedure.

31. It is the legal responsibility of the _____ to obtain the client's consent before a surgical procedure.

32. Latex allergies have become much more common since the late 1980s with the advent of _____ Precautions.

33. Positioning the client for surgery is usually done _____ induction of anesthesia.

34. _____ is a respiratory emergency caused by reflex contractions of pharyngeal muscles, causing spasm of the vocal cords.

35. To encourage maximal lung expansion following surgery, a client should use an _____ _____.

36. A nurse should assess for bladder distention in the postoperative client if the client has not voided for _____ hours.

37. _____ and _____ instructions are given to a client before discharge following surgery.

EXERCISING YOUR CLINICAL JUDGMENT

Mr. Warren, a 61-year-old Afro-Caribbean man, has come to the United States for a second medical opinion after he was diagnosed with prostate cancer. His daughter, who is a nurse, lives in Atlanta.

38. Which of the following nursing diagnoses would you be sure to consider, knowing that Mr. Warren is undergoing surgery for cancer, a potentially incurable problem?
    a. Anxiety
    b. Knowledge deficit
    c. Hopelessness
    d. Powerlessness

39. You are providing instructions to Mr. Warren about leg exercises that he can do after surgery to reduce the risk of thrombus formation in the legs. How often should you tell him to perform them?
    a. 1–2 times every hour
    b. 5–6 times every hour
    c. 10–12 times every hour
    d. 20–25 times every 8 hours

40. Before offering Mr. Warren any sips of liquids to drink following surgery, you would check to make sure that fluids are allowed and that he has:
    a. thirst.
    b. bowel sounds.
    c. a heart rate of at least 70 per minute.
    d. no crackles in any lung fields.

41. You are assisting Mr. Warren to get out of bed for the first time since surgery. Knowing he has an abdominal incision, you would be sure to use which of the following when helping him get up?
    a. cane to steady himself against
    b. walker to lean on in case of dizziness
    c. pillow to use as a splint during movement
    d. mechanical lift, since he should not stand at all

TEST YOURSELF

42. As part of client preparation just before surgery, you must obtain the client's signature on the consent form, have the client void, give preoperative medication, and assist the client onto the stretcher to go to the operating room. Which of the following would be best to do first?
    a. have the client void
    b. put the client on the stretcher for needed rest
    c. administer the ordered medication
    d. obtain the signature on the consent form

43. The preoperative nurse would alert the anesthesiologist or surgeon regarding which of the following health problems that could cause cancellation of a client's elective surgery?
    a. headache
    b. sore throat
    c. heart attack one year ago
    d. chronic lung disease

44. The circulating nurse in the operating room notes that two sponges are missing near the end of a client's surgery. Which of the following actions should the nurse take first?
    a. call for an x-ray
    b. ignore it since the sponges dissolve
    c. perform a second count
    d. search the floor around the operating table

45. The nurse would teach the client about which of the following ordered pain medication administration methods that provides for the most continuous relief of pain?
    a. patient-controlled analgesia
    b. intermittent nurse-administered IV push medication
    c. subcutaneous injections
    d. intramuscular injections

46. A postoperative client with nausea has begun vomiting. The nurse would avoid giving antiemetic medication by which of the following routes?
    a. intravenous
    b. intramuscular
    c. subcutaneous
    d. oral

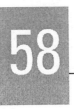

The Emergency Client

PURPOSE

This chapter introduces you to concepts related to emergency care, including triage, role of the triage nurse, and types of treatment areas. It uses the nursing process as a framework for discussing the emergency nursing care needs of clients with a change in respiratory, cardiac, or psychosocial status.

LEARNING OBJECTIVES

After studying this chapter, you should be able to:

1. describe the concept of emergency care.
2. discuss the concept of triage and the roles of the triage nurse.
3. identify factors affecting the outcome of emergency care, including lifestyle, culture, and socioeconomics.
4. describe the assessment of the emergency department client.
5. write nursing diagnoses for a client who has an emergent respiratory problem, cardiac problem, or a risk of violence directed at self or others.
6. plan for specific goal-oriented nursing intervention in emergent respiratory problems, cardiac problems, or violence directed at self or others.
7. describe fundamental emergency nursing care to the client with a change in respiratory, cardiac, or psychosocial status.
8. evaluate the outcomes of goal-oriented nursing care for the emergency client.

MATCHING

1. _____ acuity rating
2. _____ acute area
3. _____ against medical advice
4. _____ emergency
5. _____ hemodynamic monitoring
6. _____ interfacility transfer
7. _____ intrafacility transfer
8. _____ nonacute area
9. _____ nonurgent
10. _____ semiurgent
11. _____ triage
12. _____ urgent

a. the transfer of an emergency department client from one health care facility to another

b. a serious health situation that arises suddenly and either threatens life or would result in serious complications without prompt treatment

c. a classification of a problem for which the client requires timely treatment within 4–6 hours

d. a priority rating based on the severity of the illness or injury

e. the physical space where clients with life-threatening health problems are treated

(Continued on p. 236)

f. using invasive procedures and sophisticated equipment to monitor the client's cardiac output, arterial pressure, and central venous pressures

g. the decision-making process used to determine client treatment priorities based on the severity of injury and priority for treatment

h. the transfer of a client from the emergency department to another area in the same facility

i. a classification of a problem for which the client requires prompt care, although a wait of 20-60 minutes will not affect the outcome of treatment

j. a discharge that is of the client's will and is against the advice of a physician and without proper discharge instructions

k. a classification of a problem for which the amount of time a person delays treatment is not a critical issue

l. the physical space used for clients who present with problems that are not life-threatening

19. ____ Delay in seeking medical care due to financial constraints often results in a higher likelihood of more urgent problems once the client does seek care.

20. ____ Teaching proper use of safety belts and motorcycle helmets is an example of teaching done by emergency department nurses.

21. ____ The objectives of the triage assessment area are to collect baseline data and establish priorities for the client's care.

22. ____ A serum glucose level is unnecessary for any client with an altered level of consciousness.

FILL-IN-THE-BLANKS

23. The goal of an emergency department is to _____ and _____ clients with acute problems.

24. The triage nurse in an emergency department gathers assessment data primarily about the client's _____ _____.

25. Most emergency departments have a _____ _____ available to counsel clients about social and financial issues.

26. A client who needs a prescription refilled would have the classification of _____ assigned to the problem in the emergency room.

27. The triage nurse assesses the level of consciousness and the ability to _____ as the client approaches the triage desk or counter.

28. With a client under 12 years of age, the nurse would often record the client's _____ instead of a blood pressure.

29. The emergency department nurse should make sure that a _____ client has no access to hospital supplies or personal items that could be used as a weapon.

30. The nurse should find a _____ before leaving the treatment area of a suicidal client.

31. For a client with Impaired gas exchange and no previous history of lung disease, the goal would be to ensure an oxygen saturation level above _____%.

TRUE OR FALSE

13. ____ Traumatic emergencies are injuries commonly caused by blunt or penetrating impact to the body from motor vehicle collisions, knives, or guns.

14. ____ A laceration that requires sutures is appropriately classified as a semiurgent problem.

15. ____ A triage nurse must be able to function under pressure in the role of clinician, educator, and manager.

16. ____ To organize urgent nursing interventions effectively, the nurse should perform the least time-consuming ones last.

17. ____ An emergency department nurse should consolidate activities such as taking vital signs and assessing pain to make the most of each client contact.

18. ____ Cultural factors have no influence on the outcomes of emergency care.

32. For a client with Decreased cardiac output the immediate goal is to stabilize the

_____ _____.

EXERCISING YOUR CLINICAL JUDGMENT

Barry, the middle-aged homeless man identified in the chapter case study, is admitted to the acute area of the emergency department after being found unconscious on the street in 17°F weather. His oxygenation and circulatory status are impaired due to the effects of the cold. He is restrained after becoming combative with emergency medical treatment personnel in the ambulance. You are assigned to work with Barry in the emergency department after his arrival.

33. Your highest priority for Barry's care until you release his restraints is:
    a. nutrition.
    b. comfort.
    c. safety.
    d. psychosocial.

34. Before initiating oxygen therapy you should determine whether Barry has a history of:
    a. heart failure.
    b. peripheral vascular disease.
    c. chronic obstructive pulmonary disease.
    d. neurological deficits.

35. Because Barry has no home to be discharged to once his condition is stabilized, you would consult with which of the following members of the health care team?
    a. chaplain
    b. social worker
    c. occupational therapist
    d. billing clerk

36. After Barry is stabilized, he tells you that he no longer needs or wants to be in the emergency room and wishes to leave. None of your explanations about his condition and need for care help him to change his mind. At this point, you should:
    a. have him sign a form indicating he left against medical advice (AMA) and document this.
    b. ask the physician for an order for chemical restraint.
    c. ask the security guard to block the door and assume a menacing stance.
    d. call the on-call administrator.

TEST YOURSELF

37. A nurse working with a client who dies in the emergency room places highest priority on which of the following?
    a. contacting the funeral home
    b. communicating with family
    c. calling for transport to the morgue
    d. signing the death certificate

38. Before discharging a client to the home setting from the emergency room, the nurse must ensure that which of the following is in place?
    a. home health aides for one month
    b. financial resources to pay for medications for the next two weeks
    c. client bookings for the next two follow-up visits
    d. client ability to provide self-care or a competent caregiver

39. The nurse in the emergency room is trying to determine whether a client has an airway obstruction. Which of the following should the nurse assess?
    a. ability to speak
    b. ability to hear
    c. oxygen saturation
    d. adventitious breath sounds

40. A client taking warfarin (Coumadin) is being seen in the emergency room for an injury. The nurse should be sure to gather information about the results of which of the following laboratory tests?
    a. blood urea nitrogen (BUN)
    b. serum glucose
    c. sodium and potassium
    d. coagulation studies

41. The triage nurse in an emergency room would be least concerned with which of the following regarding a client approaching the triage desk?
    a. ability to breathe
    b. pallor or cyanosis of the skin
    c. number of accompanying family members
    d. motor function

The Community as a Client

PURPOSE

This chapter discusses key concepts that relate to the community as a client. It includes the factors that affect community health; methods and types of data used in assessing communities; and nursing diagnosis for groups, populations, or communities. It also describes methods used in planning care for a community, goal-directed interventions, and methods of evaluation used to measure outcomes of community health interventions.

LEARNING OBJECTIVES

After studying this chapter, you should be able to:

1. describe basic concepts of community health nursing as they apply to the community as the client.
2. discuss factors that affect community health.
3. describe several methods and types of data used in assessing communities.
4. identify two approaches to nursing diagnosis for groups, populations, or communities.
5. describe methods used in planning care for a community.
6. identify goal-directed interventions that promote health and prevent disease in a community.
7. identify methods of evaluation used to measure outcomes of community health interventions.

MATCHING

1. ____ community
2. ____ community forum
3. ____ community health nursing
4. ____ epidemiology
5. ____ focus group
6. ____ key informant
7. ____ Omaha system
8. ____ opinion survey
9. ____ parish nurse
10. ____ participant observation
11. ____ public health nursing
12. ____ vulnerable population
13. ____ windshield survey

a. a method of data collection performed through telephone interviews, mailed questionnaires, door-to-door interviews, or at clinic sites

b. a method of community assessment that examines formal and informal social systems at work; the researcher shares in life activities of the group while observing and collecting data

c. a geographic location, or an aggregate or population of individuals who have one or more personal or environmental characteristics in common

(Continued on p. 240)

d. a nursing diagnosis system developed by the Visiting Nurses Association of Omaha, Nebraska

e. a registered nurse who is employed by or volunteers at a religious or health care organization for the purpose of providing nursing care to members of a church congregation

f. a method of data collection in which 6–12 people from a group or aggregate are brought together for discussion, guided when necessary by a skilled, nonjudgmental leader

g. a synthesis of nursing theory and public health theory aimed at preserving and promoting the health of these populations

h. a subgroup of a larger population that has an increased risk of health problems because of exposure or other health or nonhealth problems

i. a community leader, professional, politician, or business person who possesses knowledge of the needs of the community and who can act as a useful source of data and a supporter of new programs

j. method of data collection in which the researcher drives through a neighborhood to conduct a general assessment of that neighborhood through observation

k. the study of the cause and distribution of disease, disability, and death among groups of people

l. the nursing practice of promoting and protecting the health of populations using knowledge from nursing, social sciences, and public health sciences

m. an open meeting where members of a community or group may come to share opinions and concerns about a particular issue

15. ____ Community partnerships are a means of participation and involvement in a community to make health changes.

16. ____ Telemedicine is the use of technologies to support the education of community members.

17. ____ Accessibility to health care refers to the availability of health services and the equality of delivery to those who have insurance.

18. ____ Assessments are the same in the types of data or information collected.

19. ____ One health care problem that migrant workers have is that the transient nature of their work makes it difficult to provide continuity of health care.

20. ____ Difficulties in defining a community diagnosis may result from differences in the definition of health among populations.

21. ____ Community activation emphasizes the involvement and coordination of major community institutions to mobilize community leadership and resources for health promotion and to improve public awareness of health issues.

22. ____ Health promotion interventions are used to decrease the health and well-being of individuals, families, and communities.

FILL-IN-THE-BLANKS

23. Home health nurses provide _____ _____ to clients and families.

24. Nurse epidemiologists are _____ of illness and disease.

25. Models of community participation include community activation, participatory action research, and _____ _____ _____ _____.

26. _____ populations are subgroups of a larger population that have an increased risk of health problems because of exposure or other health or nonhealth problems.

27. Health and the health care of individuals, families, and communities are influenced by social, cultural, economic, political, and _____ factors.

TRUE OR FALSE

14. ____ A community is defined by location, people, and social systems.

28. A community or group _____ is the initial step in the problem-solving process to promote health or prevent illness in a population.

29. Demographic data may include information collected through the _____, such as race, age, numbers of persons living in specific locations, population growth, and family statistics.

30. The three components of the Omaha System are the problem classification scheme, the intervention scheme, and the problem rating scale for _____.

31. _____ is the process of determining whether the goals or objectives of a program have been met.

EXERCISING YOUR CLINICAL JUDGMENT

32. A public health nurse was sent to investigate the outbreak of diarrhea among the ABC Day School's children and staff. This type of community health nurse is defined as one who:
    a. coordinates access and utilization of health services.
    b. helps clients in the process of moving from one health care setting to another.
    c. provides direct care to clients and families.
    d. promotes and protects the health of populations.

33. The nurse determined that ABC Day School's personnel were inadequately trained in the use of proper hand washing after changing infants' diapers. Which of the following nursing diagnoses would be most appropriate to address this problem?
    a. Knowledge deficit related to age of population
    b. Knowledge deficit related to inadequate training in personal and environmental hygiene
    c. Knowledge deficit related to state regulations
    d. Knowledge deficit related to the rules of the day care school

34. When working with the ABC Day School's staff to identify goals and interventions, the nurse needs to have certain knowledge, skills, and attitudes. Which of the following is an example of these?
    a. The nurse builds consensus and cohesiveness among the staff and assesses whether the goals, interests, and motivations of the day school are the same as those of the nurse.
    b. The nurse informs the staff of her disappointment with their lack of understanding of how the infection was spread.
    c. After the nurse assesses that the staff members were not properly washing their hands, she informs the director of the day school that she has arranged a series of educational programs for the staff.
    d. The nurse has the health officer recommend that ABC Day School's board of directors reprimand the school director for being negligent in her duties.

TEST YOURSELF

35. Which of the following definitions of *community* is the most comprehensive?
    a. a geographic location
    b. an aggregate or population of individuals who have one or more personal or environmental characteristics in common
    c. a geographic location, or an aggregate or population of individuals who have one or more personal or environmental characteristics in common
    d. a high-risk population group

36. Which of the following is *not* a key component in community health nursing?
    a. a combination of public health and nursing knowledge and practice
    b. a primary focus on restoration of health
    c. a primary focus on populations or groups
    d. a goal of primary care

37. Which type of nurse provides direct care to clients and families?
    a. home health nurse
    b. school nurse
    c. occupational health nurse
    d. care management nurse

38. A nurse interviews the city's mayor about the health concerns of the staff. This is an example of which kind of data collection?
    a. focus group
    b. participant observation
    c. opinion survey
    d. key informant

39. A parish nurse is a registered nurse employed by:
    a. the health department.
    b. a neighborhood clinic.
    c. a home health agency.
    d. a religious or health care organization.

40. Evaluation at the end of interventions or programs is called what?
    a. summative evaluation
    b. formative evaluation
    c. final evaluation
    d. outcome evaluation

The Homebound Client

PURPOSE

The purpose of this chapter is to help you understand the concepts that are important to home care nursing and the factors affecting the outcomes of home care. It identifies nursing diagnoses that are consistent with reimbursement guidelines and typical interventions used to achieve expected outcomes for homebound clients.

LEARNING OBJECTIVES

After studying this chapter, you should be able to:

1. describe concepts important to home care nursing, including accreditation, reimbursement, and scope of services.

2. describe factors affecting the outcomes of home care.

3. write effective nursing diagnoses that are consistent with reimbursement guidelines for homebound clients.

4. describe expected outcomes for homebound clients.

5. describe types of nursing interventions employed to achieve typical expected outcomes for homebound clients.

6. document evaluation data that promote the expected outcomes of home heath care.

MATCHING

1. ____ care planning

2. ____ cultural competence

3. ____ community health nursing

4. ____ environmental assessment

5. ____ functional assessment

6. ____ home care

7. ____ home care nursing

8. ____ home care provider

9. ____ public health nursing

10. ____ support services

a. cross-cultural communication, cultural assessment, cultural interpretation, and intervention

b. a focus on activities of daily living, such as when and how well the client can bathe, toilet, dress, eat, sleep, move about, cook, clean and communicate with caregivers

c. refers to any of a variety of services provided to clients and families in their place of residence for the purpose of treating illness, restoring health, rehabilitating, promoting health, and palliating

d. refers to population-focused nursing activities designed to improve quality of life, including its physical, mental, and social aspects; prevent disease; promote health; and control communicable disease consistent with available knowledge and resources

(Continued on p. 244)

e. promotes and preserves the health of populations

f. assistance with shopping, meals, and cleaning for the homebound

g. incorporates each client's sense of modesty, personal hygiene, special clothing or amulets, food beliefs, and rituals.

h. comprehensive, holistic field of nursing focused on the client and family (or support system) and delivered in the client's home

i. a person or organization (often called an agency) that delivers home care

j. identifies the client's capacity to establish and maintain a safe home environment that supports the success of treatment goals

TRUE OR FALSE

11. ____ Accreditation is important to protect the safety of the public using home care services, and it affects the nature and quality of the services offered.

12. ____ Medicare and Medicaid regulations have specific criteria for home care reimbursement and have created a shift to a holistic model of nursing practice.

13. ____ To properly plan care, your initial assessment requires a focus on both the client and the family.

14. ____ The impact of health maintenance organizations (HMOs) and telemedicine is slowly having a negative impact on the scope of reimbursed services.

15. ____ The Albrecht Nursing Model assumes that clients and their families participate actively, capably, and responsibly in their care.

16. ____ An objective observation that may indicate the client's inability to maintain his or her home is the presence of offensive odors and the accumulation of dirt, dirty laundry, or unhygienic wastes.

17. ____ The goal for a client with a long-term condition is to return to the previous level of functioning.

FILL-IN-THE-BLANKS

18. The _____ of nurses in public health, community health, or home health may overlap with the roles described for home health care nursing.

19. The nature and practice of home care is affected by the _____ and _____ forces that act on health care.

20. The referring _____ is required to write orders that outline the client's plan of treatment, including frequency and duration of services.

21. Always remember that you are a _____ in your clients' homes.

22. _____ are usually provided for home care staff who travel in high-risk communities.

23. Ongoing communication with the _____ is necessary for adjustments in the medical regimen.

24. The nursing diagnosis of _____ _____ _____ _____ is made when clients or families need assistance with cleaning their houses, insulating their homes, or paying their utility bills.

25. Compliance with your nursing care plan will be increased through client and family _____.

EXERCISING YOUR CLINICAL JUDGMENT

26. Cynthia Mullen, the 35-year-old with a history of type 1 diabetes referred to in the chapter's case study, is in need of support services. Which one of the following is an example of such a service?
    a. changing her catheter
    b. cleaning her house
    c. bathing her
    d. instructing her regarding her medications

27. Mrs. Mullen is having difficulty using her crutches. The most appropriate nursing diagnosis that reflects her functional status and is directly treatable by a prescription for the underlying medical problem is:
    a. Risk for injury related to lack of experience using crutches
    b. Risk for infection related to diabetes
    c. Activity intolerance related to diabetes
    d. Self-care deficit related to immobility

28. Mrs. Mullen agreed to learn how to change her wound dressing. The two of you agreed that she would first watch you change her dressing, and then you would supervise her changing it on the next visit. This is an example of:
    a. teaching her "survival skills"
    b. providing her teaching
    c. mutual goal setting
    d. providing quality care

TEST YOURSELF

29. The Community Health Accreditation Program does which of the following?
    a. completes an overall evaluation of home care agency programs and services, organization and administration, and strategic planning and marketing
    b. surveys client care issues, such as rights, safety, confidentiality, informed consent, etc.
    c. reviews home care organizations and their structures
    d. reviews staffing for homemakers and home health aides

30. Your 80-year-old client is under the care of a physician. The client is eligible for Medicare reimbursable home care services; this means that he has met which of the following regulation(s)?
    a. was hospitalized in acute care facility prior to your initial home visit
    b. is homebound and requires skilled nursing care
    c. requires tertiary care
    d. requires nursing and social work care

31. As a home care case manager, you are expected to:
    a. function dependently and follow directions of other health care providers.
    b. follow the RN's plan of care to help the client and family meet clearly defined, measurable, and client-centered goals.
    c. function dependently and cost effectively to save the client money.
    d. function independently and collaborate with and direct other health care providers.

32. You take an empty egg carton and label it for the client's various medications and the times they should be taken. This is an example of which nursing intervention?
    a. teaching
    b. mutual goal setting
    c. counseling
    d. ensuring quality care

33. As a home care nurse, you are responsible for supervising which staff?
    a. social workers
    b. physical therapists
    c. occupational therapists
    d. nonlicensed staff, such as home health aides

Answer Key

CHAPTER 1

1. c
2. d
3. a
4. b
5. T
6. F. Nursing practice is governed by law and standards are set forth by the profession.
7. T
8. T
9. T
10. F. A doctoral program is considered advanced practice education.
11. F. critical thinker
12. T
13. F. Politics has always permeated both the health care delivery system and the profession of nursing.
14. T
15. Middle Ages
16. Florence Nightingale
17. Civil
18. Mary Adelaide Nutting
19. public health
20. primary care, prevention, and community outreach
21. Master's degree
22. professional licensure
23. state
24. health care delivery system
25. a. The Nurse Practice Act forms the legal basis for nursing practice in a specific state. The NLN focuses on the improvement of nursing services and education. The ARN is a specialty nursing organization, while the ANA is the professional organization for nurses.
26. c. The client advocate role is one in which the nurse protects the rights of clients. In this instance, Kate is protecting the rights of the client whose privacy is being invaded.
27. b. Many states require that nurses obtain CEUs in order to maintain their professional licensure in that state.
28. b. A bachelor's degree is the minimum educational degree that must be held in order to become certified by the ANCC as a nurse generalist.
29. a. Most definitions of nursing emphasize the human response to health and illness rather than the disease processes. Although nursing interacts with other disciplines and has been influenced by the women's movement, these are not the focus of nursing.
30. c. Managed care emerged in an effort to maintain quality health care at the lowest cost. This set the stage for registered nurses to become employed as case managers, who coordinate care in various health settings.
31. b. The *American Journal of Nursing* is published by the ANA and is considered to be the "official voice" for professional nursing in the U.S.
32. d. The emerging trend in nursing is a shift away from hospitals as the most common setting for practice. Nurses are becoming increasingly employed in community settings, including short-term rehabilitation, ambulatory care, and home health agencies.
33. d. Nurse practitioners are likely to cross over medical thresholds to provide services usually provided by physicians. Clinics are more likely to be managed by nurses. Hospital stays will continue to become shorter, and there will be a continued emphasis on health rather than illness.

CHAPTER 2

1. g
2. l
3. q
4. w
5. aa
6. ee
7. a
8. f
9. m
10. r
11. x
12. bb
13. b
14. u
15. dd
16. c
17. h
18. n
19. z
20. cc
21. d
22. i
23. o
24. s
25. y
26. e
27. j
28. p
29. k
30. t
31. v
32. T
33. F. Yes, it does.
34. T
35. F. Criminal law
36. T
37. F. An individual state
38. T
39. T
40. battery
41. procedural
42. certification
43. collective bargaining
44. informed consent
45. confidentiality or privacy
46. incident report
47. date, time
48. d. This is the only option that removes the client from the area and protects the confidentiality of the information being given in report.

49. a. The CDC is the Federal agency responsible for issuing guidelines for infection control.
50. b. The other options constitute documentation errors.
51. b
52. a
53. c
54. d
55. b

CHAPTER 3

1. e
2. l
3. f
4. c
5. j
6. d
7. h
8. m
9. b
10. o
11. i
12. g
13. p
14. a
15. k
16. n
17. F. normative ethics
18. T
19. T
20. F. A terminally ill client should be told of her prognosis.
21. F. Unfavorable
22. T
23. T
24. ethics
25. moral
26. culture, life experiences
27. privacy
28. Nonmaleficence
29. rights, confidentiality
30. medical
31. c. Confidentiality means maintaining another's privacy by safeguarding information entrusted to you.
32. d. Fidelity means honoring agreements and keeping promises.
33. b. A living will is a document that provides written instructions about when life-sustaining treatment should be terminated.
34. c
35. a
36. c

37. a
38. b

CHAPTER 4

1. e
2. i
3. j
4. a
5. f
6. h
7. k
8. c
9. d
10. b
11. g
12. T
13. F. This is an example of stereotyping.
14. T
15. T
16. F. past-oriented
17. T
18. T
19. F. external
20. T
21. F. Illness is a price paid for a past or future event.
22. preservation or maintenance
23. accommodation or negotiation
24. Awareness
25. Environmental control
26. Irish
27. African
28. Hispanic
29. Chinese
30. Navajo Indians
31. space
32. c
33. b
34. a
35. d
36. d
37. b
38. c
39. a
40. d

CHAPTER 5

1. b
2. a
3. e
4. d
5. f
6. h
7. i

8. j
9. c
10. k
11. m
12. l
13. g
14. F. Health promotion and illness prevention cannot be clearly differentiated. Health promotion activities can be expected to prevent illness.
15. T. However, a shift has occurred from the hospital to other employment opportunities. It is not clear whether the shift will continue, stabilize, or shift back to the hospital.
16. F. Nurse practitioners are nurses and therefore are more likely to focus on health promotion and disease prevention.
17. F. Alternative health care is used by at least one-third of all Americans.
18. F. While there may be room for debate, many factors influence access and quality of hospital services. Among these factors, consider rural vs. urban, system of financing and types of services offered.
19. F. Seventy-five percent of nursing homes are for-profit agencies.
20. T. Emergency medical services are a means of reducing the response time to emergencies.
21. T. Respite care is designed to relieve the stress and burden of providing long-term care in the home.
22. F. The U.S. government's share of the national health care bill is 46% and growing.
23. F. An HMO establishes standards for the quality of care provided.
24. F. Managed care organizations make decisions about what services will be reimbursed, thus rationing health care.
25. T. This is also the age group with the greatest per capita expenditures for health care.
26. T. The health care system has expectations for how people will access and use the system. To the extent that these expectations are incompatible with cultural expectations, the system presents barriers.

27. T. As a nurse, you need to understand the economic forces putting pressure on the structure and function of the health care delivery system.

28. F. Cost of care and quality of care are highly interrelated.

29. health behaviors and improved environmental quality

30. Nurses

31. Pharmacists

32. inpatient

33. community general hospital

34. Rehabilitation

35. Subacute care

36. physician's office

37. Adult day care

38. United States

39. preferred provider organization

40. people over 65, disabled people, and people with end-stage renal disease

41. Canada

42. 26%

43. Gray Panthers and American Association of Retired Persons

44. b. While none of these sources may provide this service, the goal of a health maintenance organization is most in keeping with this service.

45. b. While the managed care organization will make a decision about paying for the medication, a physician must prescribe this medication and will consider his medical history in making the decision.

46. c. A dietitian is the only one specifically trained to provide dietary counseling.

47. a. Option a is a definition of *rehabilitation*. Options b, c, and d are incorrect.

48. d. While there may be elements of other types of care, supportive care is conservative care that helps the client achieve the highest level of functioning, independence, and participation in the community.

49. c. Unless you happen to know something about Ayurveda, you probably don't know whether the other answers are true or not. You do know that some alternative therapies are helpful and others are not. Therefore, option "c" is a good answer and leaves the responsibility on the client.

50. d. This definition is most consistent with a preferred provider organization.

51. c. To answer this question, you first need to choose between improving access and targeting health problems. Access is probably the better answer, since targeting health problems won't help without access. Option c is likely to include b; therefore, c is the best answer.

CHAPTER 6

1. h
2. i
3. f
4. j
5. b
6. c
7. e
8. d
9. a
10. g
11. T
12. F. not tested, but are assumed to represent reality
13. T
14. T
15. F. accepted
16. F. apprenticeship (focus on performing procedures)
17. F. Leininger
18. theoretical
19. person, nursing
20. metaparadigm
21. Nursing
22. theory
23. culturally
24. nurse
25. c. remain in the clinical area and attend continuing education programs
26. d. Leininger's influence helped stress the importance of assessing the client's cultural beliefs before planning or implementing nursing care.
27. c. Orem's theory: Health deviation self-care requisites are when the person has symptoms and is aware of a need for assessment and intervention.
28. a
29. b
30. d
31. a
32. b

CHAPTER 7

1. f
2. e
3. b
4. c
5. a
6. d
7. F. When you are making decisions in areas of uncertainty, creativity must be an element of critical thinking.
8. F. The T.H.I.N.K. model incorporates five modes of thinking used in combination or simultaneously.
9. T
10. T
11. T
12. T
13. T
14. F. Recognizing and using common patterns is at the advanced beginner level.
15. F. Routines are equated with habits. Habits are useful when they free the mind to deal with the more complex aspects of a situation. They are not useful when they substitute for thinking.
16. F. A list of assessment questions is a tool to be used as a reminder and is never intended to be complete.
17. subjective
18. discovering, making decisions
19. wellness, risk, actual
20. expected outcomes
21. direct care, teaching, counseling, coordination, collaboration, health promotion, disease prevention, health maintenance, restoration, rehabilitation.
22. data gathering
23. North American Nursing Diagnosis Association
24. inadequate knowledge, over-reliance on habits, anxiety, time, bias, lack of confidence.
25. interrelated
26. independence of thought, fair-mindedness, insight into egocentricity and sociocentricity, humility, suspension of judgment, courage, integrity, perseverance, confidence in reason, interest in related thoughts and feelings, curiosity
27. c. Shows the least evidence of thinking

28. c. Shows the most evidence of critical thinking
29. d. You will need to apply what you know and come up with new ideas.
30. b. You have decided on a course of action based on your opinion in a situation without clear guidelines.
31. a. The nursing process suggests beginning with assessment.
32. a. Critical thinking always considers that other possibilities may be present.
33. b. Unless the physician had in some way validated the belief with the client, it is an assumption.
34. a. Interpretation is the mental process of giving meaning to data.
35. a. Chances are your perspective is egocentric.
36. d. The nurse is probably an expert acting from intuition.
37. a. A nurse who cannot gather more data and make a decision to modify care is stuck in the novice stage.

CHAPTER 8

1. x
2. r
3. v
4. t
5. o
6. s
7. y
8. u
9. h
10. e
11. w
12. q
13. a
14. c
15. n
16. m
17. l
18. d
19. b
20. g
21. k
22. i
23. p
24. f
25. j
26. z
27. T

28. T
29. F. If the client wishes to maintain privacy or the family is not a reliable source you would not collect data from the family.
30. T
31. T
32. F. The purpose is never only to collect a standard set of data.
33. F. You prepare for termination when you tell the client how much time the interview will take.
34. F. Biographical data may be helpful in accurately anticipating a medical diagnosis.
35. F. The medical history helps the nurse anticipate nursing needs.
36. T
37. T
38. F. Exercise tolerance is related to the respiratory and cardiovascular systems as well.
39. F. However, subjective data is documented in an objective manner, without including your opinions.
40. T
41. thinking
42. restoration
43. potential for change, potential rate of change, evidence of change
44. location, quality, chronology, setting, aggravating or alleviating factors, associated factors
45. Rapport
46. Rapport
47. chronology
48. nutritional-metabolic
49. activity-exercise
50. self-perception/self-concept
51. d. A person's experience of stress varies with the perception of stress-producing events.
52. b. You will often use observations about self-concept as you help a client through even a short-term health care experience. However, this does not require a formal assessment.
53. b. While all these patterns could be affected, retirement is most directly related to the role-relationship pattern.
54. c. You are trying to find out if he is safe to walk unassisted.
55. a. While it is seldom true that you only can ask one question, if you had to choose, this question is the most pertinent to the

action you will take to administer pain medication.
56. b. Assessment includes the history and physical examination, is interrelated with planning and implementation, and requires analysis of the data to identify problems.
57. b. In a focused assessment you narrow your assessment to learn more about a problem that has already been identified.
58. b. Objective data is directly observable through any one of the five senses.
59. c. This is the only evidence that the wife is a reliable source.
60. c. Any of the conclusions could be true. However, all you know from the information presented is that the client has not taken the medication correctly.

CHAPTER 9

1. e
2. c
3. d
4. a
5. b
6. l
7. o
8. g
9. m
10. p
11. k
12. n
13. f
14. i
15. q
16. j
17. h
18. F. Vital signs must be evaluated compared to the client's baseline.
19. T
20. T
21. T
22. F. The oral thermometer must be placed in the pocket created by the frenulum under the tongue.
23. F. Clean from clean to dirty; that is, from the end to the bulb
24. F. A heart rate of 100 with exercise or anxiety that returns to normal with rest is normal.
25. T
26. T
27. F. Head injuries can cause bradycardia.

28. F. The blood volume is also a factor.
29. F. The carotid is not routinely used to count the pulse. Massage of the carotid can cause a reflex slowing of the heart rate.
30. T
31. T
32. T
33. vital signs
34. thermoregulation
35. glass
36. tympanic
37. metabolic rate
38. increase
39. pulsus paradoxus
40. resistance
41. contraction
42. relaxation
43. two-thirds
44. b
45. a
46. b
47. a
48. c
49. c
50. c
51. a
52. b
53. c
54. b
55. b
56. d
57. a
58. b
59. d
60. a
61. b
62. a
63. c
64. c

CHAPTER 10

1. b
2. c
3. g
4. y
5. x
6. n
7. s
8. t
9. u
10. o
11. l
12. m
13. ℓ
14. j
15. z
16. i
17. f
18. q
19. r
20. p
21. d
22. w
23. v
24. h
25. a
26. k
27. F. A good quality stethoscope has a thick wall.
28. F. A stethoscope does not amplify, it simply blocks out other sounds.
29. F. You can begin the physical exam in any position.
30. T
31. F. The heart is on the left side.
32. T
33. F. This information is a form of orientation to time, but can only be evaluated in the context of the information.
34. T
35. T
36. F. PERRLA tells you more about motor function than the ability to see clearly.
37. T
38. F. Angle the ophthalmoscope toward the nose.
39. F. The thyroid should be soft.
40. T
41. T
42. T
43. T
44. F. S_2 is associated with the aortic and pulmonic valves.
45. F. An apical radial pulse deficit usually occurs with irregular rhythms.
46. T
47. F. A grade 6 is the loudest murmur.
48. F. A bruit is never normal.
49. T
50. F. Identifying hypoactive bowel sounds is a subjective judgment dependent on your ability to recognize normal sounds.
51. T
52. T
53. light palpation
54. percussion
55. auscultation
56. affect
57. cognitive function
58. natural
59. size, consistency, shape, attachment, color, mobility
60. crepitus
61. 2, 30, 60
62. pupils equal, round, react to light and accommodation
63. Rhinne
64. gingivitis
65. Kussmaul
66. discontinuous
67. deep tendon
68. cystocele
69. Bartholin's
70. Pap smear
71. prostate
72. epididymis
73. varicocele
74. a, f, j, and k are essential

a. Essential. Assessing for adventitious sounds will help you know the seriousness of her condition, anticipate complications, and monitor progress.

b. Nonessential. However, you will probably want to gather some information about her mental status such as orientation to person, place, and time. Gather enough information that you can recognize if her condition changes.

c. Nonessential. Assess the radial and pedal pulses. Assess the radial pulse to evaluate the rate and rhythm of the heart. If the rhythm is irregular, assess the apical pulse. Assess the pedal pulses to evaluate the circulation in the feet. It would not be surprising for a 90-year-old to have diminished circulation in the feet.

d. Nonessential. However, you do want to listen for bowel sounds and assess for abdominal distention. The stress of illness can slow the bowels and cause distention.

e. Nonessential. The rectal examination is never routine for a general duty nurse.

f. Essential. Skin assessment in the elderly is important especially when the person will be confined to bed.

g. Nonessential. However, you will want to note some information about range of motion and the ability to move about safely in the environment.

h. Nonessential. However, most nurses will usually note the condition of the toenails in the elderly. Health teaching needs can be met and sometimes a podiatrist referral can be made.

i. Nonessential. However, you do want to gather some information about the client's functional level of vision and hearing and the use of glasses or hearing aids.

j. Essential. Cardiac and respiratory problems are closely interrelated and should always be assessed together.

k. Essential. Anytime you listen to the heart one of the things you are listening for is murmurs. The presence of most murmurs will not appreciably change your nursing care.

75. d. The dorsalis pedis pulse is the most distal pulse and confirms blood flow is reaching the feet. However, you might as well check the warmth and color at the same time for additional confirmation of circulation.

76. b. A pulse deficit of 20 is a significant reduction in the effectiveness of the heart to produce a pulse. Low blood pressure, pale skin, and weakness represent signs of decreased cardiac output.

77. c. All three are indicators of circulation.

78. a. Mouth breathing may take in more air thus making it easier to hear the sounds. If the person can breath out through the nose, a more natural exhalation is achieved.

79. c. Because the dorsalis pedis pulse is not palpable in about 10% of people, you should assess the warmth and color of the feet. Warm, pink feet have good circulation.

80. a. Counting an irregular pulse is often more accurate at the apex and when counted for one minute, especially when the pulse is irregularly irregular.

81. c. Bowel sounds do not necessarily occur in all four quadrants.

82. b. You probably decided to choose between b and d. Because

a positive Homan's sign is not definitive for deep vein thrombosis, b is correct.

83. b
84. d
85. d
86. b
87. c
88. c
89. c
90. b
91. c
92. b
93. b
94. a
95. b
96. c
97. b
98. b

CHAPTER 11

1. g
2. j
3. h
4. i
5. b
6. d
7. m
8. l
9. n
10. e
11. c
12. f
13. a
14. k
15. T
16. T
17. F. NANDA
18. T
19. F. exchanging, communicating, relating, valuing, choosing, moving, perceiving, knowing, feeling
20. T
21. T
22. F. qualifier
23. T
24. F. Yes, they should be.
25. second
26. four
27. Omaha
28. diagnostic label
29. wellness
30. clusters
31. differentiating
32. defining characteristic

33. libel
34. overdiagnosing
35. a. This is an actual nursing diagnosis, not "risk for," and lists specific related factors.
36. b. The client cannot retain urine with a catheter in place.
37. b. This would be a "risk for" diagnosis. The "related to" factors must relate to the client's situation.
38. d. The diagnosis would be written as Risk for infection.
39. d
40. a
41. b
42. a
43. c

CHAPTER 12

1. c
2. m
3. d
4. a
5. f
6. g
7. e
8. i
9. j
10. h
11. l
12. k
13. b
14. F. Planning is ongoing throughout the client health care experience.
15. F. Planning is interrelated with all the phases of the process.
16. F. Each care plan is individualized.
17. F. While other disciplines may in some cases assume primary responsibility for some aspects of the client's care, the nurse has a role in the provision of that care.
18. T
19. F. Nurses must plan care regardless of whether it is ever officially documented as a plan.
20. T
21. F. Physical needs may be secondary to other needs at different stages of the client's experience.
22. T
23. T
24. T

25. T
26. T
27. first client contact
28. changes
29. physiological integrity
30. adapts, alters, changes, rearranges, reorganizes, revises, varies
31. admission history, daily assessment record, nursing progress notes
32. nursing, multidisciplinary
33. graphic checklist, nursing progress notes
34. nursing progress notes, daily assessment record
35. accountable
36. sensitive
37. Likert, 5
38. functional health patterns, physiological health, psychosocial health, health knowledge and behavior, perceived health, family health
39. teaching, collaborating, managing, coordinating, monitoring, assisting, supporting, protecting, sustaining
40. communication
41. b
42. d
43. b
44. d
45. d
46. c
47. d
48. a
49. b
50. c

CHAPTER 13

1. j
2. h
3. e
4. n
5. k
6. o
7. m
8. b
9. d
10. f
11. i
12. a
13. g
14. p
15. l
16. c

17. T
18. F. Outcomes or nursing diagnoses may also be revised.
19. F. Client and family must be asked.
20. T
21. T
22. F. Standards of Professional Performance
23. T
24. F. policy
25. T
26. T
27. concurrent
28. improved
29. partially
30. resolved
31. barrier
32. external
33. indicators
34. commendation
35. protocol
36. performance appraisal
37. b. Options a and c are closed-ended questions (yes or no response) that are not likely to elicit the type of information required. Option d is not focused enough on the issue of pain relief.
38. a. The client sleeps soundly after listening to music; this indicates effectiveness of this form of therapy.
39. b. This type of record allows for review "after-the-fact;" retrospective audit.
40. c. Narcotics control is a matter of federal regulation as well as institutional policy and procedure.
41. a
42. b
43. d
44. c
45. b

CHAPTER 14

1. d
2. f
3. k
4. a
5. i
6. j
7. b
8. l
9. c
10. g

11. h
12. n
13. e
14. m
15. T
16. F. chart errors are documented
17. F. vary from geographical area or specialty
18. F. brief as possible, stripped to essential components
19. T
20. T
21. T
22. documentation, legal, nursing process, standards
23. standards
24. Black
25. client's
26. client
27. history, needs
28. observations
29. a. Narrative charting is a method of charting that provides information in the form of statements that describe events surrounding client care.
30. b. Recording of information should be sequential.
31. c. A discharge note is done when client is released from the hospital.
32. c
33. d
34. d
35. b
36. a

CHAPTER 15

1. c
2. p
3. m
4. h
5. g
6. r
7. d
8. i
9. k
10. e
11. l
12. n
13. o
14. s
15. f
16. b
17. a
18. q

19. j
20. T
21. F. Travelbee
22. T
23. F. culturally determined
24. T
25. T
26. F. ask the client to consider what might be the best thing to do
27. T
28. ethical, professional
29. Positive
30. body language
31. concrete
32. talking
33. silence
34. Active
35. a. The nurse asks "why" of the client, thereby asking for a reason for feelings and behaviors when the client may not know the reason.
36. c. The nurse lets the client know that what was said was unclear.
37. b. The nurse questions how something the client has misperceived could possibly be true.
38. a
39. a
40. d
41. a
42. d

CHAPTER 16

1. g
2. h
3. a
4. d
5. i
6. c
7. f
8. b
9. e
10. T
11. T
12. F. Clients must apply their learning.
13. F. Literacy is an important consideration when using written instructions.
14. T
15. T
16. F. Written supplemental materials reinforce learning.
17. F. Some clients prefer not to know.

18. F. Other nursing diagnoses can also apply.
19. T
20. T
21. individual
22. group
23. written
24. reinforce learning
25. active participant
26. short-term
27. long-term
28. b
29. a
30. c
31. a
32. a
33. a
34. a
35. a
36. b
37. b
38. c
39. a
40. c

CHAPTER 17

1. b
2. e
3. f
4. g
5. h
6. c
7. i
8. a
9. d
10. T
11. T
12. F. top-level
13. F. Nurse executives also hire and fire.
14. T
15. T
16. F. mission statement
17. T
18. T
19. T
20. negatively
21. flattened
22. health
23. leaders
24. organization
25. organizational chart
26. quality
27. outcomes
28. Policies, procedures

29. cost
30. a
31. b
32. c
33. d
34. b
35. c
36. d
37. a
38. c

CHAPTER 18

1. h
2. c
3. g
4. i
5. f
6. l
7. a
8. b
9. d
10. o
11. n
12. m
13. e
14. k
15. j
16. r
17. s
18. q
19. p
20. T
21. T
22. T
23. F. Ethical guidelines should still be followed.
24. T
25. F. There is a relationship, but not necessarily causation.
26. F. The abstract is a short summary only.
27. T
28. T
29. T
30. F. It can.
31. T
32. F. Valuable information can still be obtained.
33. T
34. T
35. T
36. Nursing research
37. Florence Nightingale
38. human subjects
39. case study

40. variables
41. random
42. reduction
43. extraneous
44. maturation
45. Transferability
46. a
47. d
48. b
49. a
50. d
51. a
52. a
53. b

CHAPTER 19

1. h
2. q
3. r
4. o
5. t
6. m
7. j
8. k
9. e
10. s
11. d
12. c
13. a
14. b
15. g
16. i
17. n
18. p
19. u
20. l
21. f
22. T
23. F. They usually correspond.
24. T
25. F. Tasks can derive from cultural patterns as well.
26. T
27. F. primary
28. T
29. T
30. T
31. head, heel
32. motor
33. 4
34. separation anxiety
35. walk
36. 2
37. 12
38. Phenylketonuria

39. otitis media
40. d. The other toys are best used with children less than 12 months of age.
41. b. The other strategies should be avoided.
42. c. The client cannot read (age 33 months) and has a language barrier.
43. c. A nap should be planned around lunchtime.
44. c
45. c
46. a
47. b
48. c

CHAPTER 20

1. h
2. d
3. f
4. e
5. j
6. i
7. a
8. c
9. g
10. b
11. F. gains weight slowly
12. F. rarely do new teeth erupt
13. T
14. F. many fears
15. T
16. T
17. T
18. ectomorphic, endomorphic
19. muscle
20. preschool-aged
21. Decentering accommodation
22. growth, development, prevention
23. head, collisions
24. five
25. a. Timmy's parents were expecting him to engage in sports activities that were beyond his ability, thereby adversely affecting his growth and development.
26. a. Evidence of child abuse is a clear defining characteristic of Altered parenting.
27. d. Children under age 5 are not developmentally prepared to protect themselves from injury.
28. d
29. c

30. c
31. a
32. b

CHAPTER 21

1. a
2. j
3. k
4. f
5. e
6. g
7. d
8. i
9. b
10. m
11. h
12. c
13. l
14. T
15. T
16. F. boys more than girls
17. F. heredity
18. T
19. T
20. F. Do not be afraid.
21. puberty
22. identity, identity
23. health care
24. adolescent boys
25. preventable, behaviors
26. psychosocial
27. comply
28. a. inability to identify, manage, and/or seek help to maintain health
29. c. the state in which an individual is at increased risk for being invaded by pathogenic organisms
30. b. inadequate choices of practical responses, and/or ability to use available resources
31. a
32. c
33. b
34. d
35. c

CHAPTER 22

1. d
2. h
3. b
4. g
5. j
6. e

7. f
8. i
9. c
10. a
11. T
12. T
13. F. intimacy versus isolation
14. F. one in every five deaths
15. T
16. T
17. F. health education and counseling
18. Growth, development
19. generativity, stagnation
20. seasons
21. infectious diseases
22. depressed
23. Poverty
24. ergonomic
25. individualized
26. d. Generativity versus stagnation; the individual must balance the feeling that life is personally satisfying and socially meaningful with the feeling that life is without meaning.
27. c. Midlife crisis is a stressful life period during middle adulthood, precipitated by the review and reevaluation of one's past, including goals, during which the person experiences inner turmoil and self-doubt.
28. c. To persuade clients to change their behaviors, it is first necessary to identify their beliefs relevant to the high-risk behavior and to provide information based on this foundation.
29. d
30. c
31. b
32. a
33. a

CHAPTER 23

1. b
2. d
3. a
4. c
5. T
6. F. Almost 5 million older Americans suffer food insecurity, in which the household does not always have adequate food.
7. T
8. F. It is usually difficult to detect.
9. T

10. T
11. T
12. F. Aging does not necessarily limit mobility.
13. F. It is not uncommon for an older adult to engage in ageist thinking about others in that person's cohort.
14. T
15. forties
16. range-of-motion
17. home safety
18. alcohol
19. one
20. optic
21. twenty
22. Falls
23. calcium
24. incontinence
25. a. Religion and closeness to family are values, as is caution when working with new health providers.
26. c. Nonskid soles reduce risk of falls, while the other choices either are not helpful or have other adverse consequences.
27. b. Regardless of age, BSE should be done once a month.
28. b. The client requires a balanced diet, but should cut down on empty calories due to decreased caloric needs.
29. d. Six to eight glasses of fluid per day are highly recommended.
30. c
31. d
32. b
33. b
34. a
35. c

CHAPTER 24

1. g
2. j
3. i
4. k
5. a
6. d
7. c
8. b
9. n
10. o
11. p
12. f
13. s
14. m

15. h
16. l
17. q
18. e
19. r
20. T
21. T
22. F. Health is a fundamental right of all people.
23. F. Not all diseases can be cured.
24. T
25. F. A population health perspective does not exclude consideration of individual needs and responsibility.
26. T
27. T
28. World Health Organization
29. preventive
30. quality, years
31. diagnosis
32. health-illness continuum
33. working
34. perception
35. medical
36. a. Enabling goals are to promote healthy behaviors, protect health, ensure access to quality health care, and strengthen community prevention.
37. a. When assessing community health, your nursing care plan may address broad social issues of community health, such as the following: a safe environment and cost-effective health services.
38. b. Secondary prevention consists of actions that focus on the early diagnosis and prompt treatment of people with health problems or illnesses and who are at risk for developing complications or worsening conditions.
39. d
40. c
41. a
42. b
43. a

CHAPTER 25

1. d
2. f
3. o
4. i
5. m
6. k
7. h

8. c
9. p
10. e
11. a
12. b
13. q
14. l
15. g
16. j
17. n
18. T
19. T
20. F. They do interfere.
21. T
22. F. They may conflict.
23. T
24. T
25. T
26. F. Client and family should also be involved.
27. T
28. reasoned action
29. risk factors
30. vulnerable
31. medical
32. knowledge
33. Values clarification
34. reinforcing or motivating
35. denial
36. Discharge
37. social
38. a. In this stage, the person does not intend to change a high-risk behavior in the foreseeable future.
39. b. He disliked having to go to the bathroom so frequently because of medication effects.
40. c. An educational plan must be focused on increasing awareness of the relationships between the client's specific unhealthy lifestyles and the development of health problems.
41. d. The single most influential factor in increasing participation in effective management of a therapeutic regimen is the relationship with the health care provider.
42. a
43. c
44. b
45. d
46. c

CHAPTER 26

1. d
2. z
3. p
4. y
5. a
6. o
7. l
8. b
9. k
10. u
11. m
12. e
13. q
14. t
15. x
16. g
17. v
18. n
19. c
20. i
21. j
22. f
23. r
24. s
25. h
26. w
27. T
28. T
29. F. The drugs reach the liver first, called the first-pass effect.
30. T
31. F. It varies according to facility policy.
32. T
33. T
34. F. Sufficient body fluid is needed to transport drugs and their metabolites.
35. T
36. Drug Enforcement
37. Drug tolerance
38. Enteric-coated
39. X
40. body weight
41. Constipation, diarrhea
42. superinfection
43. 30
44. c
45. b
46. d
47. a
48. a
49. c
50. b

51. d
52. b

CHAPTER 27

1. i
2. h
3. e
4. a
5. k
6. n
7. p
8. q
9. b
10. m
11. o
12. d
13. j
14. l
15. g
16. c
17. f
18. T
19. T
20. F. airborne
21. T
22. T
23. F. left
24. T
25. F. Anxiety can reduce protection.
26. T
27. T
28. convalescence
29. reservoir
30. Opportunistic
31. environmental
32. localized
33. dirty
34. handwashing
35. steam
36. feces
37. Droplet
38. a. The others are localized signs of infection.
39. c. The environment has other children, and hand-washing is a fundamental procedure to reduce transmission of organisms.
40. b. Viruses, such as influenza, require droplet precautions.
41. d. The sites should be re-cultured or new sites of infection should be looked for.
42. a
43. a
44. d

45. b
46. c

CHAPTER 28

1. f
2. e
3. a
4. h
5. i
6. g
7. d
8. b
9. c
10. T
11. T
12. F. cigarette smoking
13. T
14. F. They develop slowly over time.
15. T
16. T
17. T
18. F. Some are not.
19. T
20. falls
21. aspiration
22. Poisons
23. accidental
24. occupational
25. money
26. infants, toddlers
27. prevention
28. grounded
29. rescue, alarm, confine, extinguish
30. b
31. b
32. d
33. c
34. c
35. d
36. c
37. a
38. b

CHAPTER 29

1. q
2. m
3. e
4. c
5. o
6. p
7. a
8. f
9. d
10. b
11. j
12. k
13. i
14. l
15. n
16. s
17. h
18. t
19. r
20. g
21. T
22. F. small intestine
23. T
24. F. cereals, raw fruits and vegetables
25. F. positive, anabolism
26. T
27. T
28. F. The RDA is meant to meet the needs of healthy individuals.
29. T
30. T
31. Digestion
32. fiber
33. four
34. Vitamins
35. minerals
36. diet history
37. Food Guide Pyramid
38. protein
39. Nutrition Facts food label
40. fruits and vegetables
41. c. The client has well-fitting dentures and no evidence of neuromuscular disease.
42. b. Physical factors that can interfere with nutrition include circumstances that interfere with the ability to shop, cook, and eat. Arthritis could limit the ability to do all of these.
43. a. The family should be assessed first as a possible resource for shopping and/or food preparation. Option b could be costly, while option c may not be necessary at this time. Option d does not solve possible difficulty in shopping when the client has arthritis.
44. d. The Food Guide Pyramid uses a graphic design that is useful in teaching clients about the types and amounts of foods to include in the daily diet. It is easy to understand and follow.
45. a
46. b
47. d
48. c
49. b

CHAPTER 30

1. d
2. e
3. a
4. f
5. g
6. b
7. c
8. T
9. F. Ketones are positive and nitrogen balance is negative.
10. T
11. F. It occurs over months or years.
12. T
13. T
14. T
15. F. At least 2 pounds per month is considered successful.
16. T
17. F. They should be avoided.
18. medulla
19. B_{12}
20. iron
21. 34
22. 10
23. pharyngeal
24. 170
25. clear
26. 2
27. limited or restricted
28. c
29. a. Clients with cancer and AIDS tend to eat better in the morning.
30. b. These foods can cause further irritation.
31. d. Both hemoglobin and hematocrit will reflect increased iron intake.
32. a
33. c
34. b
35. d
36. b

CHAPTER 31

1. z
2. f
3. a
4. g
5. d
6. h

7. c
8. e
9. q
10. t
11. o
12. n
13. s
14. r
15. j
16. v
17. i
18. m
19. k
20. p
21. y
22. l
23. u
24. w
25. x
26. b
27. T
28. T
29. T
30. F. The kidneys could fail to excrete potassium.
31. T
32. T
33. F. It cannot be measured.
34. T
35. T
36. F. It's given primarily for fluid replacement.
37. F. Sodium is present in this solution (0.45%).
38. T
39. T
40. T
41. retention
42. water soluble
43. decompression, obstruction
44. third spacing
45. high Fowler's
46. Normal saline
47. distal
48. 18
49. at the site, away from
50. blood return
51. d
52. a
53. c
54. c
55. c
56. a
57. c
58. a
59. a

60. c
61. b
62. b
63. b
64. b
65. b

CHAPTER 32

1. f
2. e
3. k
4. i
5. b
6. l
7. j
8. c
9. h
10. d
11. g
12. m
13. a
14. F. may or may not be related
15. F. yellow wound
16. T
17. T
18. F. cannot heal
19. F. does not always means the wound is infected
20. T
21. Protection
22. red, yellow, black
23. pressure ulcer
24. perioperative, postoperative
25. clock
26. sutures, staples
27. enterostomal
28. b. A Stage II ulcer may look like a blister or shallow crater.
29. b. The erythrocyte sedimentation rate can help assess the client's inflammation, infectious, or necrotic processes.
30. d. Impaired skin integrity: It is a state in which an individual has altered body tissue.
31. c
32. a
33. d
34. b
35. a

CHAPTER 33

1. f
2. h
3. c

4. a
5. g
6. d
7. e
8. b
9. F. It may also be caused by inflammation without infection.
10. T
11. T
12. F. Slow wave sleep and length of sleep increases.
13. T
14. T
15. T
16. T
17. F. only if the infection has gotten in the blood stream (septicemia)
18. F. only if the central line is suspected to be the source of the infection
19. T
20. F. a temperature of 102° to 104° F
21. T
22. T
23. F. The client may have cold diuresis.
24. T
25. T
26. effervescence, plateau, defervescence
27. 10%
28. increased
29. dry skin, hypotension, seizures, vomiting, diarrhea
30. warmth, shivering, vasodilation
31. Chronic fever, fever of unknown origin
32. tinnitus, bruising
33. liver
34. conduction
35. convection
36. hyperthermia
37. Defervescence
38. hypothalamus
39. beta-blockers, phenothiazines, anticholinergics
40. abdominal distention, bowel sounds, nausea
41. b
42. a
43. a
44. a
45. b
46. a
47. d
48. b
49. c

50. a
51. c

CHAPTER 34

1. f
2. h
3. g
4. i
5. r
6. o
7. b
8. e
9. c
10. n
11. q
12. p
13. d
14. l
15. m
16. a
17. j
18. k
19. T
20. T
21. F. It can be done with a consistent bowel training program.
22. T
23. F. It can prevent constipation.
24. T
25. F. They can lead to constipation and fecal incontinence.
26. T
27. T
28. F. It can contribute by slowing bodily processes.
29. fiber
30. loosen
31. Diverticulosis
32. mastication
33. fat, fiber
34. liquid
35. 40
36. flatulence
37. person, individual
38. dependence
39. c
40. d
41. b
42. a
43. a
44. c
45. b
46. b
47. d

CHAPTER 35

1. t
2. k
3. l
4. f
5. h
6. c
7. q
8. v
9. b
10. r
11. d
12. u
13. p
14. n
15. o
16. e
17. j
18. g
19. i
20. a
21. m
22. s
23. F. voluntary
24. T
25. T
26. F. It is not normal.
27. F. No bag is worn.
28. T
29. F. sympathetic
30. T
31. T
32. T
33. F. Small amounts of blood are not visible.
34. F. 10cc
35. F. It is not always indicated.
36. vesicoureteral
37. detrusor
38. urea, creatinine, uric acid, bilirubin, metabolites of hormones
39. sodium, potassium
40. peristalsis
41. inflammation, infection, obstruction
42. frequency
43. 150, 500
44. Voiding urogram
45. Creatinine
46. Stress
47. functional or total
48. prompted voiding
49. habit training
50. Kegel exercises

51. b
52. a
53. d
54. a
55. c
56. d
57. d
58. b
59. a
60. c
61. b
62. a

CHAPTER 36

1. f
2. b
3. a
4. j
5. e
6. i
7. c
8. g
9. h
10. d
11. F. The melanocyte, which is located at the base of the epidermis, produces melanin, one of the pigments responsible for skin color.
12. T
13. F. fungal infection
14. F. dependence
15. T
16. T
17. T
18. Self-care
19. vitamin D
20. systemic
21. caries
22. blood
23. carcinomas
24. bed bath
25. b. Bathing/hygiene self-care deficit: Impaired ability to perform or complete bathing/hygiene activities for oneself
26. b. Hot-water bath: to relieve muscle spasm and muscle tension
27. d. Altered thought processes related to loss of memory
28. b
29. a
30. b
31. a
32. d

CHAPTER 37

1. j
2. h
3. g
4. l
5. m
6. i
7. o
8. f
9. c
10. b
11. e
12. d
13. n
14. k
15. a
16. T
17. F. vertebral bone decreases
18. T
19. T
20. F. A slight limitation of ROM is acceptable.
21. T
22. T
23. osteoclastic
24. atrophy
25. metatarsus varus
26. muscle weakness
27. Crepitus
28. Physical
29. Rehabilitation
30. a. Impaired physical mobility related to healing hip fracture
31. b. Physical therapist focuses on increasing mobility skills.
32. a. ROM exercises are isotonic exercises.
33. a
34. c
35. a
36. c
37. c

CHAPTER 38

1. c
2. b
3. d
4. o
5. r
6. k
7. e
8. j
9. p
10. a
11. h
12. l
13. m
14. f
15. g
16. n
17. q
18. i
19. s
20. T
21. T
22. F. The longer the person is immobile, the higher the risk of complications of disuse.
23. F. local circulation
24. F. drop in systolic blood pressure
25. T
26. T
27. Disuse
28. longer
29. energy
30. ulcers
31. orthostatic hypotension
32. calculi
33. 1, 2, hours
34. a. In a friction injury, the epidermal layer of the skin is rubbed off.
35. b. Moderate Risk for disuse syndrome: Assess and intervene every 2–4 hours.
36. c. Risk for disuse syndrome: A state in which an individual is at risk for deterioration of body systems as the result of prescribed or unavoidable musculoskeletal inactivity.
37. d
38. b
39. a
40. b
41. a

CHAPTER 39

1. i
2. h
3. d
4. c
5. k
6. j
7. a
8. e
9. b
10. w
11. g
12. l
13. r
14. m
15. n
16. q
17. v
18. o
19. t
20. p
21. u
22. s
23. f
24. T
25. T
26. F. Tidal volume is the amount of air moved with normal flow of air in and out of the lungs.
27. T
28. F. Sitting or standing straight without support is the optimum position.
29. T
30. F. Nicotine patches, along with counseling and support, have a 30% success rate.
31. F. The pain of fractured ribs restricts the chest wall movement.
32. T
33. T
34. F. In a stable client in a home environment clean technique is appropriate.
35. F. Oxygen saturation should be 95% or greater.
36. diaphragm
37. Elastic recoil
38. Surfactant
39. Sighing
40. Dead space
41. glottis
42. complete blood count
43. forced vital capacity
44. 95
45. Obtundation
46. Thick, tenacious
47. Altered breathing pattern
48. deoxygenated hemoglobin
49. Narcan (naloxone)
50. take a deep breath, hold it, force exhalation
51. b
52. a
53. c
54. a
55. a
56. d
57. d
58. a
59. c

60. a
61. d
62. a
63. b
64. b
65. d

CHAPTER 40

1. f
2. g
3. p
4. a
5. i
6. b
7. j
8. l
9. m
10. o
11. d
12. n
13. h
14. q
15. e
16. c
17. k
18. T
19. F. greater
20. T
21. F. decreased blood flow to tissues, decreased oxygen-carrying capacity of hemoglobin
22. T
23. T
24. F. They cause inflammation and scarring of cardiac tissue.
25. T
26. T
27. T
28. 5, 6
29. Cocaine, amphetamines
30. atherosclerosis
31. 140/90
32. cerebrovascular accident
33. left
34. Iron
35. aspirin
36. vasoconstriction
37. diet, exercise, smoking
38. a. Rest periods should be interspersed with activities.
39. c. Sauces often contain salt.
40. d. This will help to prevent orthostatic hypotension, a risk of this type of medication.

41. b. Any activity that tenses abdominal or chest muscles can cause the Valsalva maneuver.
42. a
43. d
44. c
45. d
46. a

CHAPTER 41

1. k
2. a
3. m
4. v
5. s
6. c
7. h
8. q
9. t
10. p
11. e
12. r
13. f
14. x
15. i
16. w
17. u
18. g
19. b
20. n
21. d
22. j
23. l
24. o
25. T
26. F. A depressed client may stay in bed an adequate number of hours but may feel mentally drained.
27. T
28. T
29. F. intrinsic
30. F. The person will return to a restful state if left alone.
31. T
32. T
33. zeitgeber
34. Melatonin
35. caffeine
36. REM
37. two
38. Narcolepsy
39. back
40. valerian
41. a
42. c

43. b. The client should go to bed only when sleepy, refrain from daytime naps, and set the alarm for the same time each day.
44. d. They are practiced for 20 minutes, can be used during the night as well, and may be enhanced with deep breathing exercises.
45. b
46. a
47. d
48. c
49. b

CHAPTER 42

1. s
2. dd
3. l
4. hh
5. m
6. u
7. y
8. t
9. ff
10. w
11. aa
12. bb
13. ii
14. v
15. n
16. h
17. d
18. b
19. c
20. ee
21. k
22. j
23. cc
24. i
25. a
26. r
27. x
28. p
29. q
30. g
31. z
32. e
33. gg
34. o
35. f
36. T
37. F. somatic pain
38. T
39. T
40. T

41. F. Pain is the same in the elderly as for any other population.
42. T
43. diagnostic, response
44. Referred
45. learned
46. Chronic
47. pain rating scale
48. neuropathic
49. neuropathic
50. c. Cultural expectations can mold the meaning of pain and the subsequent behaviors; your lack of understanding of those expectations can interfere with an accurate pain assessment.
51. d. Chronic pain related to malignant disease progression
52. d. Rescue dosing involves giving as-needed doses of an immediate-release analgesic in response to the breakthrough pain in addition to the scheduled analgesic dosage.
53. b
54. b
55. d
56. c
57. b

CHAPTER 43

1. i
2. e
3. c
4. j
5. o
6. m
7. l
8. s
9. b
10. d
11. g
12. f
13. p
14. a
15. q
16. r
17. n
18. k
19. h
20. F. older adults
21. T
22. T
23. T
24. F. conduction or sensorineural hearing loss
25. T

26. F. may be damaged from radiation
27. somesthetic
28. Exteroceptors
29. Strabismus
30. conductive
31. age
32. Snellen
33. staining
34. overload
35. a. Night blindness is one of the most distressing symptoms of cataracts because it interferes with night driving and seeing in darkened rooms.
36. c. Sensory/perceptual alterations: visual (cataract causing visual problems for her)
37. b. Risk for injury: teaching client how to care for eye to prevent it from becoming injured
38. c
39. a
40. b
41. b
42. a

CHAPTER 44

1. i
2. d
3. k
4. g
5. l
6. a
7. h
8. j
9. b
10. e
11. f
12. c
13. T
14. F. Nonverbal communication, such as eye contact, facial expression, and head movements, may have different meanings in different cultures.
15. T
16. F. Nurses should not discuss their feelings with clients.
17. T
18. T
19. T
20. F. Yes, they can.
21. T
22. T
23. neurological
24. Telegraphic

25. global
26. dysphonia
27. tracheostomy
28. Broca's
29. esophageal
30. receptive
31. Powerlessness
32. physical
33. a
34. c
35. d
36. b
37. a
38. a
39. c
40. d
41. a

CHAPTER 45

1. e
2. g
3. n
4. f
5. l
6. j
7. i
8. a
9. o
10. c
11. k
12. m
13. p
14. b
15. d
16. h
17. F. It can occur in younger people, although incidence increases with age.
18. T
19. T
20. F. The client may not be able to judge safety issues with any degree of insight.
21. T
22. T
23. T
24. F. Attention span is included in the assessment.
25. T
26. F. Bright colors or symbols should be used to identify room and/or bathroom for a client with chronic confusion.
27. frontal and temporal
28. acute
29. night

30. circadian
31. Alzheimer's
32. abstract
33. apraxia
34. fever
35. remote
36. injury
37. b. The other options could increase the risk of injury.
38. c. The other options could increase anxiety, which could worsen confusion.
39. a. The other options could impair the client's ability to get restful sleep.
40. d. Appropriate lighting and visible reminders are most helpful.
41. d
42. b
43. c
44. a
45. b

CHAPTER 46

1. e
2. c
3. b
4. a
5. d
6. T
7. T
8. T
9. T
10. F. positive
11. T
12. F. It has a direct relationship.
13. T
14. T
15. F. done only when indicated, such as with health problems that typically affect self-concept
16. body image
17. self-actualization
18. identity
19. power, control
20. emotional, cognitive, perceptual
21. parenting
22. self-esteem
23. Self-esteem disturbance
24. Chronic
25. Body image disturbance
26. b. This often results from long-standing negative evaluations or feelings about the self.
27. b. It is helpful to include people who have meaning to the client.

28. a. Shock and disbelief are the first stage of the grieving process.
29. c. It may help to talk to someone who has lived through and coped with the experience.
30. d. Encouraging choices in care promotes a sense of power and control.
31. a
32. b
33. c
34. d
35. c
36. a

CHAPTER 47

1. d
2. a
3. b
4. c
5. T
6. T
7. T
8. F. It is common.
9. T
10. T
11. F. It is a learned behavior that is a conditioned response to a specific stimulus.
12. T
13. T
14. F. compulsion
15. biological, ego
16. vulnerability
17. severe
18. pathological
19. obsession
20. Psychoanalytic
21. Powerlessness
22. environmental
23. obsessive, compulsive
24. economic
25. b. Powerlessness is associated with a perceived lack of control over situations or life events.
26. a. This is an early goal. The others would be achieved later.
27. c. Active listening involves listening to feelings as well as words.
28. b. Anxiolytics take two or three weeks to exert a therapeutic response, and the client may need reassurance and added support during this time.
29. d
30. a

31. c
32. c
33. d

CHAPTER 48

1. j
2. f
3. b
4. h
5. a
6. d
7. c
8. e
9. g
10. i
11. T
12. F. low socioeconomic status
13. T
14. T
15. F. Hope can be present.
16. T
17. T
18. risk, health
19. housing
20. Social status
21. Social
22. energy
23. control
24. self-determination
25. d
26. b
27. b
28. a
29. d
30. c
31. a
32. a

CHAPTER 49

1. e
2. j
3. a
4. i
5. b
6. c
7. g
8. f
9. d
10. h
11. F. acquired
12. T
13. T
14. F. Older adults are especially at risk.
15. T

16. F. may be objective or subjective
17. T
18. F. an intervention to improve role performance
19. prescribed
20. Altered
21. Impaired
22. perception
23. caretaker
24. Culture
25. perception, performance
26. d. Role distance is a condition in which a person carries out role behaviors that differ from those expected in the person's current cultural or societal situation.
27. c. Role strain is the condition in which a person feels unable to accomplish the tasks required of a role or of multiple roles. This results in feelings of frustration, tension, and overload.
28. a
29. b
30. a
31. a
32. b
33. d

CHAPTER 50

1. n
2. a
3. f
4. k
5. j
6. i
7. e
8. h
9. m
10. d
11. o
12. l
13. p
14. c
15. g
16. b
17. T
18. F. dysfunctional grieving
19. T
20. T
21. T
22. F. many people
23. F. uncomfortable
24. religious, condolences, burial
25. self
26. recognition

27. reflection
28. family
29. presence
30. Condemnation
31. b. Recognition: Shock and Denial: Somatic Responses: may include gastrointestinal symptoms and cardiopulmonary reactions
32. a. act of choosing when and to whom a person will give attention to a loss and allow thoughts and feeling to enter the conscious mind
33. c. an unexpected, involuntary resurgence of acute grief-related emotions and behaviors triggered by routine events
34. b
35. a
36. c
37. d
38. d

CHAPTER 51

1. f
2. m
3. j
4. b
5. c
6. e
7. h
8. q
9. i
10. o
11. n
12. l
13. p
14. d
15. a
16. g
17. k
18. T
19. F. internal or sense
20. F. may not precisely fit
21. T
22. F. At least one-third of the nurses never assessed their client's sexual health.
23. T
24. T
25. biological, cultural
26. adolescence
27. Orgasm
28. emotional, love
29. embarrassment
30. sexual

31. touch
32. a. Altered sexuality patterns: The state in which an individual expresses concern regarding his or her sexuality
33. a. Altered sexuality patterns related to change in or loss of body part and stress of anticipated results of surgery
34. a. The first step in the PLISSIT model is *permission* to discuss sexual issues.
35. a
36. b
37. b
38. d
39. a

CHAPTER 52

1. m
2. g
3. i
4. c
5. j
6. k
7. l
8. b
9. a
10. d
11. f
12. e
13. h
14. T
15. F. exhaustion stage
16. T
17. T
18. F. rationalization
19. F. year
20. T
21. F. Stress is highly individualized.
22. T
23. T
24. alarm reaction
25. eustress
26. crisis
27. 24, 48
28. projection
29. beta-endorphins
30. sympathetic
31. coping
32. adulthood
33. denial
34. b. He is drinking and does not acknowledge that his wound is infected.

35. c. A therapeutic relationship is necessary to build trust and is a precursor to other interventions.
36. d. Knowledge and control are best achieved by helping him learn how to manage his health status.
37. a. Relaxation and music can be used together. The other methods are cognitive coping methods.
38. b
39. c
40. a
41. d
42. a

CHAPTER 53

1. o
2. g
3. k
4. b
5. a
6. h
7. c
8. j
9. q
10. e
11 f
12. i
13. d
14. l
15. n
16. m
17. p
18. T
19. T
20. F. adaptation
21. F. healthy
22. T
23. T
24. F. may not be remembered or may be rejected
25. individuals, families, cultural
26. affective, socialization, health
27. parents
28. coping
29. trusting
30. data
31. overcome, goal
32. d. Nursing interventions used to establish a nurse-family relationship include establishing trust and listening actively.
33. c. Nursing interventions to change family behaviors include providing education.

34. d. Helping family members identify destructive behavior is an advanced nursing skill but is essential to help the family with destructive behaviors.
35. c
36. d
37. b
38. c
39. d

CHAPTER 54

1. c
2. f
3. g
4. a
5. h
6. e
7. b
8. i
9. j
10. d
11. T
12. F. may be minimized
13. F. inadequate social system
14. T
15. T
16. F. not considered clients; needs may go unmet
17. T
18. ambivalent
19. neglects
20. stress
21. more
22. assess, perception
23. insight
24. support
25. b. An example of an extrafamily stressor is when a caregiver quits work to care for a family member and then experiences a financial hardship.
26. a. She is vulnerable for felt difficulty in performing the family caregiver role.
27. d. Providing direct assistance helps the caregiver identify professional resources.
28. b
29. b
30. d
31. d
32. d

CHAPTER 55

1. f
2. e

3. g
4. i
5. c
6. d
7. b
8. j
9. a
10. h
11. T
12. F. not necessarily synonymous
13. F. without proof
14. F. Nurses commonly avoid addressing spirituality.
15. T
16. T
17. T
18. God
19. Hope
20. Taoists
21. denominations
22. beliefs
23. spiritual
24. prayer
25. b. Mexican-Americans have a tendency toward traditional values of family roles, including men heading the family.
26. d. Asking a client "What has bothered you most about being sick?" helps you assess the client's perceived relation between spiritual beliefs and health.
27. c. Spiritual distress: Disruption in the life principle that pervades a person's entire being and that integrates and transcends one's biological and psychological nature
28. d
29. a
30. b
31. b
32. d

CHAPTER 56

1. c
2. g
3. h
4. j
5. b
6. f
7. e
8. d
9. a
10. i
11. T

12. T
13. F. orthotist
14. F. long-term-care facilities
15. T
16. T
17. F. unilateral neglect
18. injury, mental conditions
19. physical, bowel, skin
20. coping
21. Assisted
22. Americans, Disabilities
23. Functional Independence Measure
24. maximizing, complications
25. b. The physical therapist assesses client's range of motion, mobility, strength, balance, and gait.
26. d. Respite care is a temporary service enabling informal caregivers to take a break.
27. a. Self-care deficit is applicable to people experiencing impaired ability to perform any one of the basic self-care activities.
28. b
29. c
30. c
31. c
32. d

CHAPTER 57

1. h
2. n
3. g
4. l
5. p
6. o
7. m
8. b
9. i
10. q
11. d
12. c
13. a
14. j
15. f
16. k
17. e
18. T
19. F. circulating
20. T
21. T
22. T
23. F. expected and normal
24. T

25. T
26. F. dantrolene sodium
27. T
28. elective
29. preinduction
30. general
31. surgeon
32. Standard
33. after
34. Laryngospasm
35. incentive spirometer
36. six
37. Verbal, written
38. a. Anxiety is expected due to the uncertain outcome of the surgery.
39. c. They should be done 10–12 times for best effect.
40. b. It is critical that clients have bowel sounds, ensuring that paralytic ileus has not occurred.
41. c. Splinting the incision makes movement more comfortable.
42. d
43. b
44. c
45. a
46. d

CHAPTER 58

1. d
2. e
3. j
4. b
5. f
6. a
7. h
8. l
9. k
10. c
11. g
12. i
13. T
14. T
15. T
16. F. They should be done first.
17. T
18. F. They do influence outcomes.
19. T
20. T
21. T
22. F. It is routinely done.
23. resuscitate, stabilize
24. chief complaint
25. social worker
26. nonurgent

27. breathe
28. weight
29. violent
30. sitter
31. 95
32. vital signs
33. c
34. c
35. b
36. a
37. b
38. d
39. a
40. d
41. c

CHAPTER 59

1. c
2. m
3. l
4. k
5. f
6. i
7. d
8. a
9. e
10. b
11. g
12. h
13. j
14. T
15. T
16. F. Telehealth
17. F. to all
18. F. Assessments vary.
19. T
20. T
21. T
22. F. increase
23. direct care
24. detectives
25. community partnership primary care
26. Vulnerable
27. environmental
28. assessment
29. census
30. outcomes
31. Evaluation
32. d. A public health nurse promotes and protects the health of populations.
33. b. Knowledge deficit related to inadequate training in personal and environmental hygiene is the most relevant nursing diagnosis.

34. a. For the nurse to be successful with nursing interventions, the nurse must build consensus and cohesiveness among the staff and assess whether goals, interests, and motivation of the day school are the same as those of the nurse.
35. c
36. b
37. a
38. d
39. d
40. a

CHAPTER 60

1. g
2. a
3. e
4. j
5. b
6. c
7. h
8. i
9. d
10. f
11. T
12. F. medical model
13. T
14. F. positive impact
15. T
16. T
17. F. The goal is to maintain the maximum level of functioning.
18. roles
19. political, social
20. physician
21. guest
22. Escorts
23. physician
24. Impaired home maintenance management
25. satisfaction
26. b. Examples of support services are assistance with shopping, meals, and cleaning.
27. a. Risk for injury related to lack of experience using crutches (Treatment includes teaching the client to use them.)
28. c. Mutual goal setting and compliance are increased by the use of a contract (an agreement between two or more parties that something will or will not be done).
29. a
30. b
31. d
32. a
33. d

Name _____ Specific Skill Performed _____

Date _____ Attempt Number _____

Instructor _____ PASS _____ FAIL _____

Performance Checklist 26–1.   Administering Oral Medications

		S	U	Comments
1.	Verified order and client allergies; assessed appropriate parameters (e.g., blood pressure, pulse) if applicable.			
2.	Dispensed solid medication correctly.			
	a. Selected medication, calculated dose based on labeled concentration, and rechecked dose.			
	b. Poured medication into soufflé cup if whole tablet used, or split a scored tablet with a gloved hand or cutting device for a partial dose.			
	c. Left unit-dose medications in original container and placed all in a single cup, except for medications requiring special assessments.			
	d. Removed tablet from a stock medication bottle by dropping it into bottle cap and transferring to a soufflé cup.			
	e. Poured a liquid dose by mixing medication and removing lid, placing it upside down. Held bottle with label under palm of hand. Poured dose holding plastic cup at eye level, with thumbnail at the dose mark, and used the bottom of the meniscus as the measuring guide. Wiped lip of container before closing.			
3.	Rechecked all medications and dosages after dispensing.			
4.	Identified client and performed final assessments.			
5.	Gave medications to client.			
	a. Rechecked accuracy of a medication that the client questioned.			
	b. Removed unit-dose wrappers and placed medications in the cup or client's hand per client preference.			
	c. Offered sufficient liquid for swallowing and ensured that client swallowed all medications.			
6.	Documented medications administered immediately and stated to check client response in 30 minutes.			

Additional Comments:

NOTES

Name _____   Specific Skill Performed _____

Date _____   Attempt Number _____

Instructor _____   PASS _____   FAIL _____

Performance Checklist 26–2.   Withdrawing Medication from an Ampule

		S	U	Comments
1.	Opened ampule by tapping upper chamber to drop fluid into lower chamber. Wrapped alcohol swab or gauze pad around ampule neck and snapped neck so it opened away from nurse.			
2.	Placed ampule on flat surface and withdrew medication into syringe without touching needle against ampule rim. Tilted ampule as needed to keep needle below level of medication. Did not inject air into ampule.			
3.	Ejected excess air or fluid from syringe. Recapped needle and replaced with new one, properly discarding old needle. Compared final volume to dose ordered.			

Additonal Comments:

Name_____   Specific Skill Performed_____

Date_____   Attempt Number _____

Instructor_____   PASS _____   FAIL _____

Performance Checklist 26–3.   Withdrawing Medication from a Vial

		S	U	Comments
1.	Removed plastic cap of a new vial or wiped rubber seal of an open one with alcohol swab. Used a previously-used vial only if opened within 30 days.			
2.	Prepared syringe by securing capped needle to syringe with a twisting motion and removed needle cover. Drew back on plunger to fill syringe with a volume of air equal to the medication dose.			
3.	Withdrew medication.			
a.	Inserted needle into center of rubber seal and injected air.			
b.	Inverted vial and withdrew medication slowly while holding vial at eye level. Kept tip of needle in solution at all times.			
c.	Removed excess air by tapping side of syringe with finger and pushed air back into vial. Removed additional fluid if needed to obtain correct dose.			
d.	Returned vial to upright position and removed needle by pulling back on barrel, not plunger. Removed excess air.			
4.	Recapped needle and replaced with a new one if indicated. Compared volume of fluid in syringe with ordered dose.			

Additional Comments:

Name_____   Specific Skill Performed_____

Date_____   Attempt Number_____

Instructor_____   PASS_____   FAIL_____

Performance Checklist 26–4.   Mixing Insulin in a Single Syringe

	S	U	Comments
1. Mixed insulin in suspension by rotating vial between palms of hands. Wiped vials with alcohol after checking expiration dates.			
2. Added air to both vials.			
a. Drew up volume of air equal to dose of modified (NPH) insulin and injected into NPH vial without letting needle touch solution. Removed needle from vial.			
b. Drew up a volume of air equal to dose of regular (unmodified) insulin and injected into regular insulin vial. Left needle in vial.			
3. Removed insulin from both vials.			
a. Inverted regular insulin vial and withdrew correct dose without air bubbles present.			
b. Turned vial upright and removed needle from vial.			
c. Cleansed port of NPH vial, inserted needle, inverted vial and withdrew correct dose. Turned vial upright again and removed needle. Recapped. Had another licensed nurse double-check the dose. Administered within 5 minutes of preparation.			

Additional Comments:

Name_____   Specific Skill Performed_____

Date_____   Attempt Number _____

Instructor_____   PASS _____ FAIL _____

Performance Checklist 26–5. Administering an Intradermal Injection

		S	U	Comments
1.	Checked order and noted client allergies. Withdrew medication from vial and brought dose to bedside.			
2.	Checked client identity, prepared client by explaining procedure and using proper positioning. Donned disposable gloves.			
3.	Prepared injection site and syringe.			
a.	Chose an area free from bruises, redness, or lesions.			
b.	Cleansed skin with alcohol wipe using circular motion outward from injection site.			
c.	Removed needle cap and checked that syringe was free of air and volume was correct.			
4.	Injected medication.			
a.	Held syringe in dominant hand and spread skin taut with nondominant hand.			
b.	Inserted needle bevel-up at a 10–15 degree angle into skin for 1/8-inch or until bevel disappeared from view. Needle was visible below skin surface and resistance was felt.			
c.	Injected medication slowly while watching for wheal formation. If none appeared, withdrew needle slightly and continued injecting.			
d.	Withdrew needle at same angle and patted dry, without rubbing, with gauze pad.			
5.	Observed for immediate allergic reaction. Disposed of equipment, removed gloves, and washed hands. Circled the skin site and documented appropriately in medical record.			

Additional Comments:

NOTES

Name _____   Specific Skill Performed _____

Date _____   Attempt Number _____

Instructor_____   PASS _____   FAIL _____

Performance Checklist 26–6.   Administering a Subcutaneous (SC) Injection

	S	U	Comments
1. Checked order, noting any client allergies. Withdrew medication and brought materials to bedside.			
2. Checked client identity, prepared client by explaining procedure and using proper positioning. Donned disposable gloves.			
3. Prepared injection site and syringe.			
a. Chose an area free from bruises, redness, or lesions.			
b. Cleansed skin with alcohol wipe using circular motion outward from injection site.			
c. Removed needle cap and checked that syringe was free of air and volume was correct.			
4. Injected the medication.			
a. Held syringe in dominant hand between thumb and forefinger.			
b. Pinched or "bunched up" SC tissue between thumb and forefinger of nondominant hand.			
c. Quickly inserted needle up to hub at 45- or 90-degree angle, depending on needle length.			
d. Released tissue and grasped distal end of syringe. Aspirated for blood return unless injecting insulin or heparin.			
e. Injected medication slowly and steadily if no blood return. Discarded syringe and repeated procedure if positive blood return.			
f. Withdrew needle at same angle used for insertion and massaged area with alcohol swab unless heparin given.			
5. Disposed of equipment, removed gloves, and washed hands. Documented appropriately and stated to recheck client in 30 minutes.			

Additional Comments:

Name _____   Specific Skill Performed _____

Date _____   Attempt Number _____

Instructor _____   PASS _____   FAIL _____

Performance Checklist 26–7.   Administering an Intramuscular Injection

	S	U	Comments
1. Checked order, noting any client allergies. Withdrew medication and brought materials to bedside.			
2. Checked client identity, prepared client by explaining procedure and using proper positioning. Donned disposable gloves.			
3. Prepared injection site and syringe.			
a. Chose an area free from bruises, redness, or lesions.			
b. Cleansed skin with alcohol wipe using circular motion outward from injection site.			
c. Removed needle cap and checked that syringe was free of air and volume was correct.			
4. Injected medication.			
a. Held syringe in dominant hand between thumb and forefinger.			
b. Spread skin taut between thumb and forefinger of nondominant hand, or displaced tissue using Z-track technique.			
c. Inserted needle quickly at 90-degree angle up to hub.			
d. Released skin and grasped distal end of syringe in nondominant hand.			
e. Aspirated for blood return by pulling back gently on plunger with thumb and forefinger of dominant hand. Discarded syringe and began procedure again if blood seen.			
f. Injected medication slowly at a rate of about 10 seconds per mL.			
g. Waited a few seconds, withdrew needle quickly at same angle used for injection. Applied gentle pressure to site with alcohol wipe or small gauze.			
5. Disposed of equipment, removed gloves, and washed hands. Documented appropriately and stated to recheck client at appropriate time interval.			

Additional Comments:

Name_____   Specific Skill Performed_____

Date_____   Attempt Number _____

Instructor_____   PASS _____ FAIL _____

Performance Checklist 26–8.   Adding Medication to an IV Bag

		S	U	Comments
1.	Checked medication order. Drew up medication into a syringe from vial or ampule.			
2.	Injected medication into IV solution.			
	a. Closed roller clamp on tubing if already attached to solution bag. Wiped medication port of IV bag with alcohol wipe.			
	c. Inserted needle into center of medication port and injected medication into bag.			
	d. Withdrew needle and properly disposed of needle-syringe assembly without recapping.			
	e. Rotated solution bag gently but thoroughly.			
	f. Affixed a medication label to bag with medication name, dose, date, time, and nurse's initials noted.			
3.	Primed tubing and hung solution according to standard procedure. Documented appropriately.			

Additional Comments:

NOTES

Name _____   Specific Skill Performed _____

Date _____   Attempt Number _____

Instructor _____   PASS _____   FAIL _____

Performance Checklist 26–9. Administering an IV Medication by Intermittent Infusion

		S	U	Comments
1.	Checked order and prepared and labeled IV medication.			
2.	Administered IV medication through an existing IV line.			
a.	Attached secondary tubing to IV bag using standard protocol. Ensured that nonvented tubing was attached to IV bag and vented tubing was attached to IV bottle. Primed and labeled bag, as appropriate, and brought materials to bedside.			
b.	Identified client, assessed IV site, and donned gloves if part of agency policy.			
c.	Removed cap from distal IV tubing and attached needle or needleless device.			
d.	Wiped IV additive port of primary IV line with alcohol swab and attached secondary IV tubing to primary line above the level of the regulator clamp.			
e.	Lowered primary IV solution below level of the IV medication bag using hook provided by manufacturer. Regulated IV medication drip rate or set infusion pump as ordered. Returned to reset drip rate if needed and reassessed client.			
3.	Administered IV medication through a heparin lock (intermittent infusion device).			
a.	Attached tubing as needed to IV medication bag or bottle using standard protocol. Primed tubing and attached needle or needleless device.			
b.	Withdrew 3 mL sterile normal saline solution into 3 mL syringe (vary amount according to policy) and brought all materials to bedside.			
c.	Identified client, assessed IV site, and donned gloves if part of agency policy.			
d.	Wiped port of intermittent infusion device with alcohol swab. Assessed site and flushed infusion port with sterile saline per protocol.			
e.	Wiped port again. Attached IV medication tubing to infusion port and regulated flow rate.			
f.	Returned upon completion of infusion, closed roller clamp, removed tubing from port, and flushed again with ordered solution. Assessed IV site and client response and documented.			

Additional Comments:

Name _____   Specific Skill Performed _____

Date _____   Attempt Number _____

Instructor _____   PASS _____   FAIL _____

Performance Checklist 26–10.   Administering an IV Push Medication

	S	U	Comments
1. Checked medication order and assessed client allergies. Prepared medication and brought materials to bedside. Checked client identity, assessed IV site, and donned gloves if part of agency policy.			
2. Administered medication through existing IV line.			
a. With alcohol swab, wiped IV additive port of primary line nearest to client.			
b. Inserted needle into port and pinched off tubing above injection port.			
c. Injected medication at manufacturer's recommended rate, using watch with second hand to time the injection.			
d. Released tubing, removed syringe, and assessed client tolerance of medication.			
3. Administered medication through an intermittent infusion device.			
a. Drew up normal saline into two syringes in a volume according to agency policy (often 3 mL). Labeled syringes.			
b. Wiped port of intermittent infusion device with alcohol swab.			
c. Inserted one syringe with normal saline and injected slowly. Removed needle and syringe.			
d. Wiped port again with alcohol swab. Inserted syringe with medication into port and injected at manufacturer's recommended rate. Used watch with second hand to ensure accurate timing. Assessed site during injection.			
e. Wiped port again with alcohol swab. Inserted second normal saline flush syringe into port and injected slowly. Withdrew needle and syringe and correctly disposed of all supplies.			
4. Documented medication according to policy.			

Additional Comments:

Name_____ Specific Skill Performed_____

Date_____ Attempt Number _____

Instructor_____ PASS _____ FAIL _____

Performance Checklist 26–11.   Administering an Eye Medication

	S	U	Comments
1. Checked the medication order and any client allergies.			
2. Prepared the client for medication instillation by checking the client's identity, explaining the procedure, donning gloves, and hyperextending the client's head. Assessed the condition of the eye and washed away exudate, wiping from inner to outer canthus.			
3. Administered an eye drop.			
a. Removed cap and filled medicine dropper (if used) to prescribed amount.			
b. Placed nondominant hand on client's cheekbone under eyelid and pulled downward against bony orbit to expose lower conjunctival sac. Held tissue or cotton ball under eyelid and applied slight pressure to inner canthus.			
c. Rested dominant hand against client's forehead and held medication ½–¾ inch above conjunctival sac.			
d. Asked client to look up at ceiling and instilled prescribed number of drops into lower conjunctival sac.			
e. Asked client to gently close eye and move it around. Applied gentle pressure over lacrimal duct for one minute or asked client to do so.			
4. Administered an eye ointment.			
a. Removed cap from tube and placed on its side. Squeezed and discarded a small bead of medication.			
b. Separated client's eyelids with thumb and forefinger of nondominant hand, pulling lower eyelid over bony prominence of cheek (or, drew upper lid up and away from eyeball if instilling in upper lid).			
c. Asked client to look up for instillation in lower lid (down for instillation in upper) and applied thin layer of ointment along inside edge of lower or upper lid, moving from inner to outer canthus. Asked client to gently close eye and move it around.			

	S	U	Comments
5. Administered an eye disk.			
a. Opened package and pressed tip of index finger against convex part of disk.			
b. Pulled lower eyelid away from eye with nondominant hand and asked client to look up.			
c. Placed disk horizontally in conjunctival sac between iris and lower lid.			
d. Pulled lower lid out, up and over the disk. Asked the client to blink a few times. Repeated if still visible. Had client place fingers against closed lids and press without rubbing eyes or moving disk.			
e. Removed disk by inverting lower eyelid to see disk, and used thumb and index finger of dominant hand to pinch disk and lift it from conjunctival sac. Stroked closed eyelid with fingertip in gentle, long, circular motions to lower a disk caught in the upper eye.			
6. Removed gloves, washed hands, and documented.			

Additional Comments:

Name _____   Specific Skill Performed _____

Date _____   Attempt Number _____

Instructor _____   PASS _____   FAIL _____

Performance Checklist 26–12.   Irrigating an Eye

		S	U	Comments
1.	Prepared client for irrigation and helped client sit or lie with head tilted toward eye to be irrigated. Used waterproof pad and gloves. Poured irrigant into container and drew up into syringe using aseptic technique. Cleaned eyelids and eyelashes with cotton ball moistened with irrigant or normal saline. Positioned curved basin under cheek and asked client to hold if possible.			
2.	Irrigated eye.			
a.	Used nondominant hand to hold client's upper lid open and expose lower conjunctival sac.			
b.	Held irrigation syringe 1″ above eye without touching eye and pushed fluid gently into conjunctival sac, directing flow from inner canthus to outer canthus.			
c.	Repeated irrigation until secretions or irrigant were gone. Allowed client to close eyes intermittently during procedure. Dried area with cotton balls and offered client a towel to dry face and neck.			
3.	Removed gloves, washed hands, and documented.			

Additional Comments:

NOTES

Name _____ Specific Skill Performed _____

Date _____ Attempt Number _____

Instructor _____ PASS _____ FAIL _____

Performance Checklist 26–13.   Administering an Ear Medication

		S	U	Comments
1.	Checked the medication order and any client allergies.			
2.	Prepared the client for medication instillation by checking the client's identity, explaining the procedure, helping the client lie with affected ear upward, and donning gloves. Assessed condition of ear and washed away cerumen or exudates with cotton-tipped applicators.			
3.	Administered the medication.			
a.	Removed cap from bottle and placed cap on its side. Filled medication dropper to prescribed amount.			
b.	Pulled the pinna up and back for an adult or down and back for a child.			
c.	Held dropper ½ inch above ear canal and instilled ordered number of drops.			
d.	Asked client to maintain side-lying position for 2–3 minutes. Used finger to apply gentle pressure to tragus of ear or asked client to do so. Placed a cotton ball into outermost portion of ear canal.			
4.	Removed gloves, documented, and stated to check on client in 15 minutes to remove cotton ball, assess condition, and reposition.			

Additional Comments:

Name_____   Specific Skill Performed_____

Date_____   Attempt Number _____

Instructor_____   PASS _____   FAIL_____

Performance Checklist 26–14.   Administering an Intranasal Medication

		S	U	Comments
1.	Checked medication order and noted any client allergies.			
2.	Checked identity of client, explained procedure, donned gloves, and asked client to blow nose unless contraindicated.			
3.	Administered nasal spray medication.			
	a. Removed cap from bottle and placed cap on its side.			
	b. Asked adult client to tilt head backward and supported head with nondominant hand. Kept a child's head in upright position.			
	c. Held the medication container just inside tip of nostril without touching nasal tissue. Asked client to occlude other nostril and inhale while spraying in. Positioned client for comfort.			
4.	Administered nasal drops.			
	a. Removed cap from bottle and placed cap on its side. Positioned client to accommodate intended site of action. Supported head with nondominant hand.			
	b. Held tip of dropper just above intended nostril and pointed toward midline of ethmoid bone. Instilled ordered number of drops with client breathing through mouth, and without touching nasal tissue with dropper.			
	c. Asked client to maintain head position for 5 minutes and then assisted to comfortable position. Documented care.			

Additional Comments:

NOTES

Name_____   Specific Skill Performed_____

Date_____   Attempt Number _____

Instructor_____   PASS _____ FAIL _____

Performance Checklist 26–15.   Administering a Vaginal Medication

		S	U	Comments
1.	Checked medication order and prepared client for medication instillation. Identified client, explained procedure, offered opportunity to void, provided privacy, and assisted client to supine position with abdomen and legs draped. Donned gloves, inspected area, and provided hygiene as needed.			
2.	Administered vaginal suppository.			
a.	Removed suppository from wrapper and inserted into applicator, if used.			
b.	Lubricated rounded end with water-soluble lubricant. Lubricated index finger of gloved dominant hand if not using applicator.			
c.	Separated client's labia with nondominant hand and inserted rounded end of suppository along posterior vaginal wall for entire finger length. Withdrew finger or applicator and wiped away excess lubricant from client's genitals.			
3.	Administered a foam, jelly, or cream medication.			
a.	Filled applicator with medication per package directions.			
b.	Separated labia with nondominant hand, pointed applicator toward client's sacrum and used dominant hand to insert applicator 2–3" into vagina.			
c.	Depressed plunger on applicator to push medication out of applicator.			
d.	Withdrew applicator and placed it on tissue or paper towel. Wiped away excess medication from client's genitals.			
4.	Assisted client to comfortable position and asked her to remain supine for 5–10 minutes. Offered perineal pad if needed. Washed applicator with soap and water and stored for future use. Removed gloves, washed hands, and documented.			

Additional Comments:

Name _____   Specific Skill Performed _____

Date _____   Attempt Number _____

Instructor _____   PASS _____   FAIL _____

Performance Checklist 26–16.   Administering a Rectal Medication

		S	U	Comments
1.	Checked medication order and prepared client for medication instillation. Identified client, explained procedure, offered opportunity to void, provided privacy, assisted client to left lateral Sims position with upper leg flexed, and draped client. Donned gloves, inspected area, and provided hygiene as needed.			
2.	Administered medication using clean aseptic technique.			
a.	Removed suppository from packaging. Lubricated rounded end of suppository and index finger of gloved, dominant hand.			
b.	Instructed client to breathe slowly and deeply through mouth. Separated buttocks with gloved, nondominant hand. Used dominant hand to insert rounded end of suppository 4″ into rectal canal along rectal wall (2″ for child).			
c.	Withdrew finger and wiped away any fecal material or excess lubricant from client's anus. Asked client to remain on side for 5–30 minutes depending on medication.			
3.	Removed gloves, washed hands, and gave client call bell to ring when urge to defecate was felt.			
4.	Returned after 5 minutes to see if suppository was expelled (reinserted if it was expelled). Assisted client as needed. Documented administration and results.			

Additional Comments:

Name _____   Specific Skill Performed _____

Date _____   Attempt Number _____

Instructor _____   PASS _____   FAIL _____

Performance Checklist 27–1. Hand-Washing

		S	U	Comments
1.	Turned on warm water faucet, wet hands, and lowered arms under running water with hands held lower than elbows.			
2.	Used soap to rub all surfaces of hands. Worked soap into foamy lather while rubbing hands together using circular motions.			
3.	Used care between fingers, creases, and breaks in skin, and under nails. Spent at least 15–30 seconds cleaning each hand.			
4.	Rinsed hands with warm running water, with water washing down hands and over fingertips.			
5.	Dried hands with towel, used towel to turn off faucet, and discarded towel in receptacle.			

Additional Comments:

Name _____   Specific Skill Performed _____

Date _____   Attempt Number _____

Instructor _____   PASS _____ FAIL _____

Performance Checklist 27–2.   Caring for a Client in Isolation

	S	U	Comments
Application of Barriers			
1. Washed hands. Picked up gown by collar and allowed it to unfold. Put arms through sleeves and pulled gown up over shoulders. Fastened neckties and waist ties, making sure gown lapped over itself at the back.			
2. Put on disposable gloves by pulling cuff of each glove over edge of gown sleeve, and interlaced fingers as needed to adjust fit of gloves.			
3. Donned mask by positioning over nose and mouth. Bent nose bar over bridge of nose, and fastened it in place with elastic or strings.			
4. Put on goggles after mask was in place.			
Removal of Barriers			
1. Removed goggles first without touching face or hair at the entrance to client's room. Untied gown at waist only.			
2. Removed gloves by grasping outside cuff of one glove and pulling glove inside out over hand. Held removed glove in second hand, and pulled second glove off inside out over first.			
3. Removed gown by untying gown at neck and allowing it to fall forward. Slid hands through sleeves and removed them without touching outside of gown. Held gown at inside shoulder seams away from body, turned it inside out and folded it with contaminated side to the inside. Discarded in proper receptacle.			
4. Removed mask by pulling elastic or untying strings without touching outside surface of mask. Discarded and washed hands.			

Additional Comments:

Name _____ Specific Skill Performed _____

Date _____ Attempt Number _____

Instructor _____ PASS _____ FAIL _____

Performance Checklist 27–3.   Donning and Removing Sterile Gloves

	S	U	Comments
Donning Sterile Gloves			
1. Washed hands and removed rings with stones or irregular surfaces. Grasped package at tabs above sealed edge, peeled down, and discarded outer wrapper.			
2. Placed inner package on flat surface, opened inner package at first fold, touched outside of folded edge and pulled outward. Opened next fold, pulling edge outward without touching inside of package.			
3. Put on first glove.			
a. Grasped folded edge of cuff of one glove.			
b. Lifted glove above wrapper and away from body.			
c. Slid opposite hand into glove. Did not adjust cuff or fingers at this time, or let ungloved hand touch outside of glove.			
4. Put on second glove.			
a. Picked up second glove by sliding sterile gloved fingers under cuff edge. Kept gloved thumb off cuff of second glove.			
b. Slid fingers of opposite hand into glove. Let go of edge when hand in glove. Adjusted for comfort and fit.			
Removing Sterile Gloves			
1. Grasped outside of one glove near base of thumb and removed it by pulling inside out.			
2. Discarded glove or held it in palm of gloved hand.			
3. Slid ungloved thumb or fingers inside second glove and removed pulling it inside out. Discarded appropriately and washed hands.			

Additional Comments:

Name _____   Specific Skill Performed _____

Date _____   Attempt Number _____

Instructor _____   PASS _____   FAIL _____

Performance Checklist 27–4.   Preparing a Sterile Field by Opening a Tray Wrapped in a Sterile Drape

		S	U	Comments
1.	Washed hands and removed kit from outer wrapper.			
2.	Positioned inner package in center of work surface with outer flap facing away from person.			
3.	Reached around (not over) package to open flap away from person, touching outside of flap only.			
4.	Opened side flaps one at a time, uppermost side first, and in same manner as first. Did not let hands cross sterile field.			
5.	Opened innermost flap last and stood back far enough to avoid touching person while opening.			

Additional Comments:

Performance Checklist 27–5.   Preparing a Sterile Field Using a Sterile Drape

		S	U	Comments
1.	Established a clean, dry, flat work area and checked expiration date on supplies.			
2.	Set up a drape on a surface at least 2 inches larger on all sides than area needed to work with supplies.			
	a. Opened outer wrapping of sterile cloth drape and kept drape sterile.			
	b. Picked up drape by loose corner edge and lifted drape up and away from body.			
	c. With other hand, grasped another corner edge and spread drape in air.			
	d. Decided which surface should remain sterile and spread drape on table with sterile side facing up.			
3.	Added dry sterile supplies.			
	a. Opened peel-apart package by grasping edges designed to peel open. Opened package over sterile field so material fell freely from package onto field without touching the hands.			
	b. Opened a wrapped package by holding object in one hand or by underside of wrapping. Unwrapped first corner away from body, then each side, then opened last corner toward body. Stabilized corners against wrist, turned object onto sterile field and dropped it onto field without touching sterile field.			
4.	Added sterile liquids.			
	a. Removed or loosened cap without touching inside of cap or rim of bottle. Placed cap face up on flat surface. Labeled bottle with date and time if first use.			
	b. Donned sterile glove and arranged cup to hold liquid in upright position.			
	c. Picked up liquid with ungloved hand so label was in palm of hand. Lipped bottle if not first use.			
	d. Held bottle of solution 10 cm (4 inches) above container. Poured without spills or splashes. Avoided touching field with bottle lid. Replaced lid and donned second sterile glove.			

Additional Comments:

Performance Checklist 27–6.   Performing a Surgical Hand Scrub

		S	U	Comments
1.	Applied surgical attire (shoe covers, cap or hood, face mask, protective eyewear). Opened scrub brush for ready use. Turned on water using control lever.			
2.	Wet hands and arms, keeping elbows flexed with hands higher than elbows, and allowing water to flow off arms at elbows.			
3.	Used plastic nail stick to clean under all fingernails. Removed scrub brush from wrapper and wet it. Applied antimicrobial liquid if not contained in brush.			
4.	Scrubbed nails of one hand with 15 strokes and repeated with other hand. Scrubbed palm of one hand, each side of thumbs and fingers, and back of hand with 10 strokes each. Repeated for other hand.			
5.	Divided arms mentally into thirds, and scrubbed each third with 10 strokes or by time according to agency policy. Discarded brush.			
6.	Flexed arms and rinsed each arm from fingertips to elbow in a single smooth motion, letting water run off at elbows. Released water control and walked backward into opening room with hands elevated in front and away from body.			
7.	Picked up sterile towel from sterile set-up area without dripping water onto the field. Used one end of the towel to dry one hand using rotating motion, and moving from fingers to elbow. Used other end of towel to repeat with other hand. Discarded towel into designated area.			

Additional Comments:

NOTES

Name _____   Specific Skill Performed _____

Date _____   Attempt Number _____

Instructor _____   PASS _____   FAIL _____

Performance Checklist 27–7.   Donning a Sterile Gown and Closed Gloving

	S	U	Comments
1. Donned surgical attire and scrubbed while designated person opened sterile gown and gloves.			
2. Identified inner surface of gown and picked it up beneath neckband without touching sterile field or outer surface of gown. Ensured control of all folded layers. Moved away from table, held gown away from body at arm's length, and allowed it to unfold from top down without touching floor.			
3. Held gown below neckband near shoulders and slid both hands into sleeves until fingers were at end of cuffs but not through them. Had someone tie gown.			
4. With hands covered by sterile gown cuffs, opened inner sterile glove package and picked up first glove by cuff. Positioned glove on forearm of dominant hand so cuff faced hand and fingers faced elbow.			
5. Held cuff edge of glove with sleeve cover of hand to be gloved. Grasped back of glove cuff with sleeve-covered second hand and turned cuff over sleeve. Pushed fingers into glove.			
6. Used sterile hand to pick up second glove. Positioned and donned it in same manner as first. Adjusted both gloves for comfort and fit.			

Additional Comments:

NOTES

Name _____   Specific Skill Performed _____

Date _____   Attempt Number _____

Instructor _____   PASS _____ FAIL _____

Performance Checklist 28–1.   Using Protective Restraints

	S	U	Comments
1. Assessed need for restraint, considered alternatives, and chose least restrictive restraint.			
2. Applied restraint correctly.			
a. Approached client and explained procedure in calm, reassuring manner.			
b. Padded skin under restraint, especially under bony prominences.			
c. Allowed room to place two fingers between restraint and limb or avoided constriction of client's breathing, leaving freedom to move in bed.			
d. Used a slip knot to tie restraint to bed frame rather than side rail, or, if out of bed, in a location accessible to staff but that cannot be reached by client.			
3. Took action to prevent complications.			
a. Observed client, client's skin, and client's circulatory status every 30 minutes. Reoriented client with each contact.			
b. Repositioned client, assessed respiratory status, and reassessed need for restraint every 2 hours.			
c. Provided for food and fluid intake, and toileting needs.			
4. Documented the rationale for restraint, type and time of application, any going assessments and interventions, time of removal, and client response.			

Additional Comments:

Name _____ Specific Skill Performed _____

Date _____ Attempt Number _____

Instructor _____ PASS _____ FAIL _____

Performance Checklist 30–1. Administering an Enteral Feeding

	S	U	Comments
1. Prepared the client by raising head of bed to 45 degrees and noting bowel sounds, abdominal distention, and complaints/presence of diarrhea.			
2. Selected formula at room temperature, checked expiration date, and checked the amount and pH of gastric residual.			
3. Flushed tube with at least 50 mL of water using a syringe with plunger removed.			
4. Gave a bolus feeding, verbalizing that it should take approximately 15 minutes.			
a. Filled the syringe with feeding solution and let it instill by gravity.			
b. Refilled when syringe was drained to ¼ full, and repeated until total dose given.			
c. Flushed with 50 mL water, clamped tube, covered tube with sterile gauze, and cleaned equipment.			
5. Gave an intermittent feeding.			
a. Flushed feeding tube with water; primed feeding set with formula; labeled new bag with time, date, and initials; and hung set from IV pole.			
b. Attached feeding set to feeding tube and regulated flow rate so formula infused over 20 minutes.			
c. Clamped tube, removed feeding bag, cleaned bag with tap water, and stored equipment for future use.			
6. Gave a continuous feeding as outlined in step 5a above, threaded tubing through infusion pump, and set pump at prescribed rate.			
7. Verbalized that medications given through a feeding tube must be in liquid form or finely crushed.			
8. Cleaned feeding tube site using clean technique and soap and water, dried area well, observed for signs of infection, and applied dressing if ordered using split 4 x 4 gauze and nonallergenic tape.			
9. Verbalized to tape tube securely to gown, monitor client status, tidy environment, and complete documentation.			

Additional Comments:

Name _____   Specific Skill Performed _____

Date _____   Attempt Number _____

Instructor _____   PASS _____   FAIL _____

Performance Checklist 30–2.   Administering Parenteral Nutrition through a Central Line

		S	U	Comments
1.	Confirmed order, checked the solution for correct ingredients and appearance, and assessed client (lab values, signs of inflammation at infusion site, any fears).			
2.	Prepared solution and tubing.			
a.	Connected infusion bag to IV tubing, filter, and extension tubing with clamps closed.			
b.	Opened clamp, primed and reclamped tubing, and threaded tubing through infusion pump.			
c.	Timed and dated new tubing.			
3.	Prepared central line catheter and began infusion.			
a.	Flushed catheter according to policy with heparin or saline.			
b.	Clamped tube or reminded client to perform Valsalva maneuver when accessing line or changing tubing.			
c.	Unclamped tubing and set infusion pump at prescribed rate. Verbalized to start flow rate slowly and monitor rate carefully.			
4.	Verbalized not to use single-lumen line for blood sampling or blood infusion, to avoid adding medications to TPN solution at all times, and to avoid giving IV medications in same line if possible.			
5.	Verbalized client parameters to monitor (VS, labs, weight, urine output, infusion site) and documentation to complete once infusion hung (date, time, client response, I & O).			

Additional Comments:

Name_____   Specific Skill Performed_____

Date_____   Attempt Number _____

Instructor_____   PASS _____   FAIL _____

Performance Checklist 31–1.   Inserting and Maintaining a Nasogastric Tube

	S	U	Comments
1. Prepared the equipment.			
a. Arranged efficiently.			
b. Prepared tape.			
c. Checked suction.			
2. Prepared client.			
a. Positioned client.			
b. Explained procedure.			
c. Assessed nostrils.			
3. Passed the tube.			
a. Measured length.			
b. Inserted.			
c. Checked placement.			
d. Secured to nose.			
e. Connected to suction.			
4. Documented findings.			
5. Irrigated tube.			
a. Used correct amount and type of fluid.			
b. Correctly calculated intake and output.			

Additional Comments:

NOTES

Name _____   Specific Skill Performed _____

Date _____   Attempt Number _____

Instructor _____   PASS _____   FAIL _____

Performance Checklist 31–2.   Removing a Nasogastric Tube

		S	U	Comments
1.	Prepared client.			
	a. Assessed client.			
	b. Explained procedure.			
	c. Removed tape.			
	d. Removed tube.			
	e. Documented findings.			

Additional Comments:

Name_____   Specific Skill Performed_____

Date_____   Attempt Number _____

Instructor_____   PASS _____   FAIL _____

Performance Checklist 31–3.   Initiating Peripheral Intravenous Therapy

	S	U	Comments
1. Prepared for procedure.			
a. Validated physician's order.			
b. Gathered equipment.			
c. Primed tubing.			
d. Marked tubing with date, time, etc.			
e. Primed IV loop if used.			
f. Organized equipment at bedside.			
2. Prepared client.			
a. Explained procedure.			
b. Positioned client.			
3. Identified vein and prepped skin (IV arm).			
a. Applied tourniquet.			
b. Prepped skin.			
4. Inserted IV catheter.			
a. Used standard precautions.			
b. Used correct technique.			
c. Maintained sterile technique.			
d. Released tourniquet.			
5. Attached tubing and IV loop if used; initiated flow.			
6. Secured site.			
7. Regulated flow.			
a. Calculated correctly.			
b. Counted drops or set pump correctly.			
8. Dressed site.			
9. Documented procedure.			

Additional Comments:

Name_____ Specific Skill Performed_____

Date_____ Attempt Number _____

Instructor_____ PASS _____ FAIL _____

Performance Checklist 31–4. Discontinuing Peripheral Intravenous Therapy

		S	U	Comments
1.	Prepared for procedure.			
	a. Validated order.			
	b. Gathered equipment.			
	c. Used standard precautions.			
	d. Explained procedure to client.			
2.	Removed catheter.			
	a. Stopped flow.			
	b. Removed dressing.			
	c. Applied pressure.			
	d. Applied bandage.			
3.	Documented procedure.			

Additional Comments:

Name _____   Specific Skill Performed _____

Date _____   Attempt Number _____

Instructor _____   PASS _____ FAIL _____

Performance Checklist 31–5.   Changing the Dressing on a Central Line

	S	U	Comments
1. Prepared for procedure.			
a. Validated physician's order (or agency protocol).			
b. Used sterile technique.			
c. Explained procedure to client.			
2. Removed soiled dressing.			
a. Opened tray.			
b. Donned face mask and clean gloves.			
c. Removed soiled dressing.			
d. Washed hands.			
3. Set up sterile field.			
a. Set up plastic trash bag.			
b. Donned sterile gloves.			
c. Opened Betadine and alcohol applicators.			
4. Cleaned site.			
a. Used three alcohol swabs.			
b. Used three Betadine swabs.			
5. Dressed site.			
a. Applied gauze (if used).			
b. Applied transparent occlusive dressing.			
c. Labeled dressing with date and time.			
6. Documented procedure.			

Additional Comments:

Name _____   Specific Skill Performed _____

Date _____   Attempt Number _____

Instructor _____   PASS _____   FAIL _____

Performance Checklist 32–1.   Irrigating a Wound

		S	U	Comments
1.	Prepared client and field.			
	a. Checked the wound care order and the specific order for irrigant.			
	b. Premedicated the client for pain.			
	c. Washed hands, donned protective eyewear and gown.			
	d. Placed the underpad and/or clean basin to catch the irrigant fluid.			
	e. Decided whether the procedure should be clean or sterile. Set up a clean or sterile field by opening the irrigation tray. Opened packages of sterile dressings.			
	f. Poured irrigant into the sterile basin.			
2.	Removed the old dressing using clean gloves.			
3.	Irrigated the wound.			
	a. Donned sterile gloves.			
	b. Filled the syringe with irrigant.			
	c. With the tip of the needle about 2 inches above the wound bed, flushed with slow continuous pressure.			
	d. Repeated Step 3c as needed.			
4.	Applied new dressing.			
	a. Redressed the wound with wet-to-moist packing and dried the outer dressing as needed.			
	b. Disposed of used supplies according to standard precautions.			
5.	Documented the client's tolerance of the wound irrigation and dressing change. Documented the description of the wound bed.			

Additional Comments:

NOTES

Name _____ Specific Skill Performed _____

Date _____ Attempt Number _____

Instructor _____ PASS _____ FAIL _____

Performance Checklist 32–2. Removing a Dressing

		S	U	Comments
1.	Washed hands and applied gloves.			
2.	Removed dressing.			
	a. Gently removed old dressing by pulling the tape toward the dressing and parallel to the skin.			
	b. Simultaneously applied pressure to the client's skin at the edge of the tape to prevent the skin from being pulled with the tape.			
3.	Observed the removed dressing for drainage, especially noting the amount, color, and odor (if any) of drainage.			
4.	Disposed of the dressing according to facility policy and government regulations.			
5.	Documented the odor, color, amount, and consistency of the drainage. Described the appearance of the wound.			

Additional Comments:

Name _____   Specific Skill Performed _____

Date _____   Attempt Number _____

Instructor _____   PASS _____   FAIL _____

Performance Checklist 32–3.   Dressing a Simple Wound

		S	U	Comments
1.	Answered client's questions.			
2.	Confirmed the dressing order.			
3.	Assembled supplies needed for the dressing application.			
4.	Removed the dressing from its package and applied it to the center of the wound.			
5.	Secured the edges of the dressing to the client's skin with tape.			

Additional Comments:

Name _____   Specific Skill Performed _____

Date _____   Attempt Number _____

Instructor _____   PASS _____ FAIL _____

Performance Checklist 32–4.   Culturing a Wound

		S	U	Comments
1.	Rinsed or irrigated wound thoroughly with sterile normal saline before obtaining a culture.			
2.	Swabbed the entire wound bed using a zig-zag technique starting at the top of the wound and proceeding to the bottom of the wound.			
3. a.	Placed the swab in the culture tube.			
b.	Sent swab to the laboratory after labeling appropriately.			

Additional Comments:

Name _____   Specific Skill Performed _____

Date _____   Attempt Number _____

Instructor _____   PASS _____   FAIL _____

Performance Checklist 32–5.   Applying a Wet-to-Moist Dressing

		S	U	Comments
1.	Confirmed the physician's order and assembled the needed supplies.			
2.	Opened sterile dressing supplies. Used sterile normal saline solution (or another ordered solution) to dampen the dressing.			
3.	Prepared wet dressing.			
	a. Donned sterile gloves.			
	b. Twisted the dressing so it remained wet, but not dripping.			
	c. Opened the dressing fully and fluffed it open.			
4.	Packed wound.			
	a. Gently placed the dressing into the wound.			
	b. Did not pack the wound tightly.			
5.	Completed dressing.			
	a. Covered the damp dressing with a dry sterile dressing.			
	b. Secured it with tape or Montgomery straps, if needed.			

Additional Comments:

Name_____   Specific Skill Performed_____

Date_____   Attempt Number _____

Instructor_____   PASS _____   FAIL _____

Performance Checklist 32–6.   Applying a Hydrocolloid Dressing

	S	U	Comments
1. Cleaned the wound by irrigating it or lightly swabbing it with gauze soaked in sterile normal saline solution.			
2. Selected a hydrocolloid dressing of an appropriate size.			
3. Applied dressing.			
a. Applied the dressing from one side of the wound to the other side.			
b. Used hand pressure to hold the dressing in place for 1 minute.			
4. Placed hypoallergenic tape around the edges of the dressing to secure it if needed.			

Additional Comments:

Name _____   Specific Skill Performed _____

Date _____   Attempt Number _____

Instructor _____   PASS _____   FAIL _____

Performance Checklist 34–1.   Testing Feces for Occult Blood

		S	U	Comments
1.	Taught client about purpose of test and had client defecate, without voiding, into collection container.			
2.	Put on clean gloves, obtained small specimen using applicator and smeared thin layer in first box of Hemoccult slide while noting stool characteristics. Repeated procedure using opposite end of applicator and another area of the stool specimen.			
3.	Closed slide cover and turned it over to reverse side. Opened flap on card and applied two drops of developing solution. Observed for bluish discoloration on guaiac paper 30–60 seconds after drop application.			
4.	Disposed of slide in hazardous container, removed gloves, washed hands, and completed documentation.			

Additional Comments:

Name _____   Specific Skill Performed _____

Date _____   Attempt Number _____

Instructor _____   PASS _____   FAIL _____

Performance Checklist 34–2.   Preparing and Administering a Large-Volume Enema

	S	U	Comments
1. Gathered equipment and positioned client on left side, with bedpan in place if client was unable to retain enema. Draped client to expose only buttocks.			
2. Checked that temperature of enema solution was warm (40.5° C or 105°F), lubricated tip of enema tube, inserted it 2–3 inches into rectum, held bag 18" above rectum, and allowed 500–750 mL solution to flow in slowly over 10 minutes.			
3. Encouraged client to retain enema for up to 15 minutes, then assisted client to bathroom or commode, or checked placement on bedpan for evacuation.			
4. Cleansed perineum, assisted client to position of comfort.			
5. Verbalized to consult physician if three enemas did not produce clear results, if enemas ordered until clear.			

Additional Comments:

Name_____   Specific Skill Performed_____

Date_____   Attempt Number _____

Instructor_____   PASS _____   FAIL _____

Performance Checklist 35–1.   Collecting Urine from an Indwelling (Foley) Catheter

		S	U	Comments
1.	Cleaned connection port.			
2.	Collected 10 cc urine.			
3.	Injected urine into sterile container.			
4.	Labeled specimen.			
5.	Documented.			

Additional Comments:

Name_____ Specific Skill Performed_____

Date_____ Attempt Number_____

Instructor_____ PASS _____ FAIL _____

Performance Checklist 35–2. Applying a Condom Catheter

		S	U	Comments
1.	Positioned and draped client.			
2.	Cleaned and dried genitals.			
3.	Applied skin-protecting cream.			
4.	Wrapped adhesive around penis.			
5.	Placed condom and unrolled over adhesive.			
6.	Attached to collection system.			
7.	Documented.			

Additional Comments:

Name _____   Specific Skill Performed _____

Date _____   Attempt Number _____

Instructor _____   PASS _____   FAIL _____

Performance Checklist 35–3.   Inserting an Indwelling Catheter

		S	U	Comments
1.	Explained procedure to client, provided privacy, and washed hands.			
2.	Gathered equipment.			
3.	Positioned and draped client.			
4.	Established sterile field.			
5.	Donned sterile gloves.			
6.	Set up sterile field.			
7.	Tested balloon.			
8.	Prepped perineum.			
9.	Lubricated and inserted catheter.			
10.	Inflated balloon.			
11.	Taped catheter.			
12.	Established drainage.			
13.	Cleaned area and made client comfortable.			
14.	Documented.			

Additional Comments:

Name _____   Specific Skill Performed _____

Date _____   Attempt Number _____

Instructor _____   PASS _____   FAIL _____

Performance Checklist 36–1.   Giving the Client a Bed Bath

		S	U	Comments
1.	Performed preliminary activities.			
a.	Checked physician's orders for activity and any special positioning needs or contraindications.			
b.	Assessed client for ability to participate in the bath even if on a limited scale.			
c.	Evaluated client's need for teaching relative to skin care and planned to incorporate teaching into the procedure.			
d.	Assessed for presence of IV lines, catheters, tubes, casts, and dressing.			
e.	Assessed client's ROM.			
2.	Prepared the environment.			
a.	Washed hands and applied gloves if needed.			
b.	Changed gloves after oral care, perineal care, or washing nonintact skin.			
c.	Gathered equipment and took to the bedside.			
d.	Raised bed to comfortable working height, ensured privacy by closing door or curtains, and regulated temperature.			
e.	Placed articles on over-bed table, within easy reach.			
3.	Prepared the client.			
a.	Assisted client to use bedpan, commode, or urinal.			
b.	Placed bath blanket over the client covering the top linen.			
c.	Loosened top linen at the foot of the bed and removed from under the bath blanket and placed dirty linen in a laundry hamper or bag.			
d.	Placed bath towel under head and removed pillow.			
e.	Helped client move to the side of the bed nearest you. Made sure that the side rail on the opposite side of bed is in raised position.			
f.	Removed client's gown or pajamas.			

		S	U	Comments
4.	Washed the client's face and neck.			
a.	Filled washbasin 1/3 to 1/2 full of warm water. Tested the temperature of the water with a bath thermometer or with wrist.			
b.	Put on clean gloves if there was a possibility of exposure to body fluids during the bath.			
c.	Made a mitt with the washcloth.			
d.	Washed and dried client's face using clear water.			
e.	Washed the client's eyes with clear water.			
f.	Washed forehead, cheeks, nose, and perioral areas.			
g.	Washed the postauricular area. Cleaned the anterior and posterior ear with the tip of the washcloth.			
h.	Washed the front and back of the neck.			
i.	Removed the towel from beneath client's neck.			
5.	Washed the client's arms.			
a.	Placed a towel lengthwise under upper arm and axilla. Washed the upper surface of the arm.			
b.	Grasped the client's wrist firmly and elevated the arm to wash the lower surface to the arm.			
c.	Washed the axilla.			
d.	Washed the client's hands.			
6.	Washed the client's chest.			
a.	Folded the bath blanket down to the umbilicus.			
b.	For a female client, covered her chest with a towel			
7.	Washed the client's abdomen.			
a.	Exposed only areas being washed.			
b.	Used firm strokes to wash the abdomen from side to side, including the umbilicus.			
c.	Observed for signs of distention or visible peristalsis.			
d.	Re-covered the client with the bath blanket.			
8.	Washed the client's legs.			
a.	Exposed one leg at a time.			
b.	Used firm distal-to-proximal strokes.			
c.	Placed the client's foot in the basin for a few minutes to soak. Did ROM with the toes. Inspected the feet and nails.			
d.	Dried the feet thoroughly, especially between toes.			
e.	Repeated this process with the other leg.			

	S	U	Comments
9. Provided perineal care.			
a. Changed the bathwater.			
b. Placed the client in a supine position. If the client is able to wash genitalia without assistance, placed a basin of water, washcloth, and towel within reach and provided privacy. If the client could not wash the perineal area, draped the area with bath blanket so that only genitalia exposed.			
c. Washed the perineal area.			
10. Washed the back, buttocks, and perianal area.			
a. Placed the client in side-lying position.			
b. Placed a towel lengthwise along the client's back and buttocks.			
c. Washed, rinsed, and dried the client's back and buttocks.			
d. Performed back massage with powder or lotion (this may also be done at the completion of the bath).			
11. Helped the client don a clean gown or pajamas.			
a. While the client is still on one side, placed one arm in the sleeve of the gown.			
b. Turned the client to the back and placed the other arm in the sleeve.			
12. Assisted with hair care.			
13. Assisted with oral care, as explained in the Providing Oral Hygiene procedure.			
14. Made the bed with clean linen.			
15. Left client's environment clean and uncluttered.			
16. Documented significant observations and assessment findings.			

Additional Comments:

Name_____   Specific Skill Performed_____

Date_____   Attempt Number _____

Instructor_____   PASS _____   FAIL _____

Performance Checklist 36–2.   Providing Perineal Care

		S	U	Comments
For a Female Client				
1.	Prepared for the procedure.			
a.	Organized necessary equipment.			
b.	Placed a protective pad or towel underneath the client before placing on bedpan if doing perineal care in bed.			
c.	Placed in a comfortable position on bedpan, toilet, or commode chair, or bedpan in a semi-Fowler's position if necessary.			
d.	If care was given in bed, asked client to bend her knees and separated her legs.			
e.	Draped her with a bath blanket.			
2.	Cleaned the perineum.			
a.	Poured water or prescribed solution over the perineum.			
b.	Separated the labia with one hand to expose the urethral and vaginal openings.			
c.	With free hand, wiped from front to back in a downward motion with either washcloth or cotton balls.			
d.	Washed the external labia. Turned the client to a side-lying position and washed the anal area.			
e.	Patted dry with a second towel.			
3.	Made the client comfortable.			
a.	Removed equipment.			
b.	Covered the client and positioned her for comfort.			

	S	U	Comments
For a Male Client			
1. Prepared for the procedure.			
a. Organized necessary equipment.			
b. Covered the client with a bath blanket.			
2. Cleaned the perineum.			
a. If the client was uncircumcised, retracted the foreskin to remove smegma.			
b. Held the shaft of the penis firmly but gently with one hand. With the other, washed at the tip of the penis. Used a circular motion, cleaned from the center to the outside.			
c. Washed down the shaft toward the scrotum. Did not repeat washing an area without changing to a clean area on the washcloth.			
d. After washing the penis, replaced the foreskin if necessary.			
e. Washed around the scrotum.			
3. Made the client comfortable.			
a. Removed equipment.			
b. Covered the client and positioned him for comfort.			

Additional Comments:

Name_____   Specific Skill Performed_____

Date_____   Attempt Number _____

Instructor_____   PASS _____ FAIL _____

Performance Checklist 36–3.   Helping the Client with a Tub Bath or Shower

		S	U	Comments
1.	Assessed the client's capacity for self-care. Assessed the tolerance for activity, cognitive state, and musculoskeletal function.			
2.	Made sure that the bathroom was prepared and that the tub or shower was clean. Placed a disposable mat or towel on the floor by the tub or shower. Adjusted the room temperature so the client was not chilled during the bath.			
3.	Put on clean gloves.			
4.	Assessed the client's ability to access bathroom.			
5.	Kept the client covered with a bath blanket while preparing the water.			
6.	Provided privacy for the client by placing an "occupied" sign on the door.			
7.	Tested the water temperature before the client got into tub or shower. If used the bathtub, filled it no more than 1/2 full of warm water (105° F).			
8.	Provided assistance for client while client entering tub or shower.			
9.	Assessed whether the client could safely bathe without assistance. If client could remain unattended, showed client how to use the call signal and safety bars. Placed all bath supplies within easy reach.			
10.	If the client was left unattended, checked every 10–15 minutes to determine if help was needed.			
11.	If client was not able to bathe independently, remained with client at all items. Assisted as needed with bathing.			
12.	Washed any areas that the client was unable to reach.			
13.	Watched closely for signs of dizziness or weakness while client was in the tub or shower and immediately on exiting tub or shower.			
14.	Helped the client out of the tub or shower. Assisted with drying.			
15.	Assisted with grooming and dressing in clean pajamas or gown.			

	S	U	Comments
16. Helped the client return to room.			
17. Assessed the client's tolerance for the procedure.			
18. Left the bathroom clean. Discarded soiled linen. Cleaned the tub or shower according to agency policy.			
19. Documented the client's response to the activity.			

Additional Comments:

Performance Checklist 36–4. Making an Occupied Bed

	S	U	Comments
1. Organized the environment and positioned the client to expose half the bed.			
a. Washed hands.			
b. Closed the door or curtain for privacy.			
c. Folded a full-size sheet to be used as a draw sheet.			
d. Lowered the rail on the nearest side of the bed.			
e. Positioned the bed at a comfortable working height. Moved the client toward the near side of the bed.			
f. Loosened the top linen.			
g. Removed spread, top sheet, and blanket in one movement, at the same time pulling the bath blanket over the client. If top linens are to be reused, folded and placed them in a chair.			
h. Placed any linen that was not to be reused in laundry hamper or linen bag. Avoided contact with uniform. Held at arm's length while removing from bed to linen hamper.			
i. Loosened bottom sheet on near side of bed. Had the client roll to opposite side of bed. Adjusted pillow under head.			
j. Lowered the bed position to flat unless the client couldn't tolerate it.			
2. Made half the bed from top to bottom.			
a. Fan-folded the dirty bottom sheet and draw sheet, and tucked them under the client's back and buttocks as tightly as possible.			
b. Placed the clean bottom sheet on bed. Started with the bottom edge even with foot end of bed, with the center fold in the middle of the bed. Unfolded to the top and allowed the extra length to hang over the top.			
c. Fan-folded the top layer to the middle of the bed.			
d. If contour sheets were used, fitted the elastic edges under top and bottom corners of mattress. If regular sheets were used, made a mitered corner. Tucked the sheet well under the mattress at the head of the bed.			
3. Placed the draw sheet on top of bottom sheet. The folded edge was placed at the top of the client's shoulders.			
a. Placed the center fold along the center of the bed.			
b. Fan-folded the top layer toward the client.			

		S	U	Comments
c.	Tucked the excess under the mattress along with the bottom sheet.			
d.	Smoothed out the wrinkles as much as possible.			
e.	If an incontinence pad was used, fan-folded and placed it on top of the linens near the client's back.			
4.	**Made the second half of the bed.**			
a.	Helped the client turn onto the clean sheets. Raised the side rail and moved to opposite side of the bed. Lowered the side rail on that side.			
b.	Removed the dirty linens, folded toward the center or one end of the bed. Held the linens away from body, placed them in dirty linen bag or hamper.			
c.	Pulled the clean linens over the exposed half of the bed.			
d.	Tucked in the bottom sheet.			
e.	Tucked the draw sheet, moved from the middle, to the top, to the bottom.			
5.	**Put on the top sheet and spread.**			
a.	Helped the client move back to the center of the bed.			
b.	Placed the top sheet over client with the seam side up. Unfolded the sheet from head to toe.			
c.	Had the client grasp the top sheet while you pulled the soiled sheet or bath blanket from under the clean sheet.			
d.	Placed the blanket and spread evenly over the top sheet. Made sure that they are even on both sides.			
e.	Made mitered corners at the foot of bed with the top sheet, blanket, and spread together.			
f.	Pulled the top sheet, blanket, and spread into a tent over the client's toes.			
g.	Cuffed the spread, blanket, and top sheet at head of bed.			
6.	**Changed the pillowcase.**			
a.	Grasped the closed end of a clean pillowcase at the center point.			
b.	With the other hand, held the open end of the case.			
c.	Inverted the case over hand and forearm by pulling the opening of case back toward the closed end. Maintained grasp at the closed end. Covered pillow.			
7.	Placed pillow under head. Returned the bed to its low position. Placed the call light within the client's reach.			
8.	Positioned the client for comfort.			
9.	Washed hands and documented care.			

362

Performance Checklist 36–5. Making an Unoccupied Bed

		S	U	Comments
1.	Organized the environment.			
	a. Washed hands.			
	b. Raised the bed to a comfortable working height.			
	c. Lowered the side rails.			
2.	Removed soiled linens. Folded soiled surfaces inward and placed in hamper.			
	a. Removed the bedspread and blanket.			
	b. When handling soiled linens, always held them away from body.			
3.	Made one side of the bed at a time. Then moved to the other side.			
	a. If the bottom sheet was a contour sheet, placed the elastic bands under the top and bottom corners of the mattress. If the bottom sheet was not a contour sheet, unfolded it lengthwise and placed the vertical crease at the center of the bed.			
	b. Tucked the side in along the mattress.			
	c. If the client needs a draw sheet, centered the draw sheet on the bed and unfolded toward the opposite side.			
	d. Moved to the other side of the bed. Removed linen with soiled side in. Held the bundle of linen away from body and placed in linen bag or hamper.			
	e. Pulled linen to side. Tucked the top of the sheet, bottom end of sheet, and draw sheet.			
4.	Placed top sheet, blanket, and spread over bed.			
	a. Left a cuff at the top of the spread.			
	b. Mitered the corners all together at foot of bed.			
5.	Prepared the bed for the client to return.			
	a. Made a toe pleat.			
	b. Fan-folded the linen to the foot of the bed to create an open bed.			
	c. Changed the pillowcase.			
	d. Returned the bed to its low position.			
	e. Positioned the call light.			
	f. Disposed of soiled linen.			
6.	Washed hands and documented care.			

	S	U	Comments
Making a Surgical Bed			
1. Made the bed as an unoccupied bed.			
2. Folded the bottom and top edges on the near side to the opposite side, making a triangle.			
3. Picked up the center point of the triangle and fan-folded the linen to the side of the bed.			
4. Left the bed in high position.			
5. Changed the pillowcase and left the pillow at the foot of the bed or on a chair.			
6. Moved all objects away from bedside to leave room for the stretcher.			

Additional Comments:

Name_____ Specific Skill Performed_____

Date_____ Attempt Number _____

Instructor_____ PASS _____ FAIL _____

Performance Checklist 36–6. Providing Oral Hygiene

		S	U	Comments
1.	Prepared for the procedure.			
	a. Assessed the client's ability to participate in procedure.			
	b. Washed hands and donned clean gloves.			
	c. Positioned the client in high or semi-Fowler's position or in a lateral side-lying position.			
2.	Placed a towel under the client's chin and over the upper chest.			
3.	Moistened the toothbrush with small amount of water and applied toothpaste.			
4.	Either gave the toothbrush to the client for brushing or brushed the client's teeth.			
	a. Asked the client to open mouth wide and held an emesis basin under the client's chin.			
	b. Positioned the toothbrush at 45-degree angle to the gumline.			
	c. Directed the bristles of the toothbrush toward the gum line, and brushed from the gum line to the crown of each tooth, making sure to clean all surfaces.			
	d. Used back-and-forth strokes, cleaning the biting surfaces of the teeth.			
	e. Gently brushed the client's tongue.			
	f. Had the client rinse mouth with water and expectorate into the emesis basin.			
5.	Had the client rinse with mouthwash if desired.			
6.	Removed the tooth-brushing equipment.			
7.	Flossed the client's teeth.			
8.	Removed all equipment and made the client comfortable.			

	S	U	Comments
For an Unconscious Client			
1. Prepared for the procedure.			
a. Washed hands and donned clean gloves.			
b. Placed the client in a side-lying position.			
c. Placed the bulb syringe or suctioning equipment nearby for when the client needs to be suctioned.			
d. Placed a towel or waterproof pad under the client's chin. Placed an emesis basin under chin as well.			
2. Cleaned the client's teeth and mouth.			
a. Used a padded tongue blade to open the client's mouth.			
b. Swabbed the inside of the mouth, tongue, and teeth with a moist, padded tongue blade.			
c. Brushed the client's teeth.			
d. Rinsed the client's mouth using a very small amount of water that could be readily suctioned from mouth.			
e. Lubricated client's lips with petroleum jelly.			
3. Removed equipment and documented care.			
4. Left the client dry and comfortable.			
For Dentures			
1. Prepared for the procedure.			
2. Asked the client to remove dentures. If this was not possible, placed a gauze square on the front of the denture. Grasped the front teeth between thumb and forefinger, pulled down gently until the suction that held the upper dentures in place was loosened. Loosened lower dentures by lifting up and out.			
3. Cleaned the dentures according to client's usual routine or the instructions on cleaning product.			
a. Soaked in a denture cleanser. If unavailable, used warm water and a gauze square or toothbrush to clean.			
b. Brushed the denture with a soft-bristle brush.			
c. Rinsed under warm water.			
4. Helped the client replace the denture.			
5. Used denture adhesive according to the package directions if the client desired.			
6. Cleaned work area and made the client comfortable. Documented care.			

Name _____ Specific Skill Performed _____

Date _____ Attempt Number _____

Instructor _____ PASS _____ FAIL _____

Performance Checklist 36–7.   Shampooing the Client in Bed

			S	U	Comments
1.		Prepared for the procedure.			
	a.	Placed waterproof pads under the client's head and shoulders.			
	b.	Removed pins, clips, or barrettes from client's hair.			
	c.	Placed the bed in its flat position.			
	d.	Placed a shampoo board or inflated basin under the client's head.			
	e.	Draped a towel over the client's shoulders.			
	f.	Uncovered the client's upper body by folding the linens down to waist level. Placed a bath blanket over the client's chest.			
	g.	Placed a washcloth over the client's eyes.			
	h.	Placed a receptacle in position to catch water.			
2.		Shampooed the client's hair.			
	a.	Used a water pitcher and poured water over the hair until it was thoroughly wet. Ensured that the water was comfortably warm.			
	b.	Applied a small amount of shampoo. Using fingertips, gently worked it into a lather over the entire scalp. Worked from the hairline to the neckline.			
3.		Rinsed the hair with warm water and reapplied shampoo if needed. Repeated until hair was "squeaky clean" when hair shafts were rubbed.			
4.		Applied a small amount of conditioner if desired.			
5.		Made a turban by wrapping a towel around the client's head. Patted or towel dried until the hair was free of excess moisture.			
6.		Changed the client's gown and linens if they were wet.			
7.		Dried and styled the client's hair.			
8.		Helped the client to assume a comfortable position.			
9.		Removed all equipment and left environment clean.			

Additional Comments:

NOTES

Name _____   Specific Skill Performed _____

Date _____   Attempt Number _____

Instructor _____   PASS _____ FAIL _____

Performance Checklist 36–8.   Shaving the Client

		S	U	Comments
1.	Prepared for the procedure.			
	a. Placed the client in a sitting position, either in bed or in a chair.			
	b. If using a safety razor, applied a warm, wet towel to the client's face before beginning to shave.			
	c. Applied a thick layer of soap or shaving cream to the client's face.			
2.	Shaved with even strokes in the direction of hair growth.			
3.	Used a damp washcloth to remove excess shaving cream. Inspected for areas that may have been missed. Applied after-shave lotion if desired.			
4.	Cleaned the area, made the client comfortable, and documented care.			

Additional Comments:

Name_____   Specific Skill Performed_____

Date_____   Attempt Number _____

Instructor_____   PASS _____ FAIL _____

Performance Checklist 36–9.   Performing Foot and Nail Care

		S	U	Comments
1.	Prepared for the procedure.			
	a. Washed hands. Donned gloves if necessary.			
	b. Helped the client to sit in a chair if possible. If the client could not sit in a chair, elevated the head of the bed.			
	c. Filled a basin half full of warm water.			
	d. Tested the temperature with bath thermometer or by inserting elbow.			
	e. Placed a waterproof pad under the basin.			
2.	Placed the client's foot or hand in the basin. Washed with soap and allowed to soak for about 10 minutes.			
3.	Rinsed the foot or hand thoroughly with the washcloth, removed from the basin and placed on a towel.			
4.	Dried the foot or hand thoroughly but gently, being especially careful to dry between the digits.			
5.	Emptied the basin, refilled with warm water, and repeated with the other foot or hand.			
6.	While the second foot or hand is soaking, provided nail care for the first hand or foot.			
	a. Carefully cleaned under the nails with cotton-tipped applicator. Used an orange stick to remove debris. Pushed the cuticle back with the orange stick. Was careful to avoid injury to skin under the nail rim.			
	b. Began with the large toe or thumb, clipped the nails straight across. Clipped small sections at a time, starting with one edge and working across. Filed and shaped each nail with an Emory board or nail file.			
	c. After completing the manicure or pedicure, applied lotion to the client's feet or hands. Dusted powder between the digits if desired.			
	d. Repeated the procedure with the other hand or foot.			
7.	Helped the client to a comfortable position, removed all equipment, washed hands, and documented care.			

Additional Comments:

NOTES

Name _____   Specific Skill Performed _____

Date _____   Attempt Number _____

Instructor _____   PASS _____   FAIL _____

Performance Checklist 37–1. Performing Range-of-Motion Exercises

		S	U	Comments
1.	Explained the procedure to the client and assessed the client's ability to assist with the exercises.			
2.	Used a head-to-toe approach if moving the joints of the entire body through range of motion.			
3.	Supported the client's body part by cradling or cupping about and below the joint being moved.			
4.	Put the joint through its complete ROM, but did not force it beyond where it would comfortably move.			
5.	Observed client for tolerance, including pulse rate and discomfort, if any. Did not exercise to the point of causing pain.			

Additional Comments:

Performance Checklist 37–2.   Helping the Client Get Out of Bed

	S	U	Comments
Without a Transfer Belt			
1. Placed the bed in the lowest position and raised the head of the bed.			
2. Placed the chair at a 45-degree angle to the bed. Planned for client to get out of bed on client's strongest side.			
3. Used good body mechanics, helped the client to a full sitting position while swinging the client's leg over the edge of the bed in a single, smooth motion. Supported the client's upper body as she came to a sitting position.			
4. Supported the client in a sitting position on the side of the bed with feet dangling.			
5. If client was able, had the client place hands on the nurse's shoulders or on the mattress on either side of the body.			
6. Placed hands under client's arms. Placed knees in front of the client's knees and helped client to rise to a standing position.			
7. Pivoted with the client toward the chair, being careful not to dislodge equipment or lines.			
8. Used good body mechanics, lowered the client into the chair slowly and repositioned client in proper body alignment. Made client as comfortable as possible.			
With a Transfer Belt			
1. Placed a transfer/gait belt around the client's waist.			
2. Stood in front of the client, grasped the transfer belt on both sides of the client toward the back. Assessed whether the client had strength to stand. When the client was ready, helped to a standing position by rolling body and arms upward, pulling the client with the transfer belt.			
3. Pivoted the client toward the chair and lowered client slowly into it.			
4. Had the client reach for the arm rests, if available, while lowering into the chair.			

Additional Comments:

NOTES

Name _____ Specific Skill Performed _____

Date _____ Attempt Number _____

Instructor _____ PASS _____ FAIL _____

Performance Checklist 37–3. Transferring an Immobile Client from Bed to Wheelchair

		S	U	Comments
1.	Obtained an assistant before transferring the client.			
2.	Placed the chair parallel to the bed before transferring the client.			
3.	Pulled the bed out from the wall, if necessary. One nurse got behind the client's shoulders and upper body from the other side of the bed.			
4.	In unison and using good body mechanics, nurse and colleague lifted the client's shoulders and legs.			
5.	Lowered the client into the chair and positioned in good body alignment using pillows and other devices as needed.			

Additional Comments:

Name_____   Specific Skill Performed_____

Date_____   Attempt Number _____

Instructor_____   PASS _____   FAIL _____

Performance Checklist 37–4.   Using a Mechanical Lift

		S	U	Comments
1.	Obtained a functioning lift and moved it into the client's room.			
2.	Placed the bed in its lowest position and placed the one- or two-piece sling under the client. Made sure the sling supported the client's shoulders and buttocks. Had the client cross arms across own chest.			
3.	Securely connected the sling hooks to the lift. Raised the lift to elevate the client enough to clear the bed.			
4.	Moved the lift until it aligned with the chair, locked the wheels, released the pressure valve, and lowered the client slowly into the chair. Removed the sling from the lift and stored it in a corner out of the traffic.			
5.	Kept the sling under the client and positioned the client into proper body alignment.			

Additional Comments:

Performance Checklist 37–5.   Supporting the Ambulating Client

		S	U	Comments
1.	Applied a gait belt around the client's waist and helped the client to a standing position.			
2.	Stood beside and slightly behind the client, and walked with the client while holding onto the back of belt.			
3.	If the client had an intravenous pole, asked client to push the pole while walking.			
4.	If the client was weaker on one side than the other, walked on client's weak side while grasping the belt.			
5.	If the client was especially weak or this was the first time ambulating, asked another person to walk with you to support the client.			
6.	If the client started to fall, did not try to prevent the fall by supporting client's weight with own body. Rather, helped client to fall safely, without injury to client or to self.			
7.	As the client started to fall, moved feet so stronger leg was somewhat behind you.			
8.	At the same time, used the transfer belt to pull the client toward you, allowing client to slide against you, supported, as you eased client onto the floor.			
9.	Stayed with the client until help arrived. Assessed client for injury before trying to move client. Had the client evaluated by physician.			
10.	Documented the events leading up to the fall, client's assessment, notification of the physician and any action taken.			

Additional Comments:

NOTES

Performance Checklist 37–6.   Walking with Crutches

		S	U	Comments
1.	Inspected the prescribed crutch or crutches to make sure that the rubber tips were in place.			
2.	Reinforced the importance of arm exercises, such as flexing and extending the arms, body lifts, and squeezing a rubber ball.			
3.	Checked that crutches were the correct length.			
	a. Had the client stand.			
	b. With the crutch tip about 2 inches (5cm) in front of the client and 6 inches (15 cm) to the side of client's foot, checked that the distance between the axilla and the top of the crutch was at least three fingers' width or 1 or 2 inches (2.5 to 5 cm).			
4.	Taught the client how to balance using the tripod position by placing the crutches 6 inches (15 cm) in front of the feet and out laterally about the same distance.			
5.	Checked with the physician or physical therapist to determine which gait the client needed: a four-point, three-point or two-point gait.			
	a. For a four-point gait, had the client follow this series of steps: Moved the right crutch forward about 6 inches (15 cm). Moved the left foot forward. Moved the left crutch forward. Moved the right foot forward.			
	b. For a three-point gait, had the client follow this series of steps: Moved both crutches and the weakest leg forward. Moved the stronger leg forward.			
	c. For a two-point gait, had the client follow this series of steps: Moved the left crutch and the right foot forward at the same time. Moved the right crutch and the left foot forward at the same time.			
6.	Taught the client how to ascend stairs.			
7.	Taught the client how to descend stairs.			
8.	Taught the client how to get in and out of a chair.			

Name_____   Specific Skill Performed_____

Date_____   Attempt Number_____

Instructor_____   PASS_____ FAIL_____

Performance Checklist 38–1.   Turning and Moving a Client in Bed

	S	U	Comments
Turning a Client Alone			
1. Lowered the head of the bed and the knee gatch until the bed was flat.			
2. Moved the client to one side of the bed. Slid arms under the client's hips, and slid the hips to the side.			
3. Crossed the client's arms across the chest and crossed the legs at the ankle. Positioned a pillow or wedge at the head or foot of the bed to be used behind the client's back after turning.			
4. Placed one hand on the client's shoulder and the other hand on the client's hip, and rolled the client toward self.			
5. Turned the client far enough forward so student could release one hand and positioned a pillow or wedge behind the client's back.			
6. If necessary, went to the opposite side of the bed and pulled the client's hips toward the center of the bed to make the position more stable. Checked the position.			
Turning a Client with Another Nurse			
1. Placed bed in flat position and moved client to one side of the bed.			
a. If client was on turning sheet, student and another nurse stood on opposite sides of the bed and grasped the top and bottom of the sheet.			
b. If client was not on a turning sheet, student and another nurse stood on the same side of the bed.			
(1) One nurse slid own arms under the client's shoulders while the other slid arms under the client's hips.			
(2) On the count of three, both nurses slid the client to one side of the bed.			
2. a. Bent the client's knee on the opposite side to which student turned.			
b. Folded the client's arms over the chest.			
c. Student was positioned on one side of the bed and another nurse was positioned on the other side of the bed.			

	S	U	Comments
3. Turned the client.			
a. If student did not have a turning sheet, the nurse positioned on the side of the bed toward which the client will turn placed one hand on the client's shoulder and one hand on the client's hip.			
b. The nurse on the opposite side of the bed slid hands under the client's bottom hip, pulled the hip toward self, and placed a pillow at the client's back.			
4. Placed a pillow between the client's legs.			
5. Made sure that the client was properly positioned.			
6. If the client's condition demanded that the student maintain anatomic alignment of the spine during the procedure, used three nurses.			
7. After turning the client, documented that the client was turned and the position assumed.			
Moving a Client Up in Bed			
1. Before moving a client up in bed, determined whether student could do it alone or whether student needed help from another nurse. If student planned to move client alone, determined whether to stand at the side of the bed or the head of the bed.			
a. For one nurse to move a client up in bed from the side of the bed:			
(1) Had the client bend knees and place feet flat on the bed.			
(2) Placed one hand under the client's back and one under the thighs, close to the hips.			
(3) Told the client to push legs on the count of three, and slid the client up toward the head of the bed.			
b. For one nurse to move the client from the head of the bed:			
(1) Started by removing the headboard from the bed.			
(2) Placed the bed in a slight Trendelenburg position.			
(3) Slid hands under the client's shoulders and pulled the client toward self.			
(4) If possible, used a turning sheet to perform this maneuver.			

	S	U	Comments

2. If client had good upper body strength, used trapeze to move client up in bed.

    a. Placed a trapeze over the bed.

    b. Had the client bend knees and place feet flat on the bed to push.

    c. Had the client hold onto the trapeze and pull with arms to lift hips slightly off the bed.

    d. With the hips lifted, had client push with legs.

    e. Assisted by placing hands under the client's thighs, close to the hips.

3. If client was too heavy, solicited help from a colleague.

    a. Stood on opposite sides of client's bed.

    b. Had client bend knees and place feet flat on the bed. Student and other nurse grasped the turning sheet with one hand at the level of the client's shoulders and the other hand at the level of the client's hips.

    c. On the count of three, had the client push with legs as student and the other nurse slid torso up in bed.

4. After moving the client up, raised the head of the bed and checked the position of the bed.

5. Documented that the client was repositioned and the position assumed.

Moving a Client from a Bed to a Stretcher

1.   a. Student and another nurse were positioned on each side of the stretcher.

    b. If client was unconscious, a third nurse stood at the top of the stretcher to support the client's head and a fourth stood at the bottom to support the client's feet.

2. Used a sheet to make the transfer easier.

    a. Untucked the sheet from the client's bed.

    b. Grasped the sheet under the client's shoulders while another nurse on the same side grasped it at the client's hips and legs.

    c. On a count of three, student and the other nurses lifted and pulled the client onto the stretcher.

3. As an alternative, used a transfer board.

    a. Student and another nurse standing on the same side of the bed turned the client away from the stretcher.

    b. Placed the transfer board where the client was lying and turned the client back onto the board.

    c. Pulled the board onto the stretcher with the client on it.

    d. Turned the client again to remove the board.

		S	U	Comments
4.	Raised the side rails on the outside of the stretcher, then moved between the bed and stretcher and raised the remaining side rails.			
5.	If the stretcher could not be positioned adjacent to the bed, used a three-person lift to transfer the client with three nurses on the same side of the bed.			
	a. Slid hands and arms under the client's head and shoulders. Another nurse slid hands under the client's back and buttocks, and the third nurse slid hands under the legs and thighs.			
	b. On the count of three, nurses simultaneously lifted the client.			
	c. Walked as a unit to rotate and carry the client to the stretcher.			
6.	a. Covered the client with a sheet. Supplied client with a pillow and raised the head of the stretcher if needed.			
	b. Fastened a safety strap over the client.			
	c. Put side rails up.			

Additional Comments:

Name _____   Specific Skill Performed _____

Date _____   Attempt Number _____

Instructor _____   PASS _____ FAIL _____

Performance Checklist 38–2.   Applying Antiembolism Stockings

		S	U	Comments
1.	Placed client supine in bed with his legs horizontal for 15 minutes.			
2.	Measured the client's legs to determine the correct stocking size.			
3.	Placed a stocking on the client's foot.			
4.	Pulled the stocking firmly up the client's leg, smoothing wrinkles as student worked.			
5.	Checked the client's toes for pressure.			
6.	As an alternative, turned the stocking inside-out down to the ankle. Turned it right-side out as student worked the stocking up the leg.			
7.	Repeated with the other leg.			
8.	Assessed the client to make sure the stockings were functioning properly.			
9.	Documented the size and length of the stockings, the time applied, the condition of the client's skin, any client complaints, and times the stockings were removed and reapplied.			

Additional Comments:

Name_____   Specific Skill Performed_____

Date_____   Attempt Number _____

Instructor_____   PASS _____ FAIL _____

Performance Checklist 38–3.   Using a Sequential Compression Device

		S	U	Comments
1.	Placed the client in a supine position with legs horizontal.			
2.	Applied antiembolism stockings.			
3.	Measured the circumference of the client's upper thigh.			
4.	Opened the inflatable sleeve on the flat bed, cotton side up, and placed the client's leg on the sleeve.			
5.	Wrapped the sleeve snugly around the client's leg, beginning with the side that did not contain tubes. Fastened the sleeve with the Velcro fasteners.			
6.	Connected the tubing on the sleeve to the compression controller.			
7.	Followed the physician's orders in setting the controller to the correct amount and time of compression. After turning it on, observed to make sure the unit was working.			
8.	Documented the date and time the sleeves were applied and assessment findings.			

Additional Comments:

Performance Checklist 39–1. Endotracheal Suctioning

		S	U	Comments
1.	Recognized the need for suctioning.			
2.	Gathered the equipment.			
3.	Used sterile technique.			
4.	Explained the procedure.			
5.	Set up the equipment.			
	a. Turned on suction.			
	b. Set up sterile saline.			
	c. Donned one sterile glove.			
	d. Connected suction tube to catheter and tested suction.			
6.	Hyperoxygenated client and correctly instructed partner in hyperoxygenation.			
7.	Passed catheter and suctioned.			
	a. Applied intermittent suction on removing catheter. Limited to 10 seconds.			
	b. Hyperoxygenated and assessed results.			
	c. Suctioned maximum of three passes.			
8.	Used standard precautions in disposing of equipment.			
9.	Documented procedure and results.			

Additional Comments:

NOTES

Name _____   Specific Skill Performed _____

Date _____   Attempt Number _____

Instructor _____   PASS _____   FAIL _____

Performance Checklist 39–2. Administering Oxygen

	S	U	Comments
1. Assessed need and verified order.			
2. Gathered equipment.			
3. Explained rationale for oxygen order.			
4. Explained procedure to client.			
5. Set up humidity.			
6. Correctly applied device.			
7. Reassessed client.			
8. Documented procedure and assessment data.			

Additional Comments:

Name_____   Specific Skill Performed_____

Date_____   Attempt Number _____

Instructor_____   PASS _____ FAIL_____

Performance Checklist 39–3.   Cleaning a Tracheostomy Site

		S	U	Comments
1.	Gathered equipment.			
2.	Prepared client.			
	a. Suctioned tracheostomy.			
	b. Removed soiled dressing using standard precautions.			
3.	Set up sterile field.			
	a. Opened tray.			
	b. Donned sterile gloves.			
	c. Poured hydrogen peroxide and normal saline.			
4.	Cleaned inner cannula			
	a. Removed inner cannula.			
	b. Cleaned inside and out and rinsed.			
	c. Replaced inner cannula.			
5.	Cleaned tracheostomy site.			
	a. Cleansed from clean to dirty.			
	b. Used sterile technique.			
6.	Changed tracheostomy ties.			
	a. Protected trach from accidental removal.			
	b. Protected client from discomfort.			
7.	Documented procedure and assessment.			

Additional Comments:

Name _____   Specific Skill Performed _____

Date _____   Attempt Number _____

Instructor _____   PASS _____   FAIL _____

Performance Checklist 40–1.   Administering Blood

		S	U	Comments
1.	Verbalized to check physician's order, verified that blood was ready in blood bank, and checked for allergies.			
2.	Verbalized to assess client allergies or previous reactions to blood, measured vital signs, ensured appropriate consent, prepared equipment, and obtained blood from blood bank.			
3.	Verified with another registered nurse that the following information was correct:			
a.	Client's name and identification number on the blood bank slip matched the client's identification bracelet.			
b.	Blood bank slip and the unit of blood contained the same blood type, donor number, and expiration date.			
4.	Donned gloves and primed tubing.			
a.	Closed clamp and attached bag of normal saline to arm of Y-tubing; opened clamp and primed arm, filter, drip chamber, and tubing below chamber.			
b.	Closed clamp and attached unit of blood to other Y-arm; opened clamp, primed second Y-arm, and re-clamped.			
5.	Began the transfusion.			
a.	Opened clamp on NS and infused 50 mL slowly; closed NS clamp.			
b.	Opened clamp on blood, and regulated at keep-open rate. Verbalized to maintain this rate for 15 minutes while staying with client.			
c.	Reset drip rate to rate prescribed, after verbalizing that client had stable VS and no signs of transfusion reaction. Verbalized to continue to monitor VS.			
6.	Completed transfusion by flushing the line with NS, clamped tubing, and disconnecting.			
7.	Completed transfusion record, stated to return designated portion of form and empty bag to blood bank. Verbalized to place designated portion of form in client record, and completed documentation (date, type, and identification number of product; time started and ended; client response).			

Additional Comments:

Name _____   Specific Skill Performed _____

Date _____   Attempt Number _____

Instructor _____   PASS _____   FAIL _____

Performance Checklist 41–1.   Back Massage

		S	U	Comments
1.	Gathered equipment and prepared environment for the procedure.			
	a. Adjusted light and temperature, and eliminated unnecessary noise.			
	b. Gathered lotion and extra blanket, and closed room door or bedside curtain.			
2.	Prepared client for procedure.			
	a. Raised bed to comfortable working height and lowered side rail.			
	b. Exposed client's back, shoulders, upper arms and sacral area, and covered rest of body with blanket.			
3.	Administered the back rub.			
	a. Started with firm, circular strokes at the base of the buttocks, moving hands toward shoulders.			
	b. Massaged over scapulae with firm, smooth strokes.			
	c. Without removing hands from client's skin, continued to use smooth strokes to the upper back and along sides of back down to buttocks.			
	d. Kneaded along side of spine from buttocks to scapulae and around nape of neck. Repeated kneading on opposite side of back.			
4.	Wiped off excess lotion and assisted with rearranging gown or pajamas if needed.			
5.	Lowered bed and side rails, if necessary, and made sure client did not require pain medication.			
6.	Ensured that any equipment or medications needed by the client were at the bedside.			

Additional Comments:

Performance Checklist 43–1.   Inserting and Removing Contact Lenses

		S	U	Comments
Inserting a Contact Lens				
1.	Washed hands.			
2.	Removed the lens from the container and applied wetting solution to both sides.			
3.	Assessed the lens.			
	a.	Checked to make sure it was cleaned and undamaged.		
	b.	Cleaned if necessary according to the specific type of contact lens.		
	c.	Placed the lens in the storage container marked for the correct eye.		
	d.	Rinsed the lens with sterile normal saline solution or manufacturer-recommended rinsing solution before re-inserting.		
4.	Placed the lens on the index finger of dominant hand.			
5.	Held the client's upper lid with the index finger of the nondominant hand and spread the upper and lower lid by slight downward pulling on the lower lid with the thumb. Had the client look straight ahead.			
6.	Placed the lens over the iris.			
7.	Gently rubbed the upper lid with the finger to remove air bubbles.			
8.	Asked client to blink and determined that lens was correctly placed.			
Removing a Soft Contact Lens				
1.	Washed hands.			
2.	a.	Asked client to look up and to the side.		
	b.	With middle finger, pulled down on the lid and placed index fingertip on the lower edge of the lens.		
3.	Moved the lens medially to the white part of the eye.			
4.	a.	Gently pinched the lens between thumb and index finger, allowing air to go beneath the lens.		
	b.	Grasped lens and removed it.		

	S	U	Comments
Removing a Hard Contact Lens			
1. Washed hands.			
2. Pulled client's upper and lower lids apart and to the side.			
3. Asked client to blink.			
4. Alternate methods:			
a. Put gentle pressure on the lower edge of the lens and grasped the upper edge of the lens as it fell away from the eye.			
b. Used a lens suction cup to lift the contact lens from the client's eye.			

Additional Comments:

Name _____ Specific Skill Performed _____

Date _____ Attempt Number _____

Instructor _____ PASS _____ FAIL _____

Performance Checklist 43–2.   Inserting a Hearing Aid

		S	U	Comments
1.	Checked that the battery was operating.			
2.	Inspected the hearing aid.			
3.	Turned down the volume, inserted the ear mold into the ear canal, and secured the rest of the aid in place according to the design.			
4. a.	For a behind-the-ear hearing aid, secured the battery device behind the ear.			
b.	Avoided kinking the connecting tube.			
5. a.	Slowly turned up the volume while speaking to the person in a normal tone of voice.			
b.	Asked the person to tell you when the volume was comfortable.			
6.	If feedback occurred, checked for a problem.			

Additional Comments:

Name _____ Specific Skill Performed _____

Date _____ Attempt Number _____

Instructor _____ PASS _____ FAIL _____

Performance Checklist 43–3.   Ear Lavage/Irrigation

		S	U	Comments
1.	Gathered the necessary equipment.			
2.	Examined the ear canal with an otoscope.			
3.	Explained the procedure and instructed the client to avoid any sudden movements.			
4.	Checked the temperature of the irrigant.			
5.	Selected the irrigating device.			
6.	a. Covered the client's shoulder.			
	b. Tipped the client's head to the side to be irrigated and asked the client to hold the emesis basin.			
7.	Placed the tip of the irrigation device just inside the external meatus with the tip still visible.			
8.	Directed the fluid toward the posterior wall of the ear canal.			
9.	a. Irrigation was steady.			
	b. Did not use more than 70 mL of solution at one time.			
10.	Periodically examined the ear canal with an otoscope to determine patency and cerumen removal.			
11.	a. Tilted the head to drain excess fluid from the ear.			
	b. Dried the ear canal gently with cotton-tipped applicator.			

Additional Comments:

NOTES

Name _____

Date _____

Instructor _____

Specific Skill Performed _____

Attempt Number _____

PASS _____ FAIL _____

Performance Checklist 58–1. Cardiopulmonary Resuscitation

		S	U	Comments
1.	Assessed client for responsiveness and called for help or activated emergency response system if unresponsive.			
2.	Ensured that client had an open airway.			
	a. Positioned client on his or her back on a hard flat surface with arms at sides if possible.			
	b. Opened airway using head tilt–chin lift method or jaw thrust maneuver.			
	c. Removed visible food or vomitus from mouth if present.			
3.	Determined whether client was breathing.			
	a. Looked to see if chest rose and fell.			
	b. Positioned ear over client's mouth and nose. Listened for exhaled air and felt for air movement from breathing on own cheek.			
4.	Began administering breaths if client not breathing.			
	a. Stated to use manual resuscitation bag if available. Used thumb and index finger of hand resting on client's forehead to pinch nose closed for mouth-to-mouth or used hand resting below client's chin to hold mouth closed for mouth-to-nose.			
	b. Took a deep breath and closed lips around client's mouth or nose.			
	c. Gave two breaths slowly, with each lasting 1–to 2 seconds, inhaling between breaths if not using a bag-valve mask.			
	d. After delivering each breath, turned head and positioned ear over client's mouth and nose to listen for exhaled air.			
5.	Checked for a pulse for 5–10 seconds at the client's carotid artery.			
	a. Located artery using 2–3 fingers in groove between trachea and neck muscles.			
	b. If pulse felt, continued rescue breathing at 10–12 breaths per minute (one every 5–6 seconds).			
	c. Began compressions if no pulse felt and client not breathing.			

	S	U	Comments
6. Assumed position for chest compressions.			
a. Placed heel of one hand on lower half of sternum, just above the xiphoid process.			
b. Placed second hand over first so that hands were parallel, and raised or intertwined fingers leaving only heels of hands resting on chest.			
c. Locked elbows and kept arms straight; positioned shoulders directly over client's sternum.			
7. Administered chest compressions.			
a. Used enough force to depress chest 1–2 inches on an adult.			
b. Released pressure fully on sternum between compressions to allow chest to return to normal position.			
c. Delivered compressions at a rate of 80–100 per minute, counting "one and, two and…."			
8. Began standard cycle of chest compressions and rescue breaths by administering 2 breaths after 15 compressions and reassessed client after 4 cycles of 15 compressions and 2 breaths.			
9. Coordinated efforts with a second rescuer who arrived on the scene.			
a. Opened airway after 15 compressions and began rescue breathing, giving two rescue breaths.			
b. Allowed second rescuer to deliver 15 compressions before giving 2 more breaths.			
c. Stated to interrupt CPR when emergency team arrived only for intubation and connection to 100% oxygen by bag-valve mask.			

Additional Comments: